Rock Solid Resilience

An Evidence-Based Guide to Preventing Injury, Optimizing Strength, and Enhancing Performance

Dean Somerset, CEP

Dan Pope, DPT, OCS, CSCS

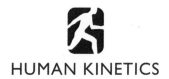

HUMAN KINETICS

Library of Congress Cataloging-in-Publication Data

Names: Somerset, Dean, 1981- author. | Pope, Dan, 1985- author.
Title: Rock solid resilience : an evidence-based guide to preventing injury, optimizing strength, and enhancing performance / Dean Somerset, Dan Pope.
Description: Champaign, IL : Human Kinetics, 2026. | Includes bibliographical references.
Identifiers: LCCN 2024038952 (print) | LCCN 2024038953 (ebook) | ISBN 9781718224155 (paperback) | ISBN 9781718224162 (epub) | ISBN 9781718224179 (pdf)
Subjects: LCSH: Weight training. | Weight training injuries--Prevention.
Classification: LCC GV546 .S655 2026 (print) | LCC GV546 (ebook) | DDC 613.7/13--dc23/eng/20241029
LC record available at https://lccn.loc.gov/2024038952
LC ebook record available at https://lccn.loc.gov/2024038953

ISBN: 978-1-7182-2415-5 (print)

Senior Acquisitions Editor: Roger W. Earle; **Senior Developmental Editor:** Cynthia McEntire; **Managing Editor:** Kim Kaufman; **Copyeditor:** Laura Magzis; **Graphic Designer:** Dawn Sills; **Cover Designer:** Keri Evans; **Cover Design Specialist:** Susan Rothermel Allen; **Photograph (cover):** Primorac91 /E+/Getty Images RF (photo) and Colors Hunter - Chasseur de Couleurs/Moment/Getty Images RF (background); **Photographs (interior):** Steve Glen & Andrew Mardon/© Human Kinetics, unless otherwise noted; **Photo Production Specialist:** Amy M. Rose; **Photo Production Manager:** Jason Allen; **Senior Art Manager:** Kelly Hendren; **Illustrations:** © Human Kinetics; **Printer:** Versa Press

We thank Evolve Strength in Edmonton, Alberta, Canada, for assistance in providing the location for the photo shoot for this book.

Human Kinetics books are available at special discounts for bulk purchase. Special editions or book excerpts can also be created to specification. For details, contact the Special Sales Manager at Human Kinetics.

Printed in the United States of America   10 9 8 7 6 5 4 3 2 1

The paper in this book is certified under a sustainable forestry program.

Human Kinetics	*United States and International*	*Canada*
1607 N. Market Street	Website: **US.HumanKinetics.com**	Website: **Canada.HumanKinetics.com**
Champaign, IL 61820	Email: info@hkusa.com	Email: info@hkcanada.com
USA	Phone: 1-800-747-4457	

E9265

Rock Solid Resilience

An Evidence-Based Guide to Preventing Injury, Optimizing Strength, and Enhancing Performance

Contents

Part I Prehab and Prevention   1

1 Preventing Injuries: What We Know   3

Current research into injury risk and prevention provides some
interesting details. Knowing the risks and mechanisms of injury
provides the opportunity to be proactive in preventing injury.

2 Athlete Assessment: Identifying Limitations in Mobility and Gross Patterns 27

Proper mobility in the gym is a key factor in performance and
longevity. Assessments identify strengths and weaknesses in
mobility and core tension to guide lifters to safer, smoother
movement.

Part II Exercise Techniques and Execution 51

3 Squat and Hinge Movements   53

We all know how to squat, don't we? But how do you squat
safety and effectively for your unique body structure?

4 Pressing and Pulling Movements   83

All lifters have had to answer the question "How much can you
bench?" Bench press, and its myriad variations, is ubiquitous
in lifting. Learn to do it properly and you can amaze when
people ask the question.

5 Core Movements   117

More than just crunches, core movements involve carries,
braces, and rotational movements. A strong core is the best
foundation for any lifter.

Exercise Finder

Athlete Assessment

Squat and Hinge Movements

Pressing and Pulling Movements

Core Movements

Level-Up and Side Quest Accessory Approaches

Preface

If you're reading this, you're probably aware of the benefits of strength training. But if you're not, know that it's amazing what strength training can do for your physical health, physique, and mental health. It has transformed my own life in a multitude of ways. The benefits of strength training are pretty astounding. Following are only a few.

Strength training is a phenomenal way to maintain and build muscle mass throughout life. Unfortunately, inactive adults will lose on average 3 to 8 percent of their muscle mass per decade of life, and this is accompanied by more body fat storage and a decrease in metabolic rate (how fast you burn calories).[3] Resistance exercise, such as strength training, helps to improve bone mineral density[3] and reduces the risk of falls in the elderly[7]—two serious issues that are quite common as we age.

Resistance exercise is a powerful tool to maintain and build health across your lifespan. It allows you to continue the activities you enjoy over your lifespan and helps to prevent osteoporosis, sarcopenia, and numerous other conditions.[1] Strength training improves insulin sensitivity and resting metabolic rate, lowers LDL cholesterol and increases HDL cholesterol, lowers triglyceride levels, and improves glucose metabolism, blood pressure, body fat percentage, and gastrointestinal transit time.[1,3]

Most of us know the benefits of endurance exercise for health, weight loss, and body composition changes, but strength training is no slouch in this regard. When resistance exercise is compared to endurance exercise, resistance exercise outperforms endurance exercise with regard to body composition changes and biomarkers for metabolic health.[6] Strength training can reduce body fat, increase muscle mass, and improve metabolic rate.[3]

Strength training can be used as an effective tool in the treatment of myriad orthopedic injuries, including the most common cause of disability in the world, lower-back pain.[1,11] Strength training can also help reduce the likelihood of injury or a new onset of pain.[12] For example, using a strength and conditioning program can help to prevent one-third of sports injuries and reduce overuse injuries by one-half.[12]

On top of all this, strength training is associated with a reduced risk of all-cause mortality (death from every cause), cardiovascular disease, and cancer mortality.[2] These benefits are even more powerful when combined with aerobic exercise. Combining these two types of training results in a 40 percent reduction in mortality, compared to 21 percent reduction with strength training alone.[4] Performing the two together is also more powerful from a mortality standpoint than performing only aerobic exercise.[5]

Another very powerful but often overlooked benefit of resistance training is the impact on your brain. Resistance training has been shown to improve cognition in older adults, those with mild cognitive decline, and even people with dementia.[9,10] Strength training has even been shown to have a positive effect on mental health, improving quality of life and sense of well-being,[8] and to help improve symptoms associated with depression and anxiety.[13]

Finally, those who perform resistance exercise regularly are less costly to the health care system, on average spending fewer health care dollars.[8] This is most likely because people who exercise tend to be healthier, which makes them less likely to need health care services and medications.

What is also very interesting about strength training is that a large majority of these benefits can often be obtained with as little as two sessions of 15 to 20 minutes per week.[1] If you needed another excuse to continue your regular strength training, there you go!

With all of these benefits in mind, it is my opinion that strength training is something that everyone should pursue for the entirety of their lives. It's one of the closest things we have to a "fountain of youth," and the benefits are astounding. It's really the main reason why we wrote this book. We want to help you on your journey to lifelong strength.

There are already a ton of workout programs on the market, so we chose not to write a new one, even if we could bring a unique perspective from our respective backgrounds. Dan could write a program to help someone limit orthopedic injuries and stay in the game. I could write something to get someone else jacked and entirely awesome while keeping the risks of major setbacks as low as possible, and together we could put together an outline to help still another person move with control and confidence and continue getting the benefits of strength training for years to come.

The challenge we found was to write programs that would benefit a wide range of people. Some might be new to working out, and some might be grizzled gym veterans who want to keep getting after it but have shoulders or knees that get cranky. Some people might be very stiff and immobile, while others might be clinically hypermobile and have a hard time building stability without winding up in tendinitis purgatory.

Given all that, we didn't want to just write a workout book. We wanted to show you, the reader, how to build a program, adjust it based on what you're feeling, and get the most from the workouts you're doing—all while ensuring you're doing the proper workouts based on how you move, your stage of training, and what you're capable of doing.

With any workout, you're likely to get to a point where something gets worked more than it can manage effectively, and an injury or even just mild discomfort is likely to happen. When something like a sore shoulder pops up, we'll show you what to do about it, whether you need to adjust your training a little and switch out an exercise or two, or whether you should talk to a medical professional. Pain is a poor coach. The deceptively simple notion of "if it hurts, don't do it" needs a heck of a lot of explanation before you can decide whether you should keep going or just change course slightly.

We want to show you not only what to do but why you should do it that way in the first place. This information gives you a serious advantage in that knowing the *why* lets you change the *how* as needed, while still being mindful of the reason for doing it. Maybe we need to adjust your positioning, stance, or range of motion to find an optimal way for you to do an exercise without it causing more discomfort than you'd like. Maybe we should explain the gradual increase of volume and load to make sure you train intensely enough to see the results you're looking for, but also include some programming breaks to let your physiology catch up to the weights you're throwing around in the gym.

This book is meant as an outline of how to train, not just a workout program to follow. Sure, we include a workout, as well as the rationale behind why and how to do things, but we want to make sure you know what to do if you get into the middle of the gym floor, try something, and it just doesn't send you the way you expected it to. A good workout gives you plan A. A great workout teaches you how to find plans B, C, and D and still get what you want out of it.

We wanted this to be a program and way of training that lets you continue successfully for decades, not just weeks. The goal isn't to run hard and simply cross the finish line but to keep pushing the finish line back further and further so you can continue getting the best benefits from strength training outlined above. There's a time to push your limits and figure out how hard you can work, but you should be able to do that, still live a life outside the gym, and then do it all over again the following week. There's nothing worse than being on the roller coaster of being injured, recovering, then getting injured again. Well, actually there are a lot of things worse than that in the grand scheme of things, but it's still pretty annoying. It's difficult to keep training hard if it's always hurting.

To do the essential service this epic undertaking requires, we had to break the book into a few parts. First, we dig into the different types of injuries you might develop through strength training and look at ways to prevent them or at least work around them. If you've had an injury before, which is likely a big reason why you're picking up this book, we wanted to start here to give you some information and clarity on what you can do about it—whether it can heal with just some rest or whether you need to adjust a few things to keep on trucking. Also, if you do things within your workout like double your working volume and then wonder why everything hurts, this book will give some insights on why it hurts and what to do to prevent the hurt. (Hint: Don't double volume overnight.)

Next, we want to see what you can do before putting together a world-class program for you, so we offer some self-assessments to figure out whether you're creaky like the Tin Man in *The Wizard of Oz* or whether you're bendy enough to get a job as an acrobat with Cirque du Soleil. There's no sense putting a bendy body on a program for a stiff sucker, and no point making Tony Tight Hips try to do a movement that requires more mobility than touching your toes.

After the self-assessments, we show you some common exercises—such as squats, deadlifts, pushes, and pulls—and explain not only how to do them properly but also how to customize them to your specific anatomy. By the way, we don't need X-ray vision to figure this out, but it can be a make-or-break consideration to successful squatting or hating your life anytime you have to hinge from the hips.

Last, we lay out all the programming ways to get jacked and awesome while also avoiding getting too beat up to enjoy the results (and avoiding the surgeon's office along the way). Want to max out every day? Try the Terminator's 50-set workouts? We'll show you why those could be great goals to build up to, but they may not be right to slide into the rotation today without enough prep to manage them. We'll also show how to include accessory exercises to maximize your specific limitations (if any) and adjust training around irritations, injuries, and other ouchies, plus varying training throughout the year to get more stress in some blocks and recover easier in others. We even put together a bunch of sample workouts you could use to get your swole on and adjust based on the outlines we provide in the book.

If you've ever worked with a good coach, you know they go out of their way to get a lot of info, assess, and then customize a plan for you while adjusting around anything that might come up along the way, and we wanted this to be the closest thing we could develop in book form that could replicate that relationship. This book won't replace working with a great coach, but while I would love to get everyone in front of someone qualified to help them with their fitness, that's just not possible for everyone, due to geography, finances, or any number of reasons, so we wanted something that could be a good option for as many people as possible.

Our hope is that you take this book and use it for years. Don't just go through the program once—refer back to it when something pops up. We hope you can do the workouts for years, but we know people change, goals adjust, and boredom creeps in. We wanted to outline a program but also explain why your other programs might work, and show how to adjust those programs as needed. This book is more about learning how to train for the long term than just learning how to go through a workout.

Enough talk—let's get into it. Read through the entire book before starting the workouts. That way you can know what's going on and what to do if something needs to change for you and your specific circumstances. Work hard, adjust as needed, and give yourself the gift of long-term strength.

Let's do this.

Acknowledgments

Writing a book has been a life-long dream, and it's been a massive undertaking. This book would have never seen the light of day without the work behind the scenes of so many individuals whom I would like to ensure get their flowers.

First to my co-author, Dan Pope. Having not met in person prior to this, I had seen your content online and tangentially known you were a great source of knowledge and passionate about what you do. Through working with you on this book, I've seen firsthand how your work ethic and enthusiasm bleed through on every page. You flew to Edmonton during wildfire season and a playoff run to make sure the photos in the book were the best possible, and during every meeting we had it felt like we had known each other since childhood. I'm grateful for the opportunity to form a strong friendship through this project and look forward to whatever else we can cook up in the future.

Second, to the publishing team at Human Kinetics. Korey Van Wyk initially reached out to see if this would be possible and slow walked Dan and me through the process of creating an appealing outline that stood a chance of getting a couple of first-time authors a shot. Cynthia McEntire, our fantastic editor who kept the project on track, made sure our words made sense outside of our own heads, and kept us organized to produce the final product in a smooth, frictionless process that can only come from someone at the helm who knows exactly what they are doing. Our undying gratitude for all assistance above and beyond.

For Jim Bowling, the Human Kinetics director of photography, your work behind the scenes on the organization for the photo shoot ensured it went off smoothly and with minimal effort. Steve Glen and Andrew Mardon, the photographers who put together the exercise pictures, ran an incredibly professional, high-quality shoot, adjusting to our whims and ensuring they got the best shot possible in every scenario. And our models, Omar Ali, Joyce Demchuk, Nolan Somerset, and Charlene Muskego were fantastically easy and fun to work with. This book wouldn't look nearly as good without any of you.

Big thanks to other Human Kinetics staff Alexis Koontz, Denise D'Urso, Tina Kinder, Laurel Mitchell, and the members of the editorial board working behind the scenes to make each component of this publication take shape and happen.

Next, thank you to all my clients, past, present, and future, who have allowed me to learn in real time what works and what might not for such a wide variety of individuals. You have helped form the entire basis of what

Acknowledgments

I do as a trainer, as it should be. To all my colleagues whom I've either worked alongside in commercial gyms or have met online or at various conferences or workshops, you have taught me even more than I could find in any course or research paper. The sharing of ideas in sidebar conversations always tends to spark new directions and in cases like this can even lead to new exciting projects together down the road.

Support doesn't just come from your work environment. My family has played such an integral part in helping me realize this dream. My parents, Leslie and Joanne Somerset, showed me not only could I accomplish whatever I set my mind to, but also how to do it through hard work and perseverance. Your unconditional love and support through every step of my development, from driving me to work to sitting in the stands while I sat on the bench as a mediocre athlete means more to me than you could imagine. My two brothers, Clint Somerset and Wade Somerset, showed me what the life of an athlete was all about and tried to involve me whenever they could. You instilled a love of sport and competition that has stayed with me since playing ministicks in the hallway and trying to figure out how to jump higher to grab the rim. Every kid needs their hero, and I grew up with two.

Last but most important, my wonderful wife Lindsay Somerset. Who knew a chance meeting at a squat rack would turn into this? You've long supported my late nights, weekends, and early mornings working with clients, writing, or traveling to who knows where to teach people about squats and deadlifts, and you stood solidly by me for any change, challenge, and celebration I've encountered over these past 20 years. You mean so much more to me than I could ever hope to put into this acknowledgment section that I may have to write another book, even if you're the only one who would ever read it.

Dean Somerset

I'm extremely grateful for the opportunity to publish a book like this and even more thankful for the supportive folks around me who helped make it happen.

To Dean, first thank you for the opportunity to be a co-author of this book. As you noted, I had never met you in person prior to collaborating on this book but had followed you anonymously (not weird or anything) and learned from you for more than a decade. Once we met, I felt like we were long time friends and that made writing that much easier and better.

Thank you to all the kind and helpful folks at Human Kinetics. You've made the journey professional and streamlined.

Thank you to my parents who raised me to pursue my dreams. Finally, the biggest thanks goes to my wife Stephanie and son Luke. Although I loved writing this book, it was a selfish act because I was unavailable for many mornings, nights, and weekends. Thank you for supporting my goals and allowing me to create this book.

Dan Pope

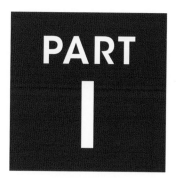

PART

I

Prehab and Prevention

Preventing Injuries: What We Know

Let's face it, injuries are terrible. Nothing is worse than getting halfway through your warm-up bench press sets and starting to experience stabbing pain in your shoulder as the weights get heavier and heavier.

Injuries keep us from doing what we love, plain and simple. For a weight-lifter, having a serious injury is the same as having an identity crisis. Lifting weights isn't just something we love doing; it is a big part of what drives our sense of self. Not being able to hit the gym and hit the programmed set of squats due to knee pain can be as bad as losing a limb. Well, maybe not that bad, but you get the point.

Rehabilitation is equally frustrating. As a physical therapist, I'll even admit that some of the exercises I prescribe are about as fun as watching paint dry. It can take weeks, months, and even years to recover from some injuries. Worse yet, time away from training is time when you are most likely getting weaker and smaller, basically the opposite of your goals.

One of the best ways to continue building strength and performance in the long haul is to stay healthy. As a physical therapist I see the opposite of this all the time. Athletes recover from an injury and jump straight back into a program they're not suited for, just to get injured again. I call it the yo-yo strategy. It's a great way to frustrate yourself so badly that you give up weights and take up bird watching.

Instead, we need a strategy that allows us to make continual gains over time—that minimizes the risk of injury and respects any sort of nagging pain you might be dealing with. It's important to understand that there is a risk of injury with any sort of activity, and strength training is no different. However, the injury rates are fairly low and the benefits are amazing.

On top of this, there is some data out there that helps us to understand what increases our risk of injury. If we can understand this data and implement some important principles in our training, we reduce the likelihood of getting hurt and taking up mushroom collecting over hitting the gym.

This chapter covers what we know so far from an injury prevention standpoint: what causes injuries and, more important, what helps to prevent them. To kick things off we'll start by talking about just how common injuries are in the gym and in strength sports such as powerlifting and Olympic weightlifting.

How Often Do Lifters Get Hurt?

To understand how common these injuries are, we first have to talk about how injuries are reported in the medical literature. "Injury rates" refers to how often people get hurt performing a specific activity, such as weight training. Injury rates are measured in the number of injuries per 1,000 hours of participation. Basically, if you trained for a total of 1,000 hours over time, how many injuries would you acquire during that time?

Let's use an injury incidence of three injuries per every 1,000 hours of participation. If an individual in this activity participates for five hours per week throughout the year, they should be injured, on average, once every 1 or 2 years or so.

It's important to understand that the research on injuries in different sports and activities varies widely from study to study. This is largely because injuries are defined differently from study to study. Injuries can be defined in several ways, for example:

- Did the injury necessitate a visit to the doctor?
- Did the injury result in forced time away from training?
- Did the injury force the athlete to temporarily modify training?
- Did the injury require surgical intervention?

In my mind an injury that forces a surgery and 6 to 12 months of rehabilitation should be ranked and recorded in a different way than an injury that forced you to modify training for a few weeks. Also, some people just don't go to a doctor despite having a fairly serious injury or aren't smart about modifying when they have pain. They may not even categorize their issue as an injury at all.

Unfortunately, injury definitions are not standard across studies, so some of the numbers need to be taken with a grain of salt. In the next few paragraphs you'll see exactly what I'm talking about. Injury rates vary widely from study to study and a lot of this is due to the factors mentioned previously.

As you know, there is an enormous amount of variation from one person's training to another. You have variety in programming, movement selection, rest, recovery, and so forth that isn't always well controlled for in these studies.

With that being said, how much risk is there in weight training and barbell sports? In a U.S. military population over a 1-year period, 4.5 percent of men and 0.6 percent of women experienced a weight training injury.[1] That equates to a 0.31 and 0.05 injury incidence per every 1,000 hours of participation for men and women. This is extremely low.

Now, on the flip side of the coin you'll find research showing injury rates as high as 9.0 per 1,000 hours of participation in group strength and endurance classes, although this is an odd finding and not in line with other literature.[4]

To compare this to adolescent sports (obviously this will depend on the study) the average injury rate was 2.64 for every 1,000 hours of participation, with soccer causing the largest amount of injuries (7.21 per 1,000 hours).[2] There is a lot of discrepancy between studies with some studies showing injury rates as high as 95.7, 64.4, and 62.6 injuries per 1,000 hours of participation in rugby, soccer, and hockey, respectively.[1] So it would appear that injury rates are substantially lower in the gym in comparison to other popular sports.

If we start looking at weight training sports (Olympic weightlifting, powerlifting, CrossFit, bodybuilding, strongman, and Highland games), the injury incidence is 2.4 to 4.5 injuries for every 1,000 hours of participation.[3] Bodybuilding comes in as the safest (0.24 per 1,000 hours), whereas the Highland games tended to cause the most injury (7.5 per 1,000 hours).

Largely, then, it seems that weight training can be quite safe. Even more competitive barbell sports seem to have, on average, similar or better rates of injury compared to other sports.[3] Lastly, the injuries are most likely going to vary greatly based on the population, training style, coaching, and so forth. We believe the benefits of strength training far outweigh the potential risk of injury and people can probably reduce the risk of injury substantially by making smart decisions in the weight room.

What Influences Injury Risk in Strength Training?

Almost every common training approach, style, or goal-specific outcome starts with the assumption that the individual is healthy, without any injuries or limitations, and isn't at a higher risk for developing a potential injury. This puts anyone with a cranky shoulder, tender lower back, or wobbly knees at a slight disadvantage, especially as the program ramps up to higher volumes and intensities.

Injured tissues tend to have a lower tolerance for loading and take longer to recover than noninjured tissues. This is a big reason why the biggest determinant of future injury is a previous injury. Injured tissues are just more susceptible and don't adapt to stress from exercise quite as quickly as uninjured tissue.[44]

Injured or previously injured tissues can still tolerate some loading and volume, and to build strength and capacity those tissues have to go through stress and recovery cycles like those found in any training program. The trick is to figure out how much stress and volume they can handle in a way that develops more of what the individual wants without pushing too hard and having tissues breaking down or increasing the risk of further injuries.

There's a concept in rehab called the law of repetitive motion, which outlines a mathematical formula for what it takes to develop an injury. The concept looks like this:

$$I = (N \times F) \div (A \times R)$$

where I is injury risk, N is the number of repetitions or number of stress exposures, and F is the absolute force applied with the stress, which could be considered the total amount of weight being lifted or the weight times the speed of movement. A is amplitude, or range of motion or distance of movement produced, or could also be considered the frequency of exposures on a training calendar. R is relative tissue recovery.

Within this framework, you can see that increasing either the number of stress exposures or the amount of force would increase the relative risk of injury of the involved tissues. Similarly, reducing the recovery time, range of motion, or frequency can increase likelihood of injury.

It bears repeating: you increase your injury risk any time you rapidly increase the volume or weight being lifted, or when recovery is significantly impaired (such as when you're fresh from travel, after a rough night shift, a few nights of terrible sleep, and maybe a bit hungover), or when you're jumping into something new without building up to specific tolerances to the activity being performed. For example, let's say you work out in the gym regularly, but decide you want to spend a day playing pickup basketball after not having done so for 20 years. You're not used to the demands of the sport, so even though you work out and are relatively fit, you're not used to those specific stressors, so your tissues will take a beating and the risk of something going wrong is higher than if you'd spent a few weeks getting used to the demands of the sport.

Understanding how to prevent injuries from a tissue load and tolerance consideration is a great starting point to making sure you can stay healthy. Another big consideration is how certain tissues tend to get injured within this framework. Muscles, tendons, ligaments, discs, and nerves all have different mechanisms of injury, symptoms, and timelines for recovery, and will be discussed in depth in the coming sections. however, there are some hard and fast rules to consider:

- The denser and less vascular the tissue, the longer the healing times.
- Within the same tissues, acute injuries require a "rest and recover" approach, whereas overuse injuries need a "load and recovery" or activity modification approach.

- The longer you've had to deal with a specific issue, the longer it's going to take to fully recover, and the slower any kind of progress in volume or load should be.
- It's crucial to work to full pain-free mobility first, then work into loading that range of motion effectively.

Muscle tissue heals fairly quickly because it has a great supply of blood to deliver nutrients and remove waste products, but it also has specialized satellite cells that work to repair and rebuild damaged tissue all the time. Bone also recovers quickly, because while it's fairly dense, the marrow has massive access to blood. Bone contains osteoblasts and osteoclasts, specialized cells that constantly break down (osteoclast) and build up (osteoblast) new bone material, which can speed up healing.

Cartilage, meniscus, and vertebral discs are very dense connective tissues, and tend not to have nearly the same blood supply as muscle or bone tissues, so their healing times can be a lot longer. A basic muscle strain might be fully back to normal in 2 to 6 weeks, but a disc injury might take upward of a year to heal on its own.

If a tissue is constantly irritated and damaged, a chronic condition can result. This might even change the physical properties of the tissue, making it harder to recover compared to not having the same irritation. Tendons that are chronically inflamed can become more brittle, reduce connective tissue density, and even see the growth of new blood vessels into the tendon to deliver nutrients to assist in healing, which also decreases how much strain the tendon can allow.

Applying the Training Continuum to Both Prehab and Rehab

One of the biggest predisposing factors to injuries is having a previous injury on the same body part. We can do a lot to reduce the risks of different injuries, but there's always a chance they can happen. Strong tissues with a larger work capacity will be less likely to become damaged than tissues with lower tolerances, so training can have a massive impact on reducing your risks of developing any kind of injury, even though exposure to exercise stress is in fact a risk.

Rehab typically involves allowing tissues to recover from damage. Damaged tissue's tolerance to loading and volume is often limited by possible recurrence of symptoms, swelling, pain or discomfort, and potential to redamage the affected tissues. The rehab process aims to gradually increase the tissue's ability to manage load and volume, just like "regular" training. The only difference is the previous history of tissue damage and the focus on allowing the affected tissues to regenerate from their damaged state.

"Prehab" as a concept essentially means trying to prevent the need for rehab with well-thought-out training programs focusing on progressive overload and increasing tissue resiliency, with the goal of increasing the amount of strain that can be managed before tissues start getting damaged. If we can prevent injuries before they happen, we're accomplishing two big outcomes: we aren't having to take time away from dedicated training, and we're not becoming more susceptible to future injuries. I call prehab "future-proofing" since the goal is to become strong enough to not get injured in the first place.

Both rehab and future-proofing work on the same muscle adaptation continuum (figure 1.1), just with different loads and volumes based on the health of the tissues being worked. A major goal of rehab is to get tissues strong enough to return to unrestricted training. A major goal of prehab is to get tissues strong enough to reduce the possible risks of tissue damage while seeing a positive training adaptation. They both involve applying stress to tissues, allowing recovery, and seeing adaptation to that stress.

Future-proofing also tries to prepare for scenarios that may expose the body to large forces or new situations. If I decide to go for a big hike up a mountain, barbell squats will help train leg muscles to develop force to push up into higher steps, but they won't build endurance or train my ankles to manage uphill and downhill angles. Activities like lunges, step-ups, step-downs, and uphill walking would be good ways to prepare for the demands of hiking, so effective future-proof training involves an element of specificity as well as a variety of activities to build resilient connective tissue.

You can also go a long way to preventing injuries with some simple programming considerations. A lot of injuries come about with sudden changes in volume, intensity, frequency, or activity, so any changes being made should be fairly gradual. A good rule of thumb is the weekly 10 percent: Make changes to volume, intensity, or frequency by no more than 10 percent a week. This gradual increase can allow time to adapt to the new

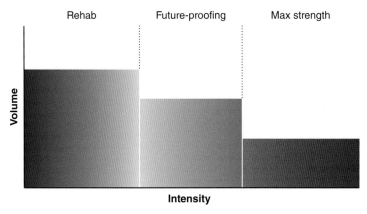

Figure 1.1 Training continuum flow.

stress without pushing into risky territory, but still allow some flexibility to program design.

For instance, a return-to-sport program involves a workout plan of 10 sets of exercises 3 times a week, for a total of 30 sets of volume. A 10 percent increase in this would bump things up to 33 sets of exercise the following week, which is only one additional set of exercise per workout. Monitor for any return of symptoms, new pain, or stuff you wouldn't want to see in recovery, and if there are any of these unwanted effects, you could either maintain the same volume for the following week to see if they reduce or return to the 30 sets of volume for another week before pushing for more.

As another example, if you were squatting 100 pounds (45 kg) for 4 sets of 5 reps, a 10 percent increase could mean either increasing the weight to 110 pounds (50 kg) for 5 reps, assuming the technique of the movement was maintained, or maintaining 100 pounds (45 kg) of loading, but completing 2 sets of 5 reps, and 2 sets of 6 reps, moving from 20 reps to 22 reps.

For any of these increases, you'd want to maintain technique, avoid pushing to maximum or to failure, and be on the lookout for any change in symptoms following the workouts or training week. Because rehab involves building up tissues, creating new proteins, and increasing blood flow and delivery of nutrients, progress can be slow, and rushing it can mean getting injured all over again.

It's important to remember that future-proof training doesn't have the same limits on how to progress, because the assumption is that the tissues aren't recovering from injury, so they can typically handle more and larger fluctuations in exercise stress. Because the tissues don't have the hindrance of a previous injury, they can manage stress and see positive adaptations without running as high of a risk of excessive stress resulting in negative adaptations (getting reinjured).

Whether you're in rehab or future-proof programming, as training stress increases, so too should the focus on recovery increase. You need to get enough sleep, eat healthy food, and manage lifestyle stress to achieve the best recovery. If you're training only once or twice a week, your recovery focus doesn't need to be too high since you have 3 or 4 days to physically recover between each workout. However, if you're training with any intensity, like 4 or more times a week, your recovery time between sessions is sometimes less than 24 hours. That means recovery time is limited and therefore more important to manage effectively. We'll discuss recovery methods in depth in later chapters.

Common Types of Injuries

If we're interested in preventing future injury, it's in our best interest to know what the most common injuries are. If I expect to prevent injuries in runners by strengthening their shoulders, I probably won't be very successful, right? Runners don't have many shoulder injuries, so I'd be wasting my time. Instead, I'd probably want to build a program to strengthen the calves and knees, given that Achilles issues and runner's knee are so common in this population.

So, returning to the gym, we ask, "What are the most common injuries in a weight training environment?" Well, we have some research to help us out here. For strength sports the most common areas of injury are generally the shoulder, lower back, and knee.[3] Most injuries reported tend to be strains, tendinitis, and sprains.[3] For powerlifters the lower back and shoulder tend to be the most problematic.[5] For Olympic weightlifters the knees and shoulders tend to be more of an issue.[5] This may simply reflect the fact that squats and deadlifts in powerlifting just tax the spine so much, whereas the knees may take more stress in Olympic weightlifters given all the deep squats. In both sports the demands on the shoulder are also quite high, which may explain the high incidence of shoulder injury.

A study by Requa et al. (1993) looking at injury rates during common gym activities found that the knee, shoulder, and lower back were the most common injury sites (in that order).[6] Grier et al. (2022) also found that the shoulder, lower back, and knee were the most common injuries, coming in at 27 percent, 27 percent, and 8 percent of all injuries, respectively.[1] Of note (more on this later), it was a very common finding that injuries consistently occurred in areas that had a previous injury.[6] Most injuries in this study required only a temporary modification of activities, with 10 to 15 percent of injuries necessitating a trip to the doctor.[6] This means most injuries were not that severe, which is good news. The most common type of injury diagnosed was a sprain or strain.[6]

Logic would dictate that injuries are simply going to be most common in the areas that take the most stress in the gym. This appears to be the shoulder, lower back, and knee. The area that is most at risk is most likely a representation of which movements you perform the most in the gym and what area those movements stress. On top of that it seems as though having a prior injury is a good indicator of which area is likely to get hurt again in the future.

Now that we know where the most common injuries generally occur, let's identify these injuries so we can start building a foundation of knowledge to stay a bit safer in the gym.

How Injuries Occur

Now that we know the most common types of injuries tend to occur in the lower back, shoulder, and knee, let's discuss some reasons why they may occur and begin a foundation for injury prevention strategies.

Injuries occur in all shapes and sizes. They can occur in the form of an acute injury like a muscular strain that occurs abruptly or an injury with a more gradual onset that starts small and slowly worsens over time.

BE AWARE OF MEDICAL RED FLAGS

Before we start going over the most common injuries in the gym, let's talk about medical red flags. This book is *not* meant to be about self-diagnosis and treatment of common orthopedic injuries in the gym. Our goal is to teach you a bit about these injuries in hopes that you'll be able to better avoid them and get the care you need if one of these issues pops up.

There's always a chance that a given injury or type of pain isn't commonplace but rather something more serious that needs medical attention right away. Some red flags[7] that indicate you may need medical attention are:

- Progressive symptoms (symptoms worsening over time)
- Thoracic (chest) pain
- Past history of cancer
- Unexplained weight loss
- Drug abuse
- Night pain
- Fever
- Night sweats

When in doubt, always get your injury checked out by a qualified professional to make sure you're not dealing with something more serious. Being seen by a qualified professional after an injury will ensure you get the best possible long-term outcome and maximize your ability to get back to training the way you want.

Lower-Back Pain

Lower-back pain may be categorized as flexion based, extension based, or compression based. Keep in mind that every individual has their own "flavor" of lower-back pain. It's rare to find someone whose pain fits into a single category. However, I think it is useful to categorize lower-back injuries this way so we can get an idea of what movements may predispose us to these types of injuries.

Flexion-based lower-back pain refers to pain in the lower back that is worse during activities that flex or round the spine, such as when performing a toe touch from a standing position. Several common exercises such as squats and deadlifts also place a large amount of load on the spine in a flexed position. Movements with potential for causing flexion-based lower-back pain are squats, deadlifts, and Olympic lifts. Visualize the bottom position of the squat or starting position in a deadlift. One example of a flexion-based injury is an intervertebral disc herniation.[8]

Extension-based lower-back pain is the opposite of flexion-based lower-back pain. People with extension-based lower-back pain experience pain while extending or arching the lower back. Several movements, such as the bench press and overhead press, load the spine into an extended position. Movements with the potential to cause extension-based lower-back pain are overhead presses, jerks, bench presses, and the backswing of kipping movements. Two injuries that cause extension-based lower-back pain are facet joint injury and spondylolisthesis.[9]

In some individuals, it's not necessarily a given position that's not tolerated but the act of compressing the spine itself. Think of what happens to the spine when you unrack a heavy barbell. This may cause compression-based lower-back pain. Many movements may compress the spine, so this can be a big challenge for folks with this issue. Movements with the potential to cause compression-based lower-back pain include overhead presses, jerks, squats, deadlifts, and Olympic lifts.

Shoulder Instability (Labral Pathology)

The shoulder is a ball-and-socket joint that is deepened and stabilized by connective tissue including ligaments and labrum. Some folks can acquire instability of those structures from a traumatic injury, such as a shoulder dislocation, that can tear the labrum and ligaments. Others can acquire instability due to repetitive activities over time, such as throwing a baseball. Lastly, some people are just born a bit "looser" than others and have some instability as a result. Exercises that challenge the shoulder in an end range of motion can be problematic for people like this due to their lack of stability.[10] Movements with the potential to cause injury include snatches, jerks, overhead presses, behind-the-neck exercises, dips, and muscle-ups.

Rotator Cuff Pain

The rotator cuff's job is to help stabilize the shoulder joint, and it is very active when we train in the gym. Over time, movements that place a large amount of stress on the rotator cuff tendons can result in pain and in some cases a torn rotator cuff.[11] Movements with the potential to cause problems like this include bench presses and overhead presses.

Biceps Long Head Pathology

The tendon of the long head of the biceps sits in the front of the shoulder inside a deep groove. Due to its role in stabilizing the front of the shoulder during movement and lack of abundant blood supply, it is theorized that this tendon can be a common source of pain in the front of the shoulder. This tendon is commonly injured together with the rotator cuff and the movements that aggravate the rotator cuff can also aggravate this tendon.[12]

Movements with the potential to cause this type of injury include bench presses and overhead presses.

Acromioclavicular Joint Pain

The acromioclavicular (AC) joint is located where the collarbone (clavicle) meets the highest point of the shoulder blade (acromion). It is a small but important joint that plays a crucial role in the mobility and stability of the shoulder. The AC joint is involved in many upper-body movements, including pushing, pulling, and overhead activities. However, it is also prone to injury, particularly in activities that involve repetitive overhead motions like those in weightlifting.[13] It is theorized that movements involving the pectoralis and deltoid muscles where the shoulder is approaching end range horizontal abduction and extension (visualize the bottom position of the bench press) place large traction forces across the joint. Therefore, people with AC joint issues often have difficulty with movements such as bench presses and push-ups. Movements with the potential to cause injury[13,14] include bench presses, overhead presses, dips, pec flys, and push-ups.

Shoulder Osteoarthritis

Shoulder osteoarthritis (OA) is a condition in which the cartilage that cushions the shoulder joint wears down over time, which may lead to pain, stiffness, and limited range of motion. Risk factors for shoulder OA include increased age, a high level of shoulder use, obesity, and smoking. Athletes and fitness enthusiasts who regularly engage in activities that place stress on the shoulder joint, such as weightlifting, may be at increased risk for developing shoulder arthritis over time.[15,16] Movements with the potential to cause problems include bench presses and overhead presses.

Patellofemoral Pain

Patellofemoral pain, commonly known as runner's knee, is a nagging discomfort felt around the kneecap during physical activities such as running, jumping, or squatting. This type of pain can be caused by overuse of the patellofemoral joint, which occurs via activities that use the quadriceps muscles for deeper degrees of knee bending, such as the bottom of a squat.[17] Movements with the potential to cause problems include squats, lunges, step-ups, jumping, and running.

Quadriceps and Patellar Tendinopathy

Patellar tendinopathy is a condition that affects the patellar tendon, which connects the kneecap to the shinbone (tibia). Quadriceps tendinopathy affects the quadriceps tendon, which attaches the quadriceps to the kneecap. It's commonly known as "jumper's knee" because it often affects athletes who do a lot of jumping, such as basketball players and volleyball players, although it can also affect weightlifters.[18] Tendinopathy is caused by overuse of these tendons, which can lead to pain in the knee, particularly around the top or bottom of the kneecap. This type of pain can be caused by overuse, especially movements that utilize the quadriceps muscles to a large degree, particularly in a plyometric fashion.[18] Movements with the potential to cause problems include squats, lunges, step-ups, and jumping.

Meniscus and Cartilage Pathology

Meniscus pathology refers to any injury or damage to the meniscus, a C-shaped piece of cartilage in the knee joint that helps cushion and stabilize the joint. Common causes of meniscus pathology include sport-related injuries, repetitive activities that stress the knee, and degenerative changes that occur with age. "Cartilage injuries" refers to any type of pain originating from or damage in the cartilage within the knee joint.[19] Meniscus injuries can occur traumatically, such as with a twisting injury of the knee during skiing. However, chronic injuries related to longer-term wear on the joint are much more common in the gym. Movements with the potential to cause injury include squats, lunges, step-ups, and jumping.

Ligamentous Injury

Ligaments are tough, fibrous bands of tissue that connect bone to bone and provide stability to a joint. In the knee, there are four main ligaments: the anterior cruciate ligament (ACL), the posterior cruciate ligament (PCL), the medial collateral ligament (MCL), and the lateral collateral ligament (LCL). Injuries to these ligaments can happen during sports that involve cutting and pivoting, and are generally traumatic.[20] Ligamentous injuries are less common in people who do weight training. Movements with the potential to cause injury include jumping, cutting, and pivoting.

Knee Osteoarthritis

Knee OA occurs when the protective cartilage that cushions the ends of the bones wears down over time. This may lead to pain within the joint.[21] Movements with the potential to cause problems include squats, lunges, step-ups, and jumping.

Mechanisms of Injury

Mechanism of injury is just a fancy term that identifies the reason why someone gets injured. If I slip and fall, breaking my hip on impact, then the mechanism of injury would be a fracture due to the impact after falling. It's important that we identify mechanisms of injury because if we have information on how we get hurt in the first place, then we can reverse-engineer a solution and reduce our risk of future injury. Let's look into these mechanisms.

Total Volume

We have quite a bit of research suggesting that the body can handle only so much stress. This is a bit of a no-brainer. If we max out our deadlift 13 times in a given afternoon, we're more likely to get injured than if we spread this effort across several months of smart training. Simply put, if we don't manage fatigue well and continue to take on more than the body is able to handle, we may be exposing ourselves to an increased risk of injury.[23]

The other thing to keep in mind is that the more often we train (more volume and or frequency) the more chances we have to get injured.[22] If you sit on the couch for the rest of your life and never enter a gym, chances are you'll never get hurt working out.

Exercise and strength training is obviously good for us, and if we're sedentary we actually open ourselves to other forms of orthopedic injury. The solution, of course, isn't to avoid the gym, but you know this. As we'll see in a moment, fitness can actually stave off injury, so things can get a little complex. More on this later.

REAL-LIFE EXAMPLE

Dan has a past hip injury that will flare up from time to time if he squats with too much volume. If Dan squats 1 or 2 times per week consistently, his hip feels great. If he pushes the volume up to 3 times per week, he notices his hip slowly starts to get more sore and irritated. In other words, if Dan keeps his volume in check the old injury doesn't become an issue.

TAKEAWAYS

- Don't take on training programs that far exceed your current level of training.
- Proceed with caution using high-volume training programs.
- Be careful not to overdo training stress on areas of the body that had a prior injury.

Spikes in Training Volume

The next idea is paradoxical to the first point. I just made the argument that *reducing* the total amount of time training in the gym will reduce your risk of injury simply because you have less exposure to lifting. Less gym time = less chance to get hurt. (Duh.) However, research from Tim Gabbett[23] has shown that having a high level of fitness is actually protective against injury. So in this model, exercising more frequently will actually reduce your risk of injury per hour of time spent training in the gym.

It all comes back to the idea of preparing your body for the tasks you plan to put it through in the future. If you are planning on running a marathon and your prep work consists of watching TV for months prior to the big day, then I'd bet some money on you getting hurt during the race. In contrast, someone who slowly builds up their run volume over time is much less likely to get injured during the race because they've increased their capacity to handle the marathon.

Compare this athlete to an ultramarathon runner who is used to regularly completing races of more than 100 miles. For this runner, a marathon—26.2 miles—is going to be a walk in the park and probably less likely to cause an injury for them in comparison to less fit runners. The ultramarathoner just has way more capacity to handle the stress of running for 26.2 miles.

Tim Gabbett has pioneered a lot of this research and way of thinking. More specifically, he found that any sort of spike in training volume consistently increases the chances of an athlete getting hurt.[23] He calculated this via the acute to chronic (A:C) workload ratio. Basically, if the training you are subjecting your body to (acute load) is much harder or greater than what your body has been prepared for in the past several weeks (chronic load), then your risk of injury in that session goes up. On the flip side, if your current training session (acute workload) is smaller and easier than what you're used to (chronic workload), your risk of injury goes down. This means two things:

1. You should always thoroughly prepare the body for upcoming training challenges (competitions, big training cycles, bear fights) slowly, over time.

2. Your training should be very consistent over time.

If you take a broad look at injury prevention programs for sport, you'll find that strength training, proprioception, and balance exercises all seem to reduce the risk of injury.[43] What these injury prevention programs attempt to do is apply exercises that are specific to the demands of a given sport and target particularly susceptible areas. For example, the FIFA 11 program to reduce soccer injuries contains strengthening, jumping, balance and change-of-direction drills to help prevent hamstring strains and ACL tears—

two injuries common to soccer players. Attempting to reverse-engineer a solution to the injury based on the mechanism of injury, these programs gradually increase the capacity or chronic training load of the area.

There are a few points at which folks get into trouble with A:C workloads:

- When first starting a training program
- When program hopping
- When working on weaknesses
- When taking time off and then returning to training
- When inconsistently training

Obviously, when we start a training program our A:C workload ratio (sometimes abbreviated ACWR) will be completely imbalanced. We're throwing stress onto the body that it may never have seen before. That's why it makes sense to go slowly and cautiously.

A second place where things can go wrong is with program hopping. This basically means switching between two very different training programs without any form of bridge or slow progression to the other. I get it—you get bored with certain training programs, and that new shiny program with 10 sets of 10 squats and high-volume Olympic weightlifting looks super fun. Trouble is, that switcheroo represents a large change in A:C workload ratio. Lifter beware!

The next place where I see this issue occur frequently is when people decide to work on their weaknesses. Don't get me wrong—I love the idea of working on your weaknesses. If you're embarrassed that your squat is weaker than your bench press (and you should be) then it makes sense to concentrate on the squat to improve your powerlifting total and build up your pencil legs. I've seen more than my fair share of folks in this situation who tried to remedy it by squatting 3 or 4 times per week when they were previously squatting once per week. This represented a 3 or 4 times increase in training volume. Now they're coming to see me because it feels like they have a hot poker on the inside of their knee cap every time they take a step down the stairs.

Another trap people fall into is taking time off and then returning to training. Sure, life gets busy and we have periods of time where we can train only once or twice a week. However, when you find the time to get back into the gym, don't overcompensate by going every single day for the next several weeks. Slowly work your way back.

Lastly, inconsistent training can really throw a wrench into your A:C workload ratio. This is especially true in group exercise classes. Let's say the group squats on Mondays, deadlifts on Wednesdays, and Olympic lifts on Fridays. If you make Mondays and Wednesdays for 2 weeks and then Wednesdays and Fridays on the following two weeks, you just spiked your volume of Olympic lifts. You've also most likely detrained or gotten worse on the squat from missing those 2 weeks of Mondays. Being consistent is key for both progress and reducing your risk of injury.

Now we know that having a spike in training can be bad. One way to combat this is simply to avoid having a spike in the acute load. However, another way we can do this is to increase the chronic workload. In other words, if injuries are occurring simply because a given area lacks capacity to handle training, then beefing up that area may be enough to reduce injury risk.

If I practice balance and plyometric exercises, it makes sense that I may be less likely to land in an awkward way and sprain my ankle. If I strengthen the hamstring it makes sense that I'll have less likelihood of injury when sprinting (which uses the hamstring a lot). We can apply this same strategy to the weight room. If the shoulders, knees, and lower back are most susceptible to injury, it makes sense to include a few exercises that target the knee, lower back, and shoulders twice per week.

As discussed earlier, a prior injury increases your risk of future injury of that given area. If we apply a strength program for this area, we may reduce the likelihood of a new injury or flare-up of pain in the future. If I have a history of shoulder pain in the gym, then it makes sense to add some rotator cuff exercises twice per week into my regular routine to reduce injury risk moving forward.

REAL-LIFE EXAMPLE

Johnny wanted to improve his ability to perform pull-ups. He bumped up his training to include pull-ups three times per week over his normal routine of once per week. Three weeks into the new program his elbow started bothering him during pull-ups. It's likely the mechanism of injury here was a large increase in pull-up volume compared to what he was accustomed to.

TAKEAWAYS

- Avoid spikes in training volume.
- Build training volume and intensity slowly over time.
- Increase chronic load in movements that could cause problems via strengthening exercises twice per week.

Exercise Technique

In the weightlifting community there is a general notion that improper technique is overall one of the largest contributors to injury. On the flip side of the coin, many in the physical therapy community believe there are probably many safe exercise techniques and the human body can over time adapt to a given training technique. In reality, the answer likely lies somewhere in between. It's likely that certain techniques minimize risk of injury compared to others. The trouble is that we don't know the answer to this question based on current evidence. However, we have some experience and perspective about what is best for the average lifter and we'll share this in subsequent chapters.

What's important to understand is that when we alter our training technique, stress is not eliminated. We're simply taking some stress away from certain structures and placing it on others. A good example is in the squat (figure 1.2). Figure 1.2*a* shows a very upright and deep squat useful for anyone looking to improve their Olympic weightlifting. Figure 1.2*b* shows a powerlifting-style squat where the trunk is inclined forward.

When the trunk is more upright and the knees translate forward of the center of mass, as in figure 1.2*a*, more of the stress is placed on the knees. Contrast this with the powerlifting-style squat (figure 1.2*b*); the hips are forced backward, with more of the load placed on the hips and spine and less on the knees.

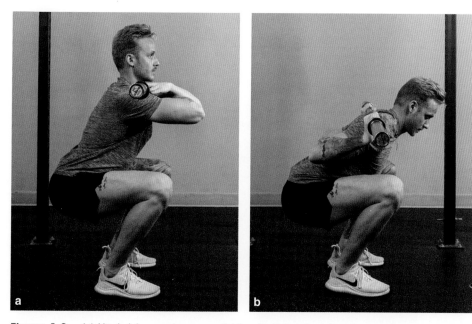

Figure 1.2   *(a)* Upright squat versus *(b)* barbell low-bar back squat.

The other point to keep in mind is that certain positions will more evenly distribute force across a given joint surface area or across muscles to share the load and hopefully result in decreased risk of injury overall. One good example is the knee-in technique during the squat (figure 1.3).

The two joints of the knee are the tibiofemoral and patellofemoral (PF) joint. Squatting places quite a bit of stress on the PF joint. The PF joint is subject to upward of 7.8 times your body weight during a squat.[24] When the knee moves inward during the squat, the surface area available to dissipate those forces gets smaller. The forces become localized to the outer portion of the joint. Now, having some knee-in from time to time isn't the end of the world. However, if we have the option to either have knee-in or not, I'd rather keep the knees straight ahead to help share those forces more evenly within the joint.

Another good example is overextension of the spine during an overhead press (figure 1.4). If we hyperextend the lower back during an overhead press (figure 1.4*a*), we focus the stress toward the posterior elements (structures toward the back) of the spine. In contrast, when we stay neutral (figure 1.4*b*) we more evenly distribute those forces across the entire joint surface and hopefully avoid overloading these posterior structures.

It's also important to understand that the body builds strength capacity—the ability to tolerate greater loads—over with training. It's common for people to want their biceps to grow due to loading, but we're also loading bones, tendons, ligaments, and joints along with the muscles. Structures that we typically don't think about stressing, like tendons and intervertebral discs, have the ability to adapt and strengthen over time.[25,26] This is good because it's often the structures that get injured during training,

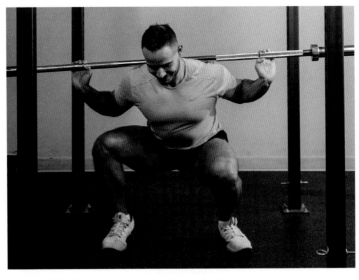

Figure 1.3 Squat with knee-in technique.

like intervertebral discs and tendons, that we want to drive these positive adaptations to make them more robust and resilient against injury.

As with most things, there is likely a sweet spot in terms of how much stress is beneficial and how much it takes to go overboard and cause harm. A good example is in runners. A large study published in 2017 in *The Journal of Orthopaedic & Sports Physical Therapy*[45] showed that only 3.4 percent of runners had hip or knee arthritis, whereas 10.2 percent of sedentary individuals had arthritis. In other words, sedentary folks were three times more likely to have arthritis than were the runners.

However, too much running may cause issues as well. In the same study, elite competitors and those who ran more than 57 miles per week had an even greater incidence of arthritis, at 13.3 percent. This is nearly a four-fold increase compared to the recreational runner. You can find similar increases in rates of patellofemoral joint arthritis in former elite Olympic

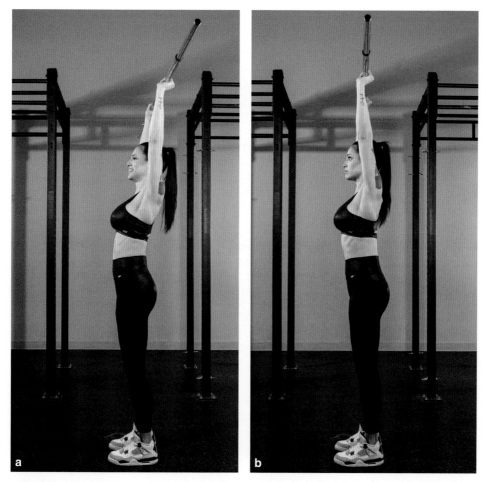

Figure 1.4 Overhead press with (a) hyperextended lower back versus (b) neutral back.

weightlifters, who were found to have higher rates of arthritis compared to sedentary people.[27] However, a modest amount of weight training doesn't seem to increase your risk of knee arthritis over time (and may potentially decrease it).[28] If the strength training program allows you to maintain a healthy body weight, then it will most likely decrease the risk of arthritis over time simply because increased fat mass appears to correlate with increased rates of arthritis.[47]

So what is the best technique for an exercise like the squat? Well, that is totally going to come down to your goals, your unique anatomy, and your past injury history. In the upcoming sections we'll give you an idea of what we consider great techniques to adopt for strength and longevity.

TAKEAWAYS

- Use the exercise technique guidance in this book.
- Use the best technique for your unique goals (Olympic weightlifting versus powerlifting versus general strength training).
- When adopting a new technique or exercise, begin increasing load and volume very slowly and progressively.

Sleep, Stress, and Nutrition

Let's first discuss sleep. Sleep is an amazing thing. It's wildly important for our health in general and actually has a pretty tight correlation with pain and injury. In university athletes, reduced sleep duration correlates with the onset of a new injury.[29] I'll say that again because it's a radical shift in thinking if you've never heard this before: Athletes were more at risk of injury during periods of time when they reported less sleep than usual.

Poor sleep is also a predictor of who goes on to develop chronic pain after the onset of a new injury.[30, 31] If you get an injury, this may mean your problem is more likely to stick around if you don't get enough sleep. How much sleep do you need? This depends on the study you read and the individual, but it appears that less than 7 hours of sleep per night is predictive of getting injured.[33] In a study published in 2021 by Huang and Ihm,[33] sleeping less than 7 hours per night for at least 2 weeks increased risk of injury by 1.7 times.

Getting adequate sleep is also a predictor of the ability to eliminate chronic pain.[30] Getting enough sleep is a critical part of the rehabilitation process after injury. Lastly, daily fluctuations in sleep are predictive of someone's level of pain the day following.[30] Put another way, if you have a night of poor sleep you're more likely to have a higher level of pain the next day.

Stress is another interesting subject. It is commonly cited as a large risk factor for developing chronic pain,[31] especially (but not limited to) in a work environment. Stress is commonly associated with headaches and pain in the neck, lower back, and shoulder.[31]

In the study mentioned earlier by Hamlin et al.,[29] perceived stress and mood was predictive of injuries in university athletes. These same athletes were more likely to be injured around examination times, when stress levels are high.[29]

Interestingly, stress management programs have been shown to be effective for reducing an athlete's risk of injury.[32] Just as stress can increase your risk of injury, stress reduction strategies also seem to be helpful to reduce your risk of injury.

Nutrition is also most likely an important factor in both injury prevention and rehabilitation from injury. Diets low in calories, calcium, and vitamin D increase risk of bone stress injury and low bone mineral density in cross-country runners.[39] Adequate dietary protein and carbohydrates are important to combat loss of muscle following injury.[40] Research about nutrition and its correlation with pain and injury is in its infancy, but I'm excited to see how it unravels over time.

In my mind, adequate sleep, low stress, and good nutrition simply represent your body's ability to recover from training. If you have poor recovery, you may be more likely to get an injury. If you already have an injury and have poor recovery, rehabilitation is going to be tougher.

TAKEAWAYS

- Sleep 7 or more hours per night.
- Consider a stress management program if you have a high level of stress.
- Eat enough macro- and micronutrients to match your level of training.
- Decrease training volume or load if sleep, stress, or nutrition levels are not optimal.

Psychosocial Influences

It may be surprising to learn that your psychology also influences your risk of injury. In a study published in 2021 by Martin et al.,[34] the researchers found that perfectionistic concerns, a strong athletic identity, and poor coach–athlete relationship all correlated with a higher risk of injury.

Perfectionistic concerns are a tendency to evaluate oneself critically. Great athletes often are very critical of their performances, both during training and competition. This pursuit of perfection is often a major catalyst to success. However, it's also important to understand that this very same variable may increase your risk of injury if you overtrain or insist on working through injury in pursuit of your goals.

Athletic identity refers to the degree to which a person identifies with the role of an athlete and looks to others for acknowledgment of that role.[34] Essentially, these athletes think their sense of value to the world is wrapped up in their athletic ability. This aspect of personality can also lead to overtraining and pushing through injury as they look for validation from the world. Those with a high athletic identity may be more apt to push through pain and injury because they see an injury as a major threat to their sense of self and their perceived value to the world. If they have to dial back in training or competition, they lose their sense of value. Sometimes these athletes use denial as a coping mechanism and train through pain.

A poor coach–athlete relationship also predisposes you to a higher risk of injury. This is theorized to occur due to a lack of communication between the coach and athlete about injury or the coach not being open to adjust training due to injury.

Lastly, a plethora of research shows a correlation between pain, anxiety, and depression.[35,36] This interaction is complex and it appears that pain can lead to anxiety and depression, and vice versa.[36] It's worth mentioning that interventions aimed at combating anxiety and depression are useful in reducing pain and risk of injury. Antidepressants have been shown to help reduce pain.[35] Behavioral interventions such as cognitive behavioral therapy have also been shown to help reduce pain[37] as well as reduce the risk of sports injuries.[38]

TAKEAWAYS

- Consider seeking professional help if you suffer from anxiety or depression.
- Understand that pushing through pain is counterproductive for long-term goals.
- Understand that optimal training often means taking into account your stress level, nutrition, and sleep and modifying accordingly.
- Check your ego at the door for every training session, prioritizing small progress over time.

Prior and Current Injury History

Generally speaking, a past history of injury is a fairly good predictor of having a future injury (in the previously injured area or elsewhere).[41] This varies, largely based on the individual and the injury sustained, but the idea is that if you sustained an injury in a given area in the past, you may be more likely to experience a similar injury or pain in the same area. For example, if you've injured your shoulder in the past during bench press, then in the future your shoulder may be more likely to start getting painful and irritated again when ramping up bench press volume or intensity.

I'm a big fan of the saying, "The body keeps the score." This is the title of a book written by Bessel van der Kolk.[46] Although the book is about healing from psychological trauma, the theme is very relevant to orthopedic injury. In our context, "the body keeps the score" means the body remembers past injuries. One of the primary goals of pain in the body is to help us stay safe (currently and in the future). If your body perceives it is going down the same path it went down in the past that created an injury, it may be more apt to start creating some pain to keep you safe. Therefore, we must be extra careful to avoid reaggravating older injuries by overdoing it in the gym.

Another interesting principle that has been more recently popping up in the literature is current injuries worsening when we try to work through them. We've all done it—a shoulder starts acting up during bench press, so you do a few painful arm circles, rub sore muscles, say a Hail Mary, and blast through the last few painful sets. Over time, three things can happen: the area gets better, it stays the same, or it worsens. I'm sure we've all been guilty of training through an injury in the past and perhaps successfully dodged the bullet of the injury worsening.

However, research published in 2019 by Whalan, Lovell, and Sampson[42] showed that working through a relatively minor injury in semiprofessional soccer players resulted in a large increase in risk of sustaining an injury that ended up sidelining the athlete from training and competition. In other words, working through pain can sometimes end up positively, but it's a risky decision that probably increases the likelihood that the injury will worsen (or cause a new injury). For the best course of action, if something hurts a bunch during your warm-up sets, it is best to modify that lift for the day.

TAKEAWAYS

- Be extra careful to keep intensity and volume moderate and avoid training spikes in areas of the body that have an older injury.
- Be quick to modify your training on days where you're experiencing pain during a given exercise.

Conclusion

We are hopeful that after reading this chapter you have a better idea of how prevalent injuries in the gym are. Luckily for us it's a low risk. On top of this, now we have a better idea of what factors may increase our risk of injury. With this knowledge we can be better prepared to avoid the yo-yo trap of recurrent injury and frustration.

Now that you know the principles, in the next few chapters we'll be giving you more practical advice on what you can do for your own training to keep doing the thing you love for the rest of your life.

Athlete Assessment
Identifying Limitations in Mobility and Gross Patterns

Before you can blaze a trail to where you want to go, you have to know where you are. It's as true when planning your strength training program as it is when hiking through the woods. The road to training success begins with assessing your starting point. In this chapter, we work through mobility assessments to determine your starting point. First, let's look at bracing.

Importance of Bracing and How to Do It

Before we dig into the nuts and bolts of assessments, we'll explore a fundamental concept that will be used consistently throughout any training program we put together: bracing and core tension. Bracing plays a couple of roles when it comes to weight training:

- Stabilization of the spine while under load
- Connecting the hips and rib cage to allow efficient force transfer between the lower body and upper body, and vice versa
- Management of blood pressure with changes in intra-abdominal pressure
- Increasing force production through the limbs compared to force production without bracing.

The spine is really just a stack of blocks held together with some ligaments and discs, so it needs a lot of muscle activity to move, hold position, and generate force when moving weights. Learning to brace effectively has two benefits: it can create better performance and also protect you against negative outcomes from training, such as injury or soreness.

There are different ways to brace depending on the loading you're using, the duration of the activity, and whether you want a max effort squeeze, rapid pulsed tension, or just a sustained hold. But regardless of which way you brace, the rules are the same. You want to find a way to get all the abdominal muscles to tense in what's known as a 360-degree brace, meaning all the muscles, from your back to your sides to your front, work together to build tension and stability through the torso. This bracing shouldn't cause you to change your posture—it should just increase tension all around. If you brace and find yourself flexing forward, you're relying on your anterior abdominal muscles and not using enough of the lateral or posterior muscles to generate that tension.

Your ability to lift heavier weights is directly related to whether you have the core strength and bracing power to lift that weight. The heavier the load, the less you want your spine to shift during the movement. This comes down to two primary factors. First, the muscles of the spine aren't massive force producers like your glutes or the muscles of your shoulders. They're designed to hold and allow small movements. Second, the vertebral segments typically have a relatively small range of motion, and exceeding this movement while under load can cause some serious issues. Small movements under load should be manageable for everyone, but as the load increases, the margin of error tends to shrink. The goal of any strength training program is to use a lot of load, so bracing is a fundamental concept for successful lifting.

Let's dig into how you can develop a strong abdominal brace and how you can apply it to your lifting, plus test out whether you have a strong brace already or need to do some work to get yours up to speed.

Bracing With and Without Breathing

There are two slightly different bracing strategies, and they relate to whether or not you plan to maintain your brace while breathing or while holding your breath. For activities with a very high threshold, you need a bracing strategy that allows you to draw from your diaphragm and pelvic floor muscles, which means you'll have to hold your breath during the reps. This technique, called a Valsalva maneuver, can be very effective when pushing very heavy loads.

If you're doing more reps or using a level of force application that isn't quite maximum but is still constant, such as carrying a load across the gym floor or carrying something up a hill, you'll want to use a bracing strategy that allows you to breathe so you don't pass out. A challenge with bracing and breathing simultaneously is that they work against each other in some ways. The harder the brace, the harder it is to get a full breath, and the reverse is also true: the easier it is to get a full breath, the less effective your bracing strategy.

Bracing While Breathing

Let's start with the easier option, bracing while breathing. Start by getting all the muscles around your midsection to flex at the same time. There should be tension, but not maximum effort. On an intensity scale of 1 through 10, where 1 is awareness that muscles are working and 10 is an out-of-body experience with a soul-ripping, earth-shattering, muscle-cramping intensity never before seen in this world, to correctly brace while breathing the level of intensity should be 2 to 4. The muscles are "on," but it's kind of a casual contraction.

Now comes the challenging part. Try to maintain this brace as you inhale, getting as much air as possible without losing that level of tension you started with. During inhalation, the diaphragm descends (figure 2.1), pushing into the abdominal cavity and possibly pushing the ab wall forward. Thus, maintaining a brace against this ab wall movement *while inhaling* is a challenge for some of us. Breathing while bracing can be achieved by switching from abdominal expansion to more rib expansion. Think of lifting the upper chest and letting the ribs expand out to the sides when you inhale versus letting the abdomen expand (figure 2.2). This will help you maintain the brace while still getting some air. When you exhale, maintain the brace and let the chest and ribs return to the starting position.

If you can maintain core bracing while completing a full breath cycle like this, you can rock a more intense brace, so try to increase how hard you squeeze the core muscles to gradually increase the intensity to a 6 or 8, and see if you can still breathe. At the lower intensity, if you can't get the breathing down without losing your bracing, spend some more time trying shallow breaths while bracing, and gradually increasing breath volume while bracing.

A good goal with your bracing and breathing is to be able to generate as much abdominal tension as possible through the 360-degree brace while still being able to draw in air without losing or adjusting the tension of the brace, and to maintain this bracing for up to 30 seconds.

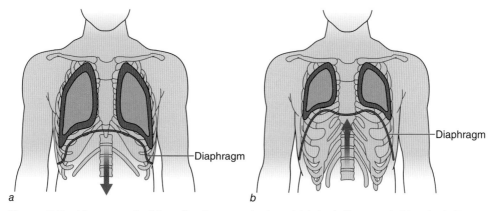

Figure 2.1 Movement of the diaphragm during (*a*) inhalation and (*b*) exhalation.

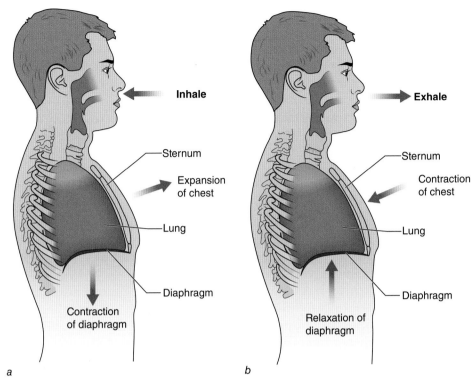

Inhale

Sternum

Expansion
of chest

Lung

Diaphragm

Contraction
of diaphragm

Exhale

Sternum

Contraction
of chest

Lung

Diaphragm

Relaxation of
diaphragm

a

b

Figure 2.2 Movement of the rib cage during (*a*) inhalation and (*b*) exhalation.

Bracing Without Breathing

For a brace without breathing, we're going to go for 360-degree bracing.
Start with the moderate level of bracing, then take in the biggest air you
can. When getting this big air, you can let the abdomen expand as far as
possible. Once your lungs are as full as possible, try to pressurize ("lock
down") your lungs by closing your mouth and squeezing your abs. The
goal is to develop the maximum amount of tension and abdominal pressure, and to hold this tension for 5 to 10 seconds. When you release, try
to exhale slowly while maintaining some core tension, rather than going
completely limp and sighing your breath away. Push the air out through
pursed lips to modulate pressure, since a rapid drop in core pressure will
also cause a fairly quick drop in blood pressure, which could leave you
feeling lightheaded, or possibly cause you to faint. Ain't nobody got time
for that.

A good starting goal when learning this form of bracing is to be able to
do 2 or 3 reps of full inhales and Valsalva holds for 5 to 10 seconds each.
If you can manage that, you're ready to rock with some heavy weights.
If you can't maintain that tension or find holding it for that long a big
challenge, just practice until you're accustomed to finding that tension and
maintaining it over time.

Now that you know the two basic bracing strategies, let's do some
assessments to see what your bracing strength is like.

Assessing Bracing Strength

There are plenty of ways to assess core strength in a clinical setting, but for someone to do it on their own takes a bit of finesse. We want to find out whether you can maintain your bracing against a force that's trying to change the positioning of the spine without putting you at risk of injury.

LEG LOWERING TEST

One of the easiest ways to assess this is with a leg lowering test.[1] This test shows whether you can control your core positioning as you lower both legs; the lower the legs get to the floor, the greater the stress to the core and the harder it is to maintain positioning.

To perform the leg lowering test (figure 2.3), lie on your back with your hands pressed into the floor by your legs. Raise both legs to ver-

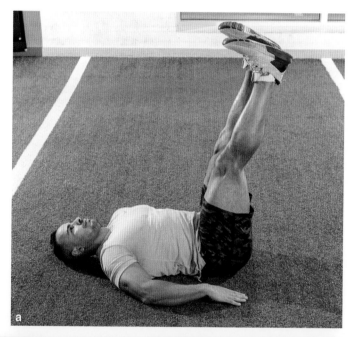

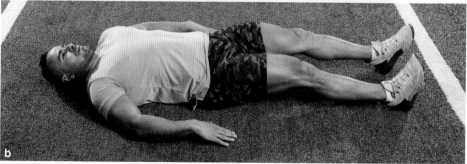

Figure 2.3 Leg lowering test: *(a)* starting position; *(b)* finish.

tical with knees straight. Focus on bracing the abs and trying to push your lower back into the floor. Slowly lower your legs while squeezing the abs. Try to keep the lower back pressed into the floor. Lower the legs as far as possible without letting the lower back lift off the floor. If you get to a position where you can no longer maintain the contact of the lower back into the floor, you've found the limit of your core control for this test. Rest with the legs down and abs soft, breathing deeply and trying to just chill for about 2 minutes, and then repeat the test 2 more times. You'll take your best effort as your final measure.

Low core strength: Legs 70 to 90 degrees when lowering

Moderate core strength: Legs 40 to 70 degrees when lowering

High core strength: Legs lower than 40 degrees when lowering

To determine what angle you get to, film yourself with a basic cell phone camera and take a screen shot of the lowest leg position you can manage with your lower back still contacting the floor. Using a simple drawing tool that has a protractor feature (there are tons of these out there, so find one that works well for you), just draw the angle between the floor and your thighs.

If you want something more specific, you could take a regular inflatable blood pressure cuff with a manual pump, put it under your lower back and inflate it with a few pumps to get a reading. As you press your lower back down into it and the floor, the pressure gauge will go up. As you lift your lower back off the cuff, the pressure gauge will go down. Lower your legs to a point where the pressure gauge shows you're not able to maintain that downward push and you'll have a more specific measurement of how well you can control your core.

Once we find the angle where you can maintain core control, we can assess your core endurance using a similar test. For this, we'll use a hollow-body hold for time.

HOLLOW-BODY HOLD TEST

To perform the hollow-body hold (figure 2.4) for time, begin with your legs vertical and lower back pressing into the floor. Lower the legs to a position slightly higher than the limit you found in the leg lowering test (2 to 4 inches [5-10 cm] higher, or roughly 10 degrees above the limit), and try to maintain this position for as long as you can without letting the lower back lift off the ground, and without letting the legs raise higher to make the position easier.

Poor core endurance: can hold the position for less than 30 seconds

Good core endurance: can hold the position for 30 to 59 seconds

Excellent core endurance: can hold the position for longer than 60 seconds

Once we have an idea of how strong your core is, as well as how good your core endurance is, we can start making an effective plan. If you scored low on the core strength or core endurance tests, include more core training exercises as part of your warm-up or do the accessory exercises in the program. You should also focus more on core strength and bracing mechanics during heavier compound lifts. If you scored high on core strength and core endurance, you could include core training exercises as activation drills or mainte-nance work, but you don't need to focus on them.

Core strength is the cornerstone of a lot of strength and condition-ing training, so set yourself up for success by knowing your bracing strength and how well you can control your spine. This way, you can improve performance while managing possible risks. There's not really any downside to having a stronger core or improving bracing strength or endurance, so this simple two-step assessment can go a long way to providing that valuable information before getting under the bar.

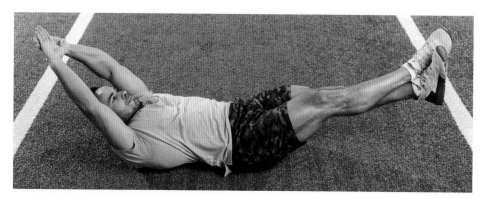

Figure 2.4 Hollow-body hold.

Assessing Mobility

One very important factor for performance and longevity in the gym is having adequate mobility to perform the lifts you desire. Just ask a creaky, stiff person how training for the snatch is going. The answer? Probably terribly.

You're simply going to need a boatload of ankle, hip, thoracic spine, and shoulder mobility to perform the Olympic lifts well. And if you don't have enough mobility in one joint, another will "compensate" (perform extra movement).

The most classic example is in the overhead squat. Someone who lacks ankle dorsiflexion mobility won't be able to maintain an upright torso in the squat. The body will need to make up for this lack of mobility somewhere, and that's often at the shoulder. A lack of ankle dorsiflexion increases the mobility demand on the shoulder and force it to stretch further in order to overhead squat.

Now, this compensation isn't always a bad thing, but you can make the argument that if you're constantly stretching your shoulder close to its limits, you may open yourself up to overuse injuries at the shoulders at a greater rate than someone who doesn't need to stretch the shoulder aggressively to overhead squat. In general, small compensations are probably fine and the body will adapt over time. But extreme limitations in mobility will often make it very challenging to get into optimal positions for the lift and may predispose us to injury.

The next important thing to talk about is that not all lifts require a tremendous amount of mobility. If all you ever want to do is squat, bench press, and deadlift for the rest of your life, then you'll be needing far less mobility than someone chasing weights on an Olympic weightlifting platform.

In the rest of this chapter, we supply you with some self-assessments to gauge your own mobility and provide some solutions for mobility restrictions. Just keep in mind that your own goals will dictate how much mobility is required for each joint.

It's important to note that we lose mobility pretty dang quickly as we age. It's actually quite frightening. Data shows that 50 percent of people over the age of 75 could not raise their arms overhead greater than 120 degrees, which is considered the minimum number for adequate function in daily life. On top of this, people lose about 10 degrees of motion for every decade of living after the age of 65.[2] Normal shoulder mobility is often designated at about 165 degrees. (If your cabinets aren't at eye level, good luck getting the coffee cups after you hit 75.) Also, some joints seem to be more affected with stiffness over time than others. For example, the knee and elbow tend to maintain mobility better over time when compared to the shoulder, hip, and spine.[3] Therefore, it makes sense to place a little more focus on the areas that tend to get stiff over time compared to others.

For this reason, if you have absolutely zero interest in performing lifts in the gym that require tremendous mobility, it probably still makes sense to include some mobility exercises as a part of your training routine. This way, when you're elderly you won't have to place all your clean coffee mugs on the countertop instead of in the cupboard because you have the shoulder mobility of the Tin Man.

Lastly, I strongly recommend taking videos or pictures of your initial assessments to track your progress. If you don't weigh yourself on the scale regularly to see if your diet is helping you lose weight, you won't know if you're making progress. The same goes for these assessments. Assess and reassess—don't guess.

Now let's break out some assessments, shall we?

Assessing Hip Mobility

Hip flexion is a very important predictor of squat depth. Those with major hip flexion mobility limitations often find it very challenging to squat to the depth they desire. On top of this, limited hip mobility will also force compensatory lower-back rounding (butt wink) during the squat. Keep in mind that it's impossible to squat without flexing the spine. One study showed that, on average, most folks have between 12 and 25 degrees of lower-back flexion (rounding) during the squat.[4]

A minimal to moderate amount of lumbar flexion probably isn't a concern unless it starts to throw off your squat technique. Too much butt wink forces the trunk to incline forward, making it challenging to maintain a strong upright position in the squat. This is especially problematic for the Olympic lifts.

The benefits of hip mobility include better squat depth, a more upright torso in the squat, and a reduction in stress at the shoulders, elbows, and wrists. Good hip mobility is especially important in squats, cleans, snatches, and pistol or single-leg squats. Hip mobility is far more important in those who squat to end range and train the Olympic lifts.

HIP FLEXION ASSESSMENT: LYING KNEE TO CHEST

Lie on your back with both legs straight out on the floor. Bend one knee, then bring your knee toward your chest and pull your thigh up against your abdomen, bending the hip maximally. Keep the same stance width and degree of toe-out you desire to use in the squat. Stop when the end range of motion is attained. Do not allow the lower back to roll up off the floor. Lower the leg and repeat on the other side.

You should be able to easily touch most of your thigh to your abdomen with the help of your arm (figure 2.5). If not, you've got a hip flexion mobility limitation.

Note: Assess to see if more range of motion can be attained with more hip external rotation (more toe out) and horizontal abduction (wider or narrower stance). This is a sign that you may increase your squat depth with more toe out or a wider stance.

If you can easily touch your thigh against your midsection fully, you've passed the test, congrats! If not, you have some work to do. It's also common to find one hip more limited than another, which means you probably will need to spend more time mobilizing the stiffer hip.

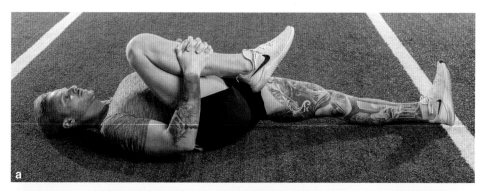

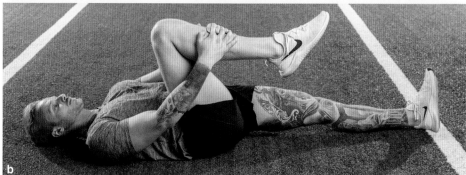

Figure 2.5 Lying knee to chest: *(a)* pass; *(b)* fail.

Assessing Ankle Mobility

Ankle mobility is also tremendously important for depth in the squat. It allows the trunk to be upright during the squat, which is advantageous when catching cleans and snatching. In strength training, adequate ankle mobility also allows us to move our knees over our toes during exercises, which allows us to better engage the quads. Contrary to popular belief, allowing the knee past the toe is not only safe but absolutely mandatory for success during Olympic lifts as well as building big, strong quads in the gym. Adequate ankle mobility ensures we don't end up with excessive compensation at the knees, hips, lower back, spine, and shoulders during squats, Olympic lifts, and other lower-body exercises.

Good ankle mobility permits a deeper squat while maintaining an upright torso. It improves the ability to use the quads and reduces stress at the shoulders, elbows, and wrists. This is especially important in lifts such as squats, cleans, snatches, lunges, step-ups, and pistol or single-leg squats. Ankle mobility is far more important in those who squat to end range and train the Olympic lifts.

ANKLE DORSIFLEXION ASSESSMENT: HALF-KNEELING ANKLE DORSIFLEXION WALL TEST

Start in a half-kneeling position with the toes 4 inches (10 cm) from the wall. Keep the front foot flat and the arch in neutral. Drive the knee as far as you can toward the wall over the second toe (figure 2.6). Don't allow the heel to pop up or lose the arch in the foot; these would be compensations. Press to the end range of the joint, attempting to tap the knee to the wall.

If you can easily touch the wall without compensation, you've passed the test, congrats! If not, you probably have some work to do. If the heel pops up, your toes spin out, or it takes all your might to press toward the wall, that's a sign your ankle mobility isn't what is could be.

I am a fan of measuring your ankle mobility regardless of whether or not you passed this test. To do this, simply bring your toe farther from or closer to the wall until you find the measurement where your knee can just barely tap the wall without the heel popping up or compensation in the arch.

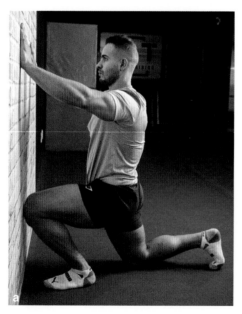 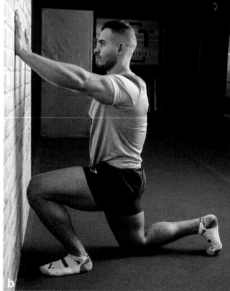

Figure 2.6 Half-kneeling ankle dorsiflexion wall test: *(a)* pass; *(b)* fail.

Those pursuing Olympic lifting or deeper squats may want to have more mobility than the standard 4 inches (10 cm). I often advise these athletes to shoot for 5 inches (12 cm). Keep in mind that taller athletes will probably need a greater number to squat well, while shorter athletes won't need as much. Those under 5 feet, 8 inches (172 cm), may do well with 4 inches (10 cm). Those over 5 feet, 8 inches (172 cm), may need closer to 5 inches (12 cm).

Assessing Thoracic Spine Mobility

The thoracic spine is the set of vertebrae that sits between the bottom of the neck and the bottom of your ribcage, just above the lower back. Being able to extend fully from this area is paramount for full overhead mobility. A lack of thoracic spine mobility is going to make it really difficult to hit solid positions in overhead lifts such as military presses, push presses, and the jerk.

With poor thoracic spine mobility, you'll also have an ice cube's shot in hell for completing snatches (figure 2.7) and overhead squats. Basically, anything overhead will be a big challenge with limited thoracic mobility.

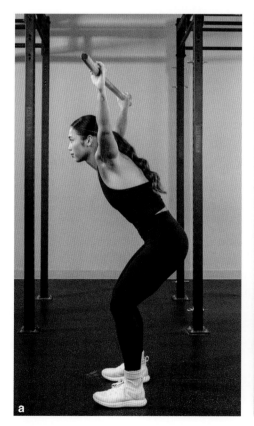
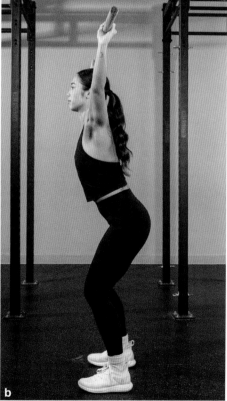

Figure 2.7 Snatch: *(a)* limited thoracic mobility *(b)* optimal thoracic mobility.

A lack of thoracic mobility forces the shoulders, elbows, and wrists to make up for that lack of movement upstream from the T-spine (thoracic spine). Other joints will be forced to compensate, potentially straining those structures excessively and leading to suboptimal lifting technique.

On top of this, poor thoracic mobility during the overhead press and the Olympic lifts will drive issues "downstream," such as compensatory lumbar extension. This can potentially lead to the lower back getting a bit cranky during overhead movements.

Limited T-spine extension can also be an issue even further downstream, during squats and snatches. If you're missing the motion in the T-spine, you'll have to make it up at the hips or ankles. The task of performing an overhead squat or snatch simply requires an enormous amount of mobility and if one section is not contributing, another will have to make up for this.

Lastly, having poor thoracic extension can make staying upright a huge challenge during front squats and when coming out of the hole in the clean. If you have trouble keeping the elbows high in the front rack during cleans and front squats, you may be dealing with some thoracic spine stiffness.

Proper thoracic mobility allows better overhead positions. With this mobility, you will be able to maintain a more upright torso during front squats, overhead squats, and Olympic lifts. This means reduced stress upstream, at the shoulders, elbows, and wrists, and reduced stress downstream, at the lumbar spine, hips, and ankles. Good thoracic spine mobility is especially important for lifts that feature overhead pressing such as military lifts, push presses, jerks, and handstands, as well as front squats, cleans, and snatches.

THORACIC EXTENSION ASSESSMENT: PRONE PRESS-UP

For this assessment, you'll need a friend to help you. Lie on your abdomen with your hands under your armpits. Extend your elbows fully to press up (figure 2.8). Relax, allowing gravity to extend your spine. Have your friend feel along your thoracic spine. Someone with thoracic spine stiffness won't extend throughout the thoracic spine and actually may stay in flexion despite relaxing and being pulled by gravity. Your partner is looking to see that the spine extends all throughout the thoracic area. If the spine remains flexed, the spine is stiff.

If you have a uniform spinal curve that is either flat or extends in the thoracic region then congratulations, you've passed! If you still have some flexion in the spine despite fully relaxing, then you have some work to do!

Also keep in mind that almost everyone has some restriction in the thoracic spine (which can worsen as we age) and could benefit from some regular thoracic spine mobility.

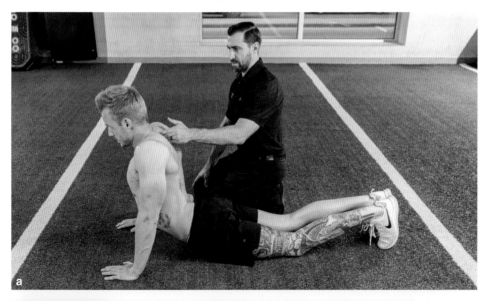

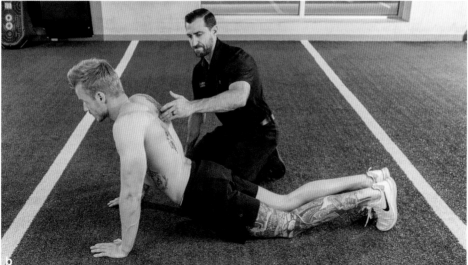

Figure 2.8 Prone press-up: *(a)* pass; *(b)* fail.

Assessing Shoulder Mobility

Overhead shoulder mobility is equally as important as thoracic spine mobility for the gym. Both areas of mobility actually aid one another during overhead movements. You can make up for a lack of thoracic motion with extra shoulder mobility. On the flip side, if you have limited shoulder mobility, you can make up for it with additional thoracic spine movement. Obviously, it's even better when both players are on board.

As with thoracic spine mobility, a lack of shoulder mobility is going to make it really difficult to hit solid positions in overhead lifts such as military presses, push presses, and the jerk. This is particularly true regarding shoulder flexion, which is the act of bringing your arm straight overhead. Snatches and overhead squats suffer the same consequences, as does any other overhead lift.

Lacking overhead shoulder mobility will drive compensatory lower-back extension during overhead lifts and force the elbows and wrists to make up for that lack of movement upstream from the shoulder.

Limited shoulder mobility can also be an issue further downstream during squats and snatches. If you're missing the motion in the shoulder, you have to make it up at the hips or ankles. The other problem is simply not being able to hit depth without the barbell falling forward.

Good shoulder mobility permits better overhead position for overhead presses, jerks, snatches, and overhead squats. It reduces stress upstream, at the elbows and wrists, and reduces stress downstream, at the lumbar spine, hips, and ankles. Shoulder mobility is especially important in lifts that require overhead pressing, such as military lifts, push presses, jerks, and handstands, as well as snatches and overhead squats.

SHOULDER MOBILITY ASSESSMENT: OVERHEAD TEST AGAINST A WALL

Lie on your back with your feet up against the wall, knees bent in a deep squat. Ensure your lower back stays flat to the floor during the entire test. Reach both arms to the ceiling, straightening the elbows fully. Touch your thumbs together. Maintaining the elbows locked out and thumbs together, lower your arms behind your head and attempt to touch your arms fully to the floor (figure 2.9). Your knuckles, backs of the wrists, and elbows should all come into contact with the floor.

If you can keep your back flat to the floor and touch the entirety of your arms to the floor without your thumbs separating or your elbows bending, you've passed! If not, you have some work to do. As with other joints, it is possible (and common) for one side to be more mobile or stiffer than the other. This just means you'll have to devote some additional time to loosening up the stiffer side.

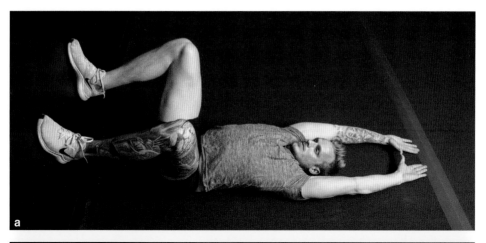

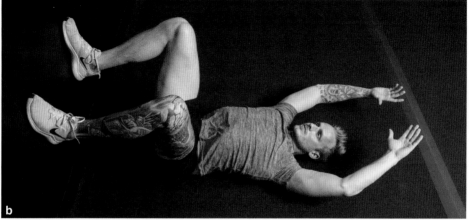

Figure 2.9 Overhead test against a wall: *(a)* pass; *(b)* fail.

Putting It All Together

So now that we've gone through an assessment and found what's limited, it's time to put a plan in action to start moving a bit better. I know some of you are going to have some big mobility issues and others will pass every test easily. Obviously, this means the stiff folks will have their hands full and the mobile folks will probably just skip this next section.

You may find that some areas are much stiffer than others. If you're really close to passing the shoulder assessment but your ankles are stiff as a board, then focus on the ankles first. Maybe you'll want two mobility exercises for the ankles but just one for the shoulders. Lastly, if you found one side stiffer than the other, you can simply put more effort on the stiff side. If one side passes but not the other, then you can make the argument for only mobilizing one side when able.

Generally, gaining new mobility is a battle won by frequency and not intensity.[5] Max effort shoulder stretches once per week probably won't do much besides dislocate your shoulder (we're mostly kidding). You're better off performing lower-level, less intense stretches and mobility drills more often throughout the course of the week instead of intensely performing them less often.[6] I recommend performing mobility exercises 5 times per week for optimal improvements in mobility.

I also recommend just 1 set of each mobility drill. Some research shows just 1 set is similar in outcome to multiple sets,[5,6] so for the sake of efficiency that's what I currently recommend. If you enjoy stretching or find you make faster progress with multiple sets, then by all means perform multiple sets. You probably don't need to start with multiple sets to make progress.

We can also use some additional weight with our stretching to improve our mobility. Some research shows adding load to stretches improves mobility more than stretching without load.[5] Interestingly, strength training into a full stretch has also been shown to be an effective way to improve mobility.[6] For this reason, you'll see several mobility exercises included that look just like regular strength training movements with a stretch at the end range of the movement.

Here's another important consideration: building this new mobility doesn't mean you'll always use it during your training. Think about it: You've been squatting or performing overhead lifting with a specific technique for years. Your old way of moving is a strong habit and tough to change. On top of this, new ranges of motion that are unlocked over time will undoubtedly be weak and unfamiliar to your body. For this reason, it's important that you begin to train into these new ranges of motion (i.e., using your full range in the squat or full overhead mobility during push press) and that you reduce the weight temporarily to ensure you don't overdo it in these fresh, underdeveloped ranges. Your body can take several weeks or even months of reduced-load training to adapt. During this time, make sure you prioritize technique over load. If the loads are too much, you may find yourself simply reverting to old habits and not using that new range of motion you've worked hard to build. Slow down, drop some of the load, and make that new mobility permanent.

Now that we've gotten the basics out of the way, here are the specific mobility drills.

HIP MOBILITY

QUADRUPED POSTERIOR HIP STRETCH

Get into position on your hands and knees. Reach one leg maximally behind and across your body (figure 2.10). Hold the stretch for 60 seconds.

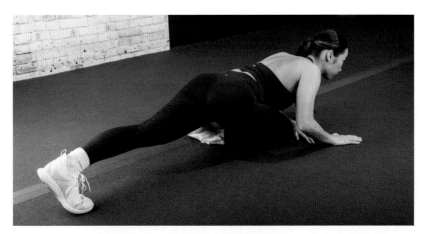

Figure 2.10   Quadruped posterior hip stretch.

GOBLET PRY SQUAT

Hold a kettlebell in a goblet position. Begin in a squat stance with feet slightly wider than shoulder width and toes turned out slightly. Descend to the bottom of the squat. Pry your elbows into the sides of your knees (figure 2.11), emphasizing one side at a time and repeating back and forth. "Pry" side to side for 60 seconds.

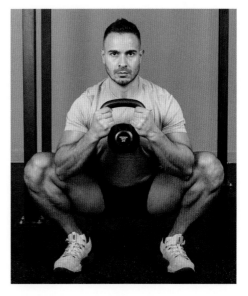

Figure 2.11   Goblet pry squat.

ANKLE MOBILITY

TOE TO WALL SOLEUS STRETCH

Place your toe against the wall with the heel flat on the floor. Bend the knee slightly on the side you're stretching (figure 2.12). Drive your knee maximally to the wall. Hold the stretch for 60 seconds.

ECCENTRIC CALF RAISE WEIGHTED STRETCH

Stand on a step with the balls of the feet in contact with the stair, heels hanging off the edge. Perform a double-leg calf raise. At the top of the movement, remove one leg and slowly lower with only one side working (figure 2.13). Sink maximally and slowly into a full stretch. Switch to the other side on the next repetition and repeat. Perform 8 reps with a full stretch held for 2 seconds at the bottom of each rep.

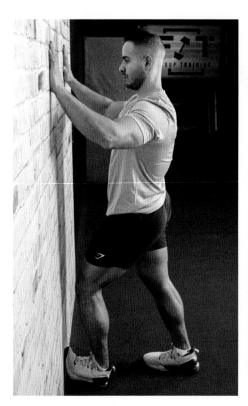

Figure 2.12 Toe to wall soleus stretch.

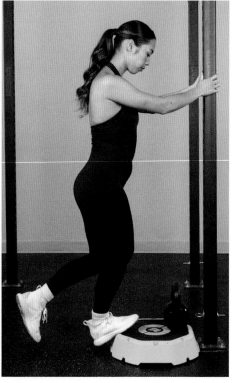

Figure 2.13 Eccentric calf raise weighted stretch.

THORACIC MOBILITY

FEET ON WALL WEIGHTED
THORACIC EXTENSION OVER ROLLER

Lie on your back with your feet against the wall in a deep squat position. Place a foam roller in the middle of your thoracic spine. Take a light kettlebell or dumbbell and hold it behind your neck for additional stretch (optional). Slowly extend over the roller as if lowering from the top of a crunch, extending maximally (figure 2.14). Attempt to get your spine to take the contour of the roller. Crunch back to the starting position. Perform 8 reps with a full stretch held for 2 seconds at the bottom of each rep.

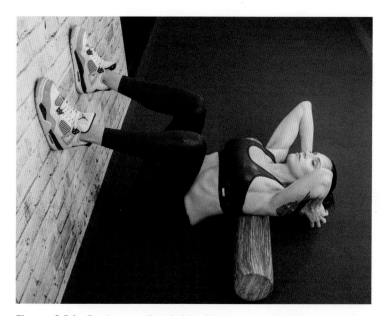

Figure 2.14 Feet on wall weighted thoracic extension over roller.

SHOULDER MOBILITY

CLOSE GRIP CHIN-UP STRETCH

Grasp a pull-up bar in a narrow grip with palms up (supinated). Place a bench under your feet so that you can support your body weight throughout the entire movement. Slowly descend maximally into the bottom of the chin-up, assisting as needed with the feet (figure 2.15). Attempt to sink as deep as possible, lowering the ribs toward the floor. Narrowing the grip intensifies the stretch. Perform 8 reps with a full stretch held for 2 seconds at the bottom of each rep.

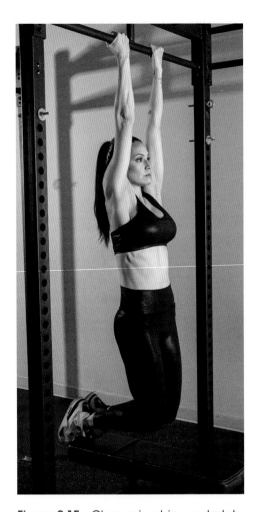

Figure 2.15 Close grip chin-up stretch.

FEET ON WALL DUMBBELL PULLOVER OVER ROLLER

Lie on your back with your feet against the wall in a deep squat position. Place a foam roller in the middle of your thoracic spine. Using a light dumbbell or kettlebell, press your arms fully over your shoulders. Keeping the elbows locked out, slowly lower the weight to a deep stretch position with the arms fully overhead (figure 2.16). Return to the start position with the weight over your shoulders. Perform 8 reps with a full stretch held for 2 seconds at the bottom of each rep.

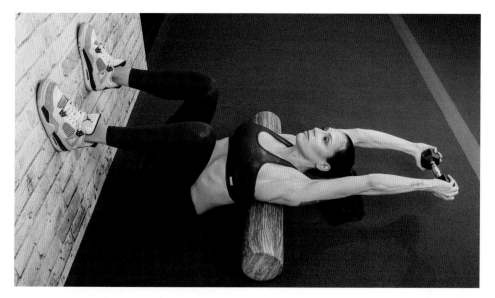

Figure 2.16   Feet on wall dumbbell pullover over roller.

Sample Mobility Program

Here is a sample program to help it all come together. Let's say you perform the assessments and are quite stiff, failing every test, and need mobility in all areas. Let's also say that no area is stiffer than another. We've got some work to do! Perform this routine 5 times a week to help improve your mobility.

Mobility Routine

Feet on wall weighted thoracic extension over roller: 8 reps

Close grip chin-up stretch: 8 reps

Calf raise weighted stretch: 8 reps

Goblet pry squat: 60 seconds

In terms of exercise ordering, I recommend performing mobility exercises as part of your warm-up before you do your strength training. This is because doing mobility exercises prior to training allows you to get into better positions during the training session and helps to build and strengthen new habits and better technique in the gym.

Finally, I recommend reassessing your mobility every 4 weeks to see if you've made progress. Four weeks is enough time to see some progress[7] and if you check too early you may get frustrated. It takes time and perseverance. Just as you don't build a 400-pound squat in 2 weeks, you won't be doing full splits in the same time frame. If you perform the reassessment and you aren't making the progress you'd like, I simply recommend adding another mobility exercise or adding another set of stretching to your next 4-week mobility routine.

Conclusion

Now you have an idea of whether you're a stiff person or a mobile person and have a plan of action to get into safer and more effective positions during your lifts in the gym. Try not to get discouraged if you're especially stiff; time and effort can work wonders for improving your motion. Also keep in mind that even surprisingly stiff national-level and Olympic-level weightlifters can excel despite their issues.

Lastly, for the super-stretchy Gumbys in the audience, you don't need to mobilize and your time is probably better spent with more training! The next few chapters explain how to perform our favorite movements in the gym and how to tailor them appropriately for your individual needs and body type.

Exercise Techniques and Execution

Squat
and Hinge
Movements

It's sort of clichéd to say that everyone is unique, but when it comes to how people squat, there's some truth to that. Some people perform better using a relatively narrow stance, with feet closer than shoulder width. Some people can find success only when using a very wide stance, with the feet outside of shoulder width. Some can squat without issues if their toes are pointing forward at 12 o'clock, and some need to turn out their toes to 10 and 2. Others may need a bit of an offset with one foot slightly forward of the other or one foot turned out more than the other. Everyone has different joint mechanics, limb length and proportions, and relative stiffness of joint capsules and muscles that might limit squatting in a certain way but would make squatting another way their absolute jam.

Is there one best way to squat? No! The best way is the one that works for the person doing the squats, where they get the best force production, can maintain positioning effectively, and feel like they're strong, solid, and not hurting during or after the movement. This means the often prescribed "feet shoulder-width apart and toes pointing forward" stance may not work for everyone and may in fact create more challenges than it solves. There's a ton of evidence that many people have a notable amount of hip structural differences[1] and asymmetry between left and right hips[2] and would benefit from a different type of setup that's tailored to their specific needs.

As with squats, when doing deadlifts some lifters prefer a conventional stance and some make absolute magic happen in a sumo or modified sumo stance. We'll break down those two options in this chapter, but suffice it to say they're both valid and offer a host of training benefits to whomever uses them. It just comes down to preference and feel, especially if someone isn't looking to compete in powerlifting but still wants to lift a lot of weight safely and comfortably.

Torso and Femur
Length and Positioning

Some people are just naturally better at squatting than at deadlifts, while others are seemingly able to pull a house off the foundation but can't squat comfortably or effectively at all. This could be due to training, motor pattern proficiency, personal preference, or any number of factors. But it could also be due to the length of their limbs: An individual with long legs and a relatively short torso might have an easier time performing a deadlift, whereas someone with shorter legs and a relatively longer torso might have a better time performing squats.

The torso is considered relatively short if it's one-third of your total height or less[8] and considered long if the torso is greater than one-third of your total height or more. To measure your torso, extend a tape measure from the upper portion of your collarbone to your groin.

Shorter legs can make it easier to maintain a vertical position and reduce the moment arm length of the working muscles. Shorter legs also require a shorter range of motion to go from start to finish than longer legs. Compared to someone with a longer torso, an individual with a shorter torso and longer legs has a shorter spine with less torque being applied to the vertebral segments during a deadlift and reduced force requirements for the spinal muscles. In addition, they have a reduced moment arm length for completing the movement compared to someone with a longer torso and shorter legs. People with shorter torsos and longer relative leg lengths also tend to excel at sumo deadlifts compared to conventional ones.[9]

Some people are just genetically built to perform certain lifts. This shouldn't stop you from training all movements or focusing on getting better at ones you may struggle with, but it could explain why progress on some movements seems slower than progress on others.

Let's say you have a long torso and shorter femurs and want to do a great deadlift. You can still accomplish a lot, but you will have to work within the challenges of your specific structure. Spend extra time working on getting set through your back and shoulders, make sure you build up as much strength as possible through the spine, brace, and develop a strong wedge to reduce the torso angle relative to the floor for an easier setup and completion of the deadlift.

If you have a short torso and longer femurs and struggle to squat to any notable depth without losing your balance, you can adjust your stance to alter your leverages. Take a wider stance and elevate your heels on some plates or wedges for more forward knee translation, and allow the hips to move closer to the vertical line of the bar so your torso angle doesn't have to be as horizontal to maintain your balance. You could also switch from back squat to either front squat or goblet squat to shift the load to your front and allow you to maintain a slightly more vertical torso compared to the back squat.

Hip Structure Differences and Asymmetry

Before we talk about hips, let's talk about eyes. When you have your vision checked, the optometrist puts a big machine in front of your eyes and flips a bunch of lenses as you stare at a chart. With each different lens pairing, they ask you which one gives you clearer vision, and after a bunch of options they come up with a relative prescription for what kind of lens helps that eye see the most clearly. Then they do the same with the other eye. If you wear glasses for anything, you likely have a different prescription for your left and right eye. It's common to have a dominant eye, one that sees better and normally takes the lead. Similarly, we have a dominant hand as well as a dominant leg. This is partially due to how our brains are wired, and part of it is structural.

Let's talk a little about the structure of the hip and how that can affect how you squat. We will dig into four main components of the hip:

- Hip socket front-to-back placement on the pelvis (anteversion or retroversion; figure 3.1)
- Hip socket center-edge angle, or how far to the side the hip socket extends over the head of the femur
- Femoral neck vertical angle (coxa, or shaft angle; figure 3.2)
- Femoral neck horizontal angle (retroversion or anteversion)

A hip socket that's oriented more to the front of the pelvis is in an anteverted position, whereas a socket that's oriented more to the back or side of the pelvis is in a retroverted position. The placement affects how much hip flexion, extension, and rotation can occur before bone-on-bone contact as well as the best positions for maximum strength and torque development. An anteverted hip allows for more hip flexion, adduction, and internal rotation but allows less hip extension and external rotation, whereas a retroverted hip is the opposite.[3] A retroverted hip allows more extension and external rotation but less flexion, internal rotation, and adduction.

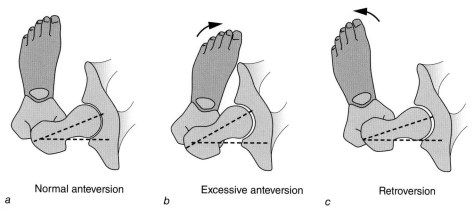

Normal anteversion   Excessive anteversion   Retroversion

a   b   c

Figure 3.1 Relative position of the femoral neck and femoral condyles: (*a*) normal anteversion, (*b*) excessive anteversion, and (*c*) retroversion.

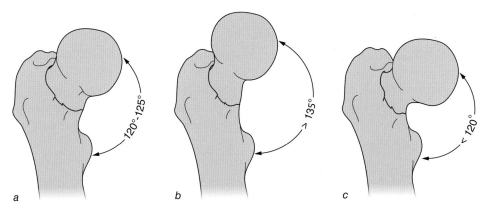

Figure 3.2 Angle of inclination: *(a)* normal, *(b)* coxa valga, and *(c)* coxa vara.

A larger center-edge angle, where the hip socket has more of a lateral bony angle overhanging the femoral head, is going to create earlier bone-to-bone contact during hip abduction or internal rotation.[4] Someone with a larger center-edge angle will have trouble hitting the splits like Jean-Claude Van Damme and might also find wider-stance squats or sumo deadlifts to be more troublesome than narrower-stance movements.

A more vertical femoral neck angle (coxa varus) allows for more hip abduction, as well as easier internal rotation, but less external rotation. A more horizontal femoral neck angle (coxa valgus) allows more adduction, internal rotation, and hip flexion.[3]

The horizontal angle of the femoral neck can be neutral but also pointing forward (retroversion) or pointing backward (anteversion). An anteverted femoral neck angle allows much higher internal rotation than external rotation but also more available hip flexion than extension. A retroverted femoral neck angle allows more external rotation and higher hip extension.[5]

What does this mean for how you squat? Because certain structural elements permit easier movements such as flexion and external rotation, which are a big part of squatting, having those structural orientations can make squatting easier than if you have a different combination of joint structures. This is why some people can squat super easily even with no training or coaching and some people have trouble even getting to a chair without maxing out their range of motion. For squatting, the easiest orientations seem to be an anteverted hip socket with a low center-edge angle and a femoral neck that is less vertical and more retroverted. But this doesn't mean you can't squat effectively with a different combination of joint orientations, and you should still continue squatting as long as the movement isn't uncomfortable or painful.

Without X-ray vision or access to a suite of medical professionals who could accurately assess these joint orientations, you can't really know what your setup may look like, so we have to approach it in detail, playing with different stances and foot positions to see what works best.

Asymmetric Stances

Finding your ideal squat stance comes down to figuring out where to position your hips, knees, and feet to get the best balance of front and back muscle tension, and of left and right muscle tension and to balance without falling over. In some people, this means putting one foot into an asymmetric position compared to the other. Some people have a dominant leg that has a slightly different structure, which requires different positioning to find that front-to-back muscle balance position, as well as to get relatively similar left and right activity.

A stance that allows the femoral head to sit squarely in the hip socket (acetabulum) allows for the best balance of musculature around the joint as possible, much like a golf ball sitting squarely on the tee gives the best chance for the ball to stay on the tee and not fall off. The muscles that surround and operate the hip work in an ideal length–tension relationship. If the muscles that direct flexion, extension, rotation, and all the other movements of the hip are in a relatively balanced length–tension relationship, we can say that the positioning and stability of the hip is relatively balanced.

If we stand in a way that stretches one group of muscles and shortens another, the tension is imbalanced. Thus, standing in a way that produces relatively equal tension, even if that stance is asymmetrical, could be the best option for producing relatively equal muscle activity throughout the hip. Standing in a way that produces unequal relative tension through the muscles of the hip, even if the stance is symmetric and lined up textbook perfect, suggests that this stance produces imbalanced muscle activity and so isn't as beneficial for the individual. In summary, standing in a forced symmetric stance might actually produce more muscle imbalances during a squat than it can correct.

Just as we can have a dominant hand with differences in structure associated with upper-body positioning and alignment, we can have a dominant leg, with differences in structure associated with lower-body positioning and alignment.[6] It's not uncommon for athletes who were involved in throwing sports as kids to develop a positional deformation to the upper arm bone that allows them more range of motion in their throwing arm, but that deformation is not present in their nonthrowing arm.[7] The forces the arm is exposed to while training and playing adapted the structure to accommodate the activity. This asymmetric structure sticks when they become adults and their growth plates fuse, meaning they will always have a degree of asymmetry that can't be corrected and has to be worked around as best as possible.

Lower-body asymmetry is also fairly common in active kids, especially if they engage in any one-sided activities or repetitive-motion activities. The dominant leg takes more loading, is used more, and adapts to that force more consistently, meaning it's not uncommon for the dominant leg to present with a larger range of motion than the nondominant leg. Should that be corrected or forced into symmetry with the nondominant side? Not if the structure, muscle balance, and relative strength of both sides are also different.

This is where the beauty of an asymmetric stance may come into play. It helps accommodate an individual's structural uniqueness while also letting them train like an absolute animal. It can also help fix some common technical issues with the movement, such as lateral hip slide when coming out of the bottom of the rep or twisting during any part of the movement.

If you squat with an asymmetric stance, how do you avoid developing muscular imbalances? To be fair, there's always a chance that using a different setup will make certain muscles work more and cause others to not come to the party. This could be said for a symmetrical setup as well, so it's not inherently different but still is worth exploring. As with any training program, the goal is global strength and not just isolated performance, so including a variety of different exercises—with different ranges of motion, positions, and loading parameters—can help to develop the best, most robust strength profile. If you only ever did one exercise, with only one position and one stance, you would likely develop some form of imbalance, regardless of what that activity entailed, so as with many things, variety is the spice of life.

A squat stance can start with feet shoulder-width apart and toes forward but may require deviating from that position to find the optimum for the individual. In the next section, we'll outline how to find your optimal squat stance, explore what that means to you and your performance, and explain how to take advantage of your own unique structural requirements.

Squat

So now that I've completely ticked off many squat technique and positional purists, let's dig into how to find your best stance. Similar to the trip to the optometrist, we're going to try a bunch of different setups to see which one feels best. It will either be a hard "Yes, this is awesome!" or "No, I absolutely hate it!"

Squat Technique

First, a few words on what we're looking for in a squat movement. Ideally, the squat movement comes from the ankles, knees, and hips and relies on a slight forward lean of the torso as the movement progresses through the eccentric (lowering) phase. The squat depth should be the maximum the individual can achieve from their hips and should stop at the point where further depth achievement comes from lower-back flexion. To begin the movement, you will be standing upright, and when viewed from the side you'll stand with a straight line down through the ear, shoulder, hip, and middle of the foot (figure 3.3). The foot is your base of support, so maintaining balance will rely on keeping your body balanced centrally over the midline of the foot. As you squat down, your head should go in front of that midline, with your hips pushing back behind, and you should attempt to keep your shoulders vertical over the midline of the foot to maintain balance.

When viewed from the front (figure 3.4), the straight line should run through your nose, sternum (breastbone), belly button, middle of your hips, and exactly between your feet. Vertical alignment should be maintained throughout the movement without leaning to the side or pushing

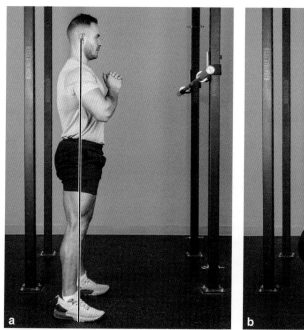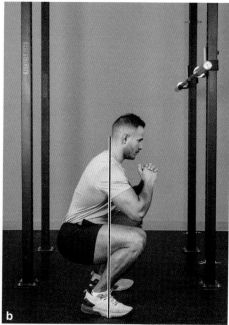

Figure 3.3 Side view of the squat: *(a)* standing position and *(b)* squat.

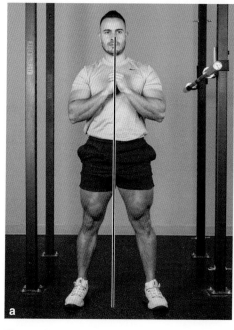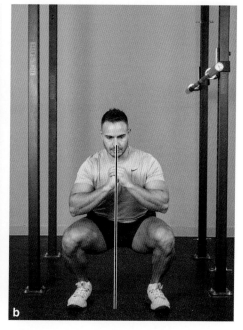

Figure 3.4 Front view of the squat: *(a)* standing position and *(b)* squat.

your hips, shoulders, or head to either side. It should look like you have equal weight on each foot, so don't lean on either foot.

Each foot should be an active participant during the squat. Think of your foot as a tripod, with the three main points of contact being the heel and the outer edges of the ball of each foot. These three points also correspond to the three arches of your foot and are essentially the anchors of your strength and balance. (The three arches of the foot include the one typically thought of as between the heel and ball of the big toe but also one from the heel to the ball of the baby toe and one across the ball of the foot itself.) When doing any squat or deadlift movement, think of standing so that all three points are pressing into the floor with equal pressure. Then think of using the muscles of your foot to draw those points closer together. This will ensure the arches of your feet are strong and supportive of your body weight and any additional weight you are planning to move.

If you tend to pronate, meaning you roll your feet in and stand mostly on the big-toe side of the foot, it would be worthwhile to adjust your stance more toward the baby-toe side to maintain a more balanced arch and ankle positioning (figure 3.5). To do this, just think of pushing the baby-toe side of the foot into the ground with more pressure, but make sure you keep the big-toe point of the tripod in contact with the ground so you aren't just standing entirely on the outside edges of your feet.

To begin the squat, inhale, brace the abs lightly, and try to grip the floor with all your toes (focus on pressing down without curling the toes) and foot arches prior to lowering into the movement, making sure you have some level of foot and core tension to pull into the bottom of the squat movement. Bend from the hips, knees, and ankles at roughly the same time and think of pushing the hips back slightly, then lowering your bum down toward your heels. Stop when you get to the end of the available range of motion for the hips, knees, and ankles and before you start needing to round your lower back to achieve a deeper positioning.

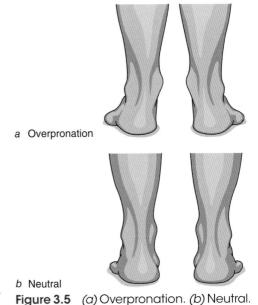

a Overpronation

When you press up, think of pushing through the floor and pushing the hips forward to return to a standing position, exhaling as you stand tall. If you're lifting a weight, make sure you don't relax your bracing while you're under load. Making sure you are strong and stable enough to support that additional weight is important.

When performing a squat, you should feel like the muscles of your

b Neutral

Figure 3.5 *(a)* Overpronation. *(b)* Neutral.

glutes, hamstrings, and quads are doing the majority of the work, with honorable mention to your calves and feet. Ideally, left and right sides should feel like they're working about the same, without one side feeling like it's carrying most of the load or getting the most sore following the reps. Now let's learn how to find your ideal squat position.

Finding Your Squat Position

First, start with feet parallel, roughly shoulder-width apart, and toes pointed out slightly. (Think 11 and 1 on a clock face.) Perform a few bodyweight squats, paying attention to feeling weight in the middle of your feet, assessing whether there's equal loading through both legs and equal tension through both hips, moderating any leaning to one side, feeling how low you can go before rounding your lower back, and noting any inability to maintain your balance.

Next, take a slightly wider stance and repeat the few squats. Then narrow your stance a bit until you find the width that feels best for you. From that new width, try turning your left toe out a little further (figure 3.6), so now it points to 10 o'clock instead of 11, and repeat the bodyweight squats. Compare how that feels with the previous observations. Did it feel easier, harder, more balanced, or less balanced? Any pinching on either hip or restriction to movements, or did it feel like a better stance? Now turn the left toe back to 11 o'clock and turn the right toe out to 2 o'clock and repeat. If turning either toe out worked better for you, set up with that stance and with your desired width for the next few adjustments.

Next, stand with the right foot slightly behind the left foot (figure 3.7), regardless of which toe is turned out. Repeat the few bodyweight squats here. Then return the right foot to the original position and repeat on the left side. You could also do these both again with the opposite toe turned out and see which feels the most at home.

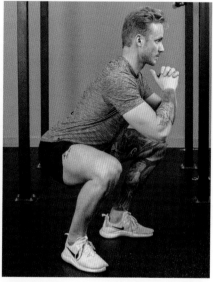

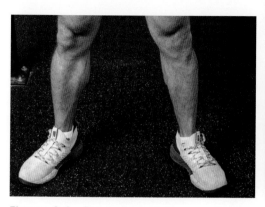

Figure 3.6 Front view of the squat, toes turned out.

Figure 3.7 Side view of the squat showing the offset stance.

Whichever front-to-back setup feels best, try putting your foot a little farther back to see what happens. Does it make the squat feel better or worse?

This process can help you figure out which stance width, rotation, and front-to-back positioning works best for you. Some people might feel right at home with feet shoulder-width apart and toes parallel, whereas others might feel best with a very asymmetrical setup. The goal is to find your best stance, regardless of how that may look or feel.

Now that you've found your ideal squat stance, we can try some different loading techniques and positions. The easiest place to start is with a dumbbell goblet squat.

DUMBBELL GOBLET SQUAT

For the dumbbell goblet squat (figure 3.8), use a single dumbbell held at your chest with the dumbbell in a vertical position. Having the weight in front of your torso allows you to maintain a slightly more upright torso position and thus achieve depth while balancing your weight over your feet versus without the weight or with a barbell on your back. The movement will be the same, but with an anterior load, there will be more movement from the knees and ankles and a slightly lower movement required from the hips, plus less likelihood of rounding the lower back at the bottom of the movement.

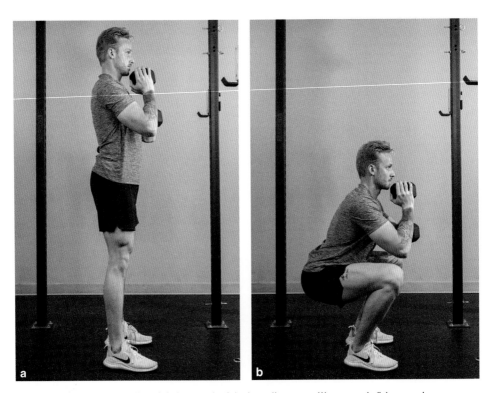

Figure 3.8 Dumbbell goblet squat: *(a)* standing position and *(b)* squat.

Follow the same approach as outlined for the bodyweight squat: find your stance; work on gripping the floor, bracing the abs, and pulling down into the movement; and then press through the floor and push the hips forward to stand tall. If the addition of weight to the front of your body changes how the squat stance feels, you're free to adjust as needed to find that best fit for you.

BARBELL BACK SQUAT

Next is a back squat with a barbell (figure 3.9), assuming you have access to a bar and a squat rack. Set up the rack so that the hooks for the bar are slightly below shoulder height. With the bar on the hooks, you should have to bend your knees slightly to get under the bar and lift it out of the hooks. Grab the bar with your hands wide enough to put your pinkie fingers on the clear rings of the bar, outside of shoulder width and in the middle of the knurling. If this grip isn't comfortable once you move under the bar, you can open your grip a bit more or move your hands in closer to your torso. However, you need to find a good grip and comfortable position for your shoulders.

Move under the bar so that you can set it on your upper back and shoulders, ideally putting the bar under your upper traps and with your shoulders slightly shrugged into the bar so that there is a shelf of your shoulder blades and upper back muscles to hold the bar in

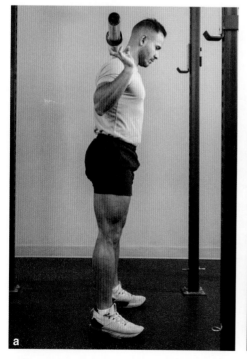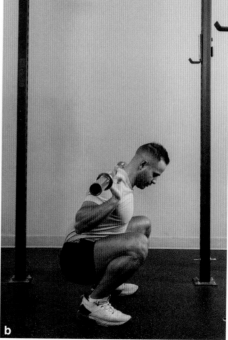

Figure 3.9 Barbell back squat: *(a)* standing position and *(b)* squat.

place. With the bar in position on your upper back, think of pulling the bar into your shoulders with your arms, targeting the lat muscles to gain some additional tension to hold the bar more securely. Brace the abs and stand up, moving the bar out of the hooks. Take a step back and set up your feet as we've discussed previously and as you've found works best for you.

Because the weight is now behind your torso versus in front like the goblet squat, your torso angle will be more forward, and as a result you won't be able to bend the ankles or knees as much to complete the reps, but the more forward torso angle also enables greater hip flexion. This greater requirement for hip flexion and forward torso angle will make the depth you can hit in this position slightly greater than with the goblet squat, since starting in more hip flexion will cause you to hit end-range hip flexion earlier in the movement.

If you're very limited in your depth with a back squat, you can some-times find success by elevating your heels over the height of your toes, allowing easier ankle movement and greater knee excursion than is possible with heels flat on the ground. You can accomplish this by wearing squat shoes, putting small plates on the ground to rest your heels on, or using wedges or slant boards to create a heel-to-toe drop. Regardless of how you find your best squat, the takeaways remain the same: Feel like work is even in both hips and thighs, weight balance front to back is solid, the joints you want to move are moving, and the joints you don't want to move aren't.

ZOMBIE SQUAT AND BARBELL FRONT SQUAT

The front squat is more challenging because the barbell is sitting on your shoulders in front of your neck instead of behind it. This is commonly used for Olympic lifting—it's the catch position following a clean—and also for a number of athletic training programs that benefit from a more anterior load compared to posterior.

To do a successful front squat, you have to protract your shoulders forward far enough to support the bar. A good learning tool for this is a zombie squat (figure 3.10), where you use an unloaded barbell or dowel, placed on the shoulders and across the collarbone, with hands extended in front of you to prevent you from holding on to the bar. If you have trouble maintaining the bar position on your shoulders because it keeps falling forward, reach the shoulder blades forward as far as possible to allow a larger shelf for the bar to sit on, or try to limit how far forward you lean during the squat movement.

Once you can manage the zombie squat positioning without your hands, you can hold onto the bar to add more weight to the move-ment. Two of the most common grips are the clean grip, with hands positioned on the bar slightly greater than shoulder width, but if you don't have the wrist or elbow flexibility to manage this position you can also go with a cross grip, where you hold the bar with your hand over your opposite shoulder (figure 3.11).

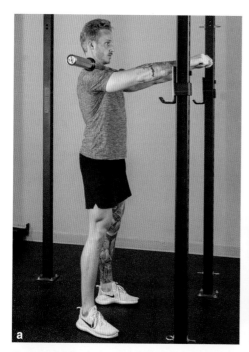
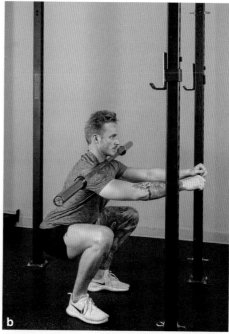

Figure 3.10   Side view of the zombie squat: *(a)* standing position and *(b)* squat.

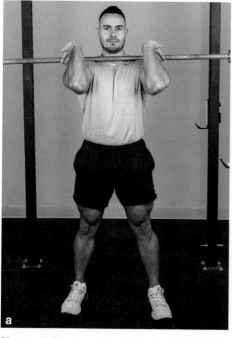
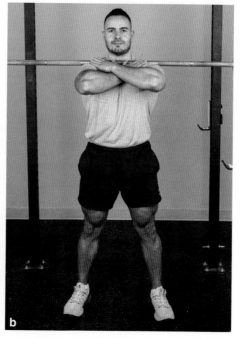

Figure 3.11   Front squat grips: *(a)* clean grip and *(b)* cross grip.

The process for a front squat is the same as for the other variations mentioned previously. The only difference is the location of the load, and how relatively stable or controlled it is compared to the others. For most people it's the hardest variation to learn, simply because it's harder to maintain correct position than a back squat or goblet squat, but it can still allow you to lift a significant amount of weight if you can learn the positioning to hold the bar and keep it stable.

COACHING CUES FOR THE SQUAT

- **Grip the floor.** Create tension through the arches of the feet and work on maintaining tension through the foot tripod to stay anchored to the floor and prevent pronation.
- **Use a 360-degree squeeze.** Brace the core muscles all the way around the waist—lower back, obliques, rectus abdominis, top and bottom. Keep that tension consistent through the entire movement.
- **Unlock and drop.** Push the hips back slightly to begin the movement, then lower your hips to your heels as far as possible without rounding your lower back.
- **Spread the floor.** Think of creating tension as if you're trying to rip the floor apart between your feet. This lateral tension comes from the hips.
- **Drive out of the hole.** From the bottom position, use a forceful movement to push the feet into the floor and push the hips forward to return to the starting position of the movement.
- **Find your heels.** Make sure the entire foot is in contact with the ground throughout the squat movement, and don't squat and raise the heels to access depth or tip forward as you press up out of the bottom of the rep.
- **Pull into the bottom.** Actively increase tension in the loaded muscles as you lower into the bottom of the movement. Don't just flop into the bottom without using any tension.

Troubleshooting the Squat

The squat has a few common technical issues that are relatively easy to fix or at least work through with either specific cues or adjustments to technique or positioning. Let's dig into a few of them.

Issue: Rounding Back at the Bottom

Rounding at the bottom of the squat is commonly referred to as a butt wink (figure 3.12) and happens when you run out of hip flexion but can still go lower with more knee, ankle, and lower-back flexion. It has been blamed on tight hamstrings or weak hip flexors, but it's much more of an end-range hip flexion issue rather than a hamstring stretch issue. As you lower into the squat movement, the knee flexes and allows the hamstring tension to reduce. The knee flexion angle in a squat is consistently greater than the knee flexion angle in a deadlift, which requires much more hamstring flexibility without lower-back flexion. Plus, the bottom of a squat that produces a butt wink often doesn't include feeling tight or stretched hamstrings.

One easy fix is to simply not squat quite as low. Descend to the point where the lower back begins to flex and stop there. Again, unless you're a powerlifter, there is no reason to squat to a specified depth, especially if it changes the exercise to something that doesn't produce the specific benefits you're looking for. It may also be a sign that the core bracing into the bottom position has reduced or let go entirely, allowing the spine to shift in the bottom position. Focus on maintaining and even increasing the bracing tension into the bottom position, especially maintaining lower-back erector tension, to reduce this lack of stability. Another fix is to wear squat shoes or Olympic lifting shoes or put a small wedge or plate under your heels when squatting. Lifting shoes have a heel-to-toe drop that elevates the heel and allows easier positioning of your center of mass over your base of support as you go through the squat movement and allows you to reduce the hip flexion requirement at different depths of your squat compared to not having the same foot positioning. The trade-off is a bit more knee pressure and quad stress with less lower-back and hip stress.

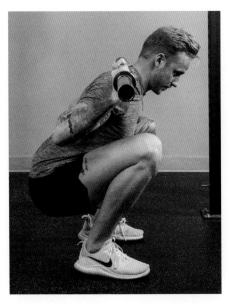

Figure 3.12 Side view of a back squat with butt wink.

Issue: Shifting Weight to One Side When Standing

The issue of shifting weight to one side (figure 3.13) usually comes down to a left–right strength issue or a dominant leg trying to do all the work. As you have a dominant hand that throws or writes more effectively, you have a dominant leg that is stronger and more stable.

A big portion of this fault is trying to rise out of the bottom of the squat too quickly and losing the ability to push through both legs equally while defaulting to using the dominant leg. Or maybe you're not focusing on pushing hard through the leg you're shifting away from. To correct this error, imagine you have a scale under each foot and you want to make the reading the same, all the way from the start to the finish of the rep. Make sure you're loading onto the less dominant leg and pushing it into the floor.

Issue: Hips Coming Out of the Hole Early

Bringing the hips out of the hole early (figure 3.14) strains the lower back and hips more than you want. In this fault, the individual squats down normally, but on the way up their hips shoot up and back. Essentially the lifter has to good morning the weight to get it back to the starting position. The knees extend but the weight doesn't go up, which causes the hips to push back and up. Another possibility is the individual is balancing their weight over the balls of the foot rather than the heels, so the hips shoot back and up to counterbalance and prevent falling over.

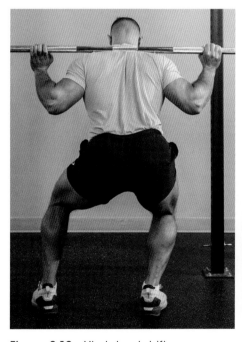

Figure 3.13 Hip lateral shift.

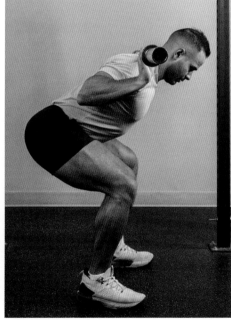

Figure 3.14 Early hips.

You can counter this error with a few cues. First, make sure your heels are in contact with the floor throughout the movement, but especially as you drive up out of the bottom position. If you use heel lifts, set the lift in the same position where you would normally place your feet for a squat. Make sure there is a downward angle from the heels to the toes, keeping in mind that you must maintain balance and not tip the plate, lift, wedge, or other device. Shifting the weight forward toward the balls of the feet will affect how you balance the weight; making sure you have contact with the heels can help reduce that shift.

Second, think of pushing the legs into the ground while simultaneously pushing the hips forward hard as you drive up out of the bottom position. The combined effort of pushing the hips forward while pushing the legs down causes you to stand. Don't simply shift your hips forward and drive your knees further in front of your toes.

Issue: Twisting When Coming Out of the Bottom

What if the lowering phase looks good, but when you transition to coming up there's a twist in the hips to find a different line of action (figure 3.15)? This is sort of a combination of a lateral shift coupled with a forward movement of one hip and a backward movement of the other. It's typically an indicator that you may need to adjust your foot positioning.

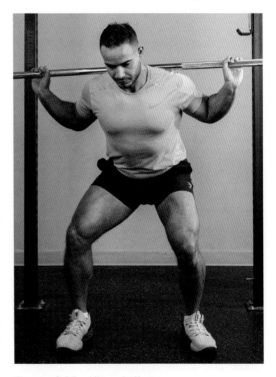

Whichever hip moves forward is put into more external rotation, so try to start the movement with that hip in more external rotation and see what happens. Try the movement with that toe turned out slightly and see if that reduces the rotation. If it does, you've found your better stance. If it doesn't, refer to the section on shifting weight when standing and see if it helps to slow the movement and keep weight shift minimal with a reduced load.

Figure 3.15 Hip rotation.

Deadlift

Deadlifts also are something that everyone does differently for greatest effectiveness. Some people lift best in what's known as a conventional stance, where the feet are hip-width apart and the hands hold the weight with the arms outside of the legs, and some lift best in what's known as a sumo stance, where the feet are wider than hip width and the hands hold the weight with the arms inside of the legs. Some people require a weight that's positioned a bit higher, and some people can lift a weight that's positioned relatively low. Some people deadlift with high hips and a lower torso angle, and some lift with a more upright torso positioning and lower hips.

All these stances and positional differences are valid, and some work better than others for specific limb lengths and joint geometries. Similar to the squat stance, you might benefit from an asymmetric stance with your deadlifts, so playing with your setup to find what works best for you is a great investment to make before lifting heavier weights. Because your hips are the same whether you squat or deadlift, an asymmetric stance for one will likely be required for the other, so follow the same foot positioning sequence for both lifts to find your best stance—the one where you feel strong, stable, and most comfortable.

Deadlift Technique

Picture a deadlift from the front (figure 3.16). The same midline balance points should be made as in the squat: through the middle of the nose, sternum, belly button, and hips, and between the feet. When the deadlift is viewed from the side (figure 3.17), you can see a definite shift in hip positioning compared to the squat.

During a deadlift, most joint movement comes from the hips, with some coming from the knees and very little flexion coming at the ankles. Compared to a squat, the torso angle during a deadlift is decidedly more horizontal and the hip displacement is much further back. The shin angle is close to vertical during a deadlift; during a squat, the shin angle tends to be forward of the ankles. This positioning during the deadlift results in a movement that is more of a horizontal back and forth from the hips than an up and down. As the hips drive forward to lift the load, the torso angle increases toward vertical. As the hips move back to lower the load, the torso returns to a more horizontal angle.

During this hip movement, the core muscles should brace hard and the shoulders should be tensed against the ribs, with the lats tight to help make the spine a rigid lever that allows force transfer from the hips to the arms and into the weight being lifted. A spine that isn't as rigid will reduce the force transfer from the lower body to the upper body and could result in either poor lift performance or a potential strain as working tissues of the spine are loaded and elongated, a recipe for tissue failure and possible damage or injury. The movement should primarily be from

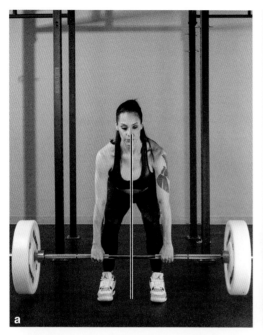 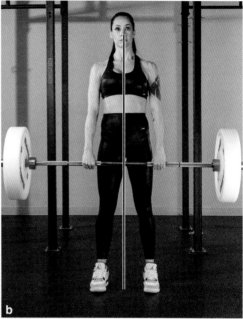

Figure 3.16 Front view of the deadlift: *(a)* start position and *(b)* finish position.

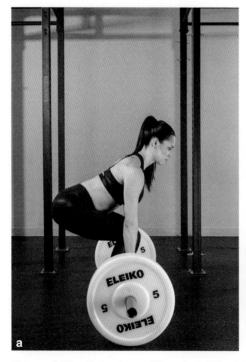 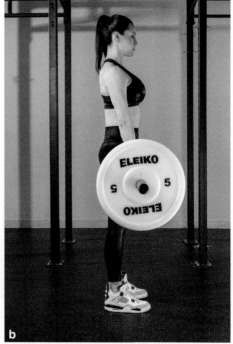

Figure 3.17 Side view of the deadlift: *(a)* start position and *(b)* finish position.

the hips and some from the knees, with as little as possible through the spine or shoulders.

Before lifting, take in a big breath and do a 360-degree brace hard on top of it to create stiffness through the spine. Make sure the brace is 360 degrees, using all muscles of the torso to add stability. Now hinge from the hips and bend the knees slightly to get down to the implement you're planning to lift, all while maintaining your strong 360-degree brace. Grab the implement, using all your fingers and not letting any slide off the implement or be uninvolved. Focus on making the movement to the implement come from the hips with as little spine movement as possible, and keep your brace as strong as possible. Squeeze your shoulder blades into and down on your ribs to add more tension to the spine, and then push the floor away and drive the hips forward to stand tall. Exhale slightly and slowly as you reach the top of the rep, making sure you maintain your brace. Lower the weight to the floor, reversing the movement used to stand up, then relax the tension you created to lift the weight.

Finding Your Deadlift Position

To find the best stance and position the weight, we can do a similar sequence as we followed with the squat, using either a barbell or broomstick, or even a light kettlebell. Using the implement of your choice, perform a few basic deadlift hip hinges, starting with your feet hip-width apart and toes pointing forward. Note how they feel, what muscles you feel working, whether you feel like your spine needs to flex, and how deep into the hinge movement you get before feeling any spine movement.

Turn your left foot out about 20 to 30 degrees and repeat the hinge movement, noting how things feel, what's different, good, or bad, and whether you can get into more or less hinge range of motion before spine movement occurs. Return the left foot to face forward, then repeat this sequence with the right turned out. If one side turned out felt better, return to that turned-out position, and then hold that foot about 3 to 6 inches (8-15 cm) back compared to the other foot, and repeat the hinge.

Now try with the other foot about 3 to 6 inches (8-15 cm) behind the back or implement, and repeat. Your goal is to find the position that feels best to you and allows you the best range of motion without spine movement.

Open your stance to shoulder width or even slightly wider. Try the hinge with the same foot positioning you previously identified as preferable. If things feel better or worse, or if you can get into more or less range of motion, make a note and use that as your preference. If you can hinge with enough range of motion to get down to a barbell positioned with plates on the floor without using any lower-back flexion to get there, you can successfully pull a weight from the floor. If you can't quite get to this bar position but you can from a little higher, you can pull from blocks, a rack, or even a trap bar with elevated handles.

KETTLEBELL DEADLIFT

When first learning to deadlift, a kettlebell deadlift (figure 3.18) is a good place to start. The kettlebell can be set between your feet, which makes it easier to position relative to your center of mass and lets you feel your back tension more effectively than starting with a barbell that's positioned slightly in front of your center of mass. To begin, place the kettlebell between your feet. Follow the setup and execution described in the previous section, using a kettlebell of a comfortable weight, one you can safely and confidently lift. If you're fairly tall or have limited hip mobility, you can put the kettlebell on a small riser to reduce the range of motion needed to lift it.

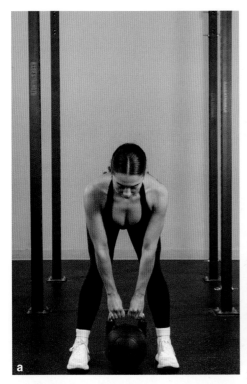 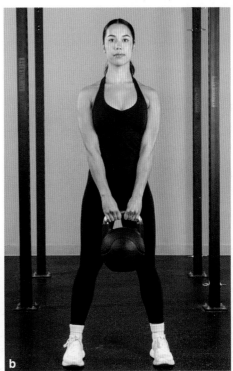

Figure 3.18 Kettlebell deadlift: *(a)* start position and *(b)* finish position.

TRAP BAR DEADLIFT

A more challenging implement for deadlifts is a trap bar. The trap bar is a bit more cumbersome than a barbell or kettlebell, but learning to use it is easy for most people. Since you don't have to bend as low to grab a trap bar as you do for a kettlebell, you can angle your torso angle in more vertically. The trap bar also allows you to grab the handles outside of your feet versus inside of your feet. It's common when using a trap bar to experience more knee flexion than with a kettlebell or a barbell, so it's important to allow only a small amount of knee flexion on a trap bar deadlift (figure 3.19) and not let it turn into a version of a squat if it's a deadlift you're looking to train.

Because the trap bar handles are usually a fixed width, it's difficult to get as much upper-back and lat tension to hold the upper body in place during the trap bar deadlift compared to a barbell or kettlebell deadlift, but efforts should still be made to maximize the tension you can achieve to limit spine torque during the movement.

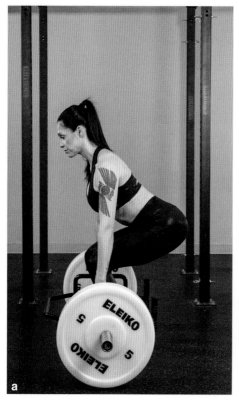 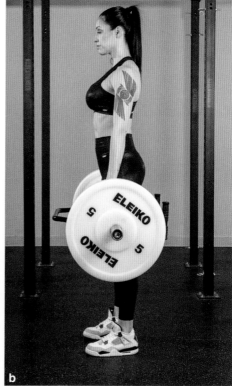

Figure 3.19 Trap bar deadlift: *(a)* start position and *(b)* finish position.

BARBELL DEADLIFT

A barbell is used most often for deadlifts, but the barbell deadlift (figure 3.20) also has the strictest requirements for successful completion. Start by standing with the bar over the midfoot and fairly close to the shins. Some people stand at a point where the bar slides up the shins the entire way and wind up looking like a character in a horror movie by the time they're done from the knurling of the bar ripping the skin apart. You don't need to stand that close unless you're looking to save every millimeter of movement for a successful lift in a powerlifting meet or unless you have some Kevlar-lined workout leggings.

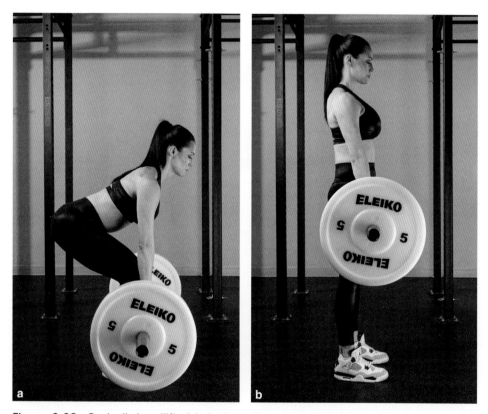

Figure 3.20 Barbell deadlift: *(a)* start position and *(b)* finish position.

Creating Tension for the Deadlift

Creating tension before you lift is massively important and can be done in one of two ways. To gain this tension in the standing position, focus on getting your air, bracing, and tensing before you bend to grab the bar and lift. Alternatively, you can create the tension in the bottom position by grabbing the bar, getting your air, and bracing before you lift. In either case, create as much spinal stiffness as possible, breathe in, and hold your breath as you begin the movement.

Holding your breath against pressure is known as a Valsalva maneuver. This maneuver can help maintain core stiffness and also modulate blood pressure during heavier exertions. If you've ever tried to lift without doing something like this, you likely felt a bit lightheaded or even passed out afterward from a drop in blood pressure. It's common, but avoidable. As you stand with the weight, you can exhale a little air slowly, to gradually reduce pressure, but maintain your bracing and tension until you set the weight down.

Completing the Deadlift

During the eccentric or lowering phase, reverse the movement to lower the weight, maintaining tension through the shoulders and core to control your body segments. You can lower the weight more quickly than you raised it, so make sure any lowering is done with a degree of control. Fast and in control is different from dropping or bouncing or slamming the weight into the ground. In addition, your gym may have a rule against dropping weights. Even if you think it's no big deal, other gym members may disagree. Besides, it's not worth getting thrown out of your training facility

Should you drop a deadlift? I know there are people who prefer to avoid doing any of the eccentric phase of a deadlift entirely, but doing so reduces the training benefits that can come from the movement. Dropping is half of the rep, so why cheat yourself out of a portion of your development? That being said, I have a relatively simple rule about dropping: you can drop bumper plates on a platform but not iron plates anywhere else. If you're using plates specifically designed to be dropped, go for it, especially if the bar is an Olympic lifting bar that can tolerate the impact. If you're using iron plates and care about the flooring not being dented, dropping it might not be the best idea.

Fine-Tuning the Deadlift

The conventional deadlift described here involves standing with your feet narrower than shoulder width and your hands gripping the bar outside the width of your feet. A sumo stance involves a wider foot positioning and hand positioning inside your knees. Some lifters take a stance as wide as the plates, while others may find a bigger benefit by standing with the feet slightly wider than their regular squat stance. Major benefits of the sumo stance deadlift versus the conventional deadlift are that it allows the hips to get closer to the bar, the hand positioning makes it easier to develop upper- and mid-back tension, and the range of motion required to get to lockout at the top of the rep is slightly less. Some detriments of the lift are that a wider stance can put more rotational pressure on the knees; the externally rotated and abducted hip position may be more challenging or uncomfortable for those without much joint space in the hips and could cause irritation with continued use; and—perhaps worst of all!—people on the internet hate it for some reason. As with anything, the pros have to outweigh the cons, and if you prefer one lift over the other, make use of it and crush your training.

Regardless of the implement used, the primary focus should be on developing and maintaining tension throughout the lift. You want everything from the arches of your feet up to the base of your skull to be flexed and tensed to generate as much strength and power as possible into the implement being lifted, while also ensuring the joints you're using to perform the lift are moving and the joints not meant to be producing the movement remain steady.

One way to generate this tension is to do what's known as taking the slack out of the bar and developing a wedge prior to lifting. When you set up to begin the lift with either a trap bar or barbell, the bar is sitting on the bottom of the plate opening. Taking the slack out of the bar involves lifting the bar into the top of the plate opening and generating pressure into the weight, but not to the point of lifting the weight off the floor. Just feeling the pressure of the bar being pulled into the top of the plate opening will increase muscle activity and help you to feel where in your feet your balance may be, as well as whether your lats, core muscles, hamstrings, and glutes are working and ready to complete the lift.

Creating a wedge (figure 3.21) expands on this concept by not just pressing the bar into the top of the

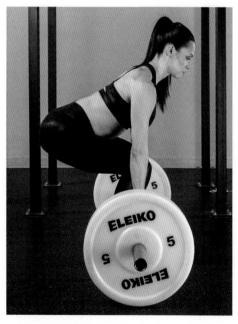

Figure 3.21 Proper wedge.

plate opening but by trying to push the hips forward toward the barbell (or, on a trap bar, toward the vertical line under your shoulders). Lifting the implement into the top of the plate opening while pushing the hips forward begins the movement and sets the stage for the kind of tension needed throughout the entire body to successfully complete the lift. This vertical lift and horizontal push creates a movement that helps to compress the spine and pull it more into a vertical position prior to lifting than if this tension wasn't present, essentially allowing you to wedge your body into the movement. A proper wedge will feel like you're almost pulling the bar off the floor as you create tension through the shoulders, torso, and hips, and that level of tension pulls you toward and almost under the bar with your hips. If you feel like getting into position lifts half the weight before you even begin your pull, you're doing it right.

With deadlifts, grip is a specific concern, especially as the weight gets heavier. One thing I try to get my clients to do is to involve every finger into the lift. It's not uncommon for someone to grab a bar and engage only with the thumb, index, and middle fingers, leaving the ring and pinkie fingers to their own devices. Not using your smallest two fingers can limit the strength of your grip significantly, since almost half of the muscles of your hands aren't involved in holding onto the bar. To counter this, set up your grip by wrapping your pinkie finger around the bar first, then working into your ring, middle, index finger, and thumb to ensure you're using your whole hand to hold onto the bar.

Another option for improving grip is to set the bar deeper into your hand rather than where the fingers meet the palm. Try to set the bar into the transverse crease, across the width of your hand, which will allow more of a squeeze. This way, individuals with smaller hands and shorter fingers will get more contact with the bar and have a better chance of hanging on as the weight comes off the floor.

As the weight gets heavier, grip tends to be the limiting factor over lower-back strength or leg strength. With a trap bar, there isn't the issue of the bar rolling out of your hands as it can with a barbell. When training hard, it is possible to use straps or other devices to help hold the bar in spite of grip weakness, but doing this will ensure that you don't actually train your grip, which kind of misses the point of the exercise. With a barbell, the bar can roll out of your hands if you have both hands facing in the same direction, so to prevent this it's common to use an alternating grip, where one hand goes over the bar and the other goes under. This can allow the individual to lift more weight without the bar rolling out of their hands.

My preference has always been to lift to the limit of the individual's grip with a double overhand position. This way, you can manage injury risk while still developing total system strength from the hands through to the feet. (We won't get into hook grip because that's an easy way to hate your life and your thumbs at the same time.)

In each of these deadlift variations, a major element for success is learning to generate total body tension. Involving every muscle in your body is a great way to limit movement of joints you don't want to move and to control the positioning of the joints you do want to move. Plus, more muscles working can allow you to move more weight through summation of force. Learning how to simultaneously tense the upper back, shoulders, lower back, core, glutes, legs, and even the arches of your feet is the most powerful tool you can develop for deadlift success.

COACHING CUES FOR THE DEADLIFT

- **Squeeze oranges in your armpits to make orange juice.** Pull the shoulder blades back and down and try to generate enough tension through that squeeze that if there were oranges in there you would crush them.
- **Find your hamstrings.** During the hip hinge to get to the bar, reach the hips back and try to maximize the hamstring stretch you feel versus just bending down to grab the bar.
- **Wrinkle the back of your shirt.** Don't round the lower back. Instead, think of extending your back to make the shirt wrinkle. Rounding would stretch out the shirt and flatten the wrinkles.
- **Take the slack out of the bar.** Start the movement by pulling the bar up into the top of the plate opening.
- **Create a wedge.** Take the slack out of the bar and push the hips forward to maximize the tension at setup.
- **Push the floor away.** Don't think of standing up or lifting the bar, think about pushing down through your feet to make the weight move off the ground.
- **Use 10 fingers.** Use the entire hand to grab the bar with all your fingers.

Troubleshooting the Deadlift

Let's look at some common technique faults that might come out of deadlift training and how you might be able to fix them.

Issue: Rounding the Back as the Weight Leaves the Floor

You lower to grab the bar, get set, everything looks perfect, and then as soon as you start to pull on the bar your spine looks like a drawn bow or a cat that's just been scared (figure 3.22). While there's conflicting research on whether a rounded back is good or bad for a deadlift, or whether it's something to worry about, I believe that if the movement should be coming from the hips, you want to make sure they're doing the work not the spine, so it's preferable to get into a position where you're not using the spine.

Often the back will round if you lose tension through the muscles of the spine and shoulders as you begin to lift the bar. The correction often requires cueing to squeeze those muscles hard and maintain that tension throughout the lift. It can also result from thinking of pulling up versus pushing the hips forward and driving down. Altering your focus during the reps can have a big impact on eliminating spine rounding as you begin the movement.

Issue: Booping the Bar

Booping the bar is a term I use with clients who set up close to the bar, then as they bend down to grab on, their shins wind up pushing the bar forward over their toes (figure 3.23). Setting the bar too far in front of the arches of the feet makes it harder to maintain a center of gravity over your

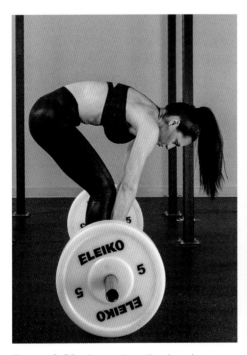

Figure 3.22 Rounding the back.

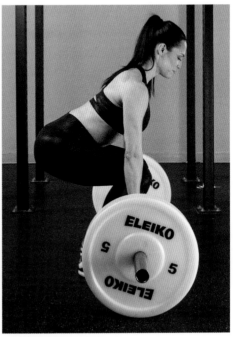

Figure 3.23 Booping the bar.

base of support; it often results in the initiation of the lift being very slow and requires moving the bar back over the arches before vertical movement can happen. These individuals fail at the floor or else have the slowest grind possible before shooting through the rest of the rep.

A way to combat the boop is to focus on reaching back with the hips, trying to maintain that vertical shin angle as you bend to grab the bar. Forward knee movement will push the bar forward or, at best, require you to lift the bar forward and around your knees. Keeping the knees behind the vertical line of the foot arches and the bar can reduce this forward movement and help reduce the amount of bar travel required to make a successful lift.

Issue: Knee Caves In During Initiation

Having the knee cave in (figure 3.24) is a common error in a deadlift but also during the concentric phase of a squat. The knee drops in toward the midline of the body and then eventually (we hope) regains the vertical line of action required at the starting position and lockout.

The two main culprits of knee cave are the foot and the hip. If the foot has a fallen arch or limited arch tension, the knee will be pulled toward the midline as pressure builds during the lift. This also happens if an individual relies on pushing through the big toe side of their foot versus through the full tripod foot discussed earlier. Knee cave can be avoided by working on developing tension through the arch prior to lifting and also ensuring pressure is maintained on the baby toe side of the foot through the lift.

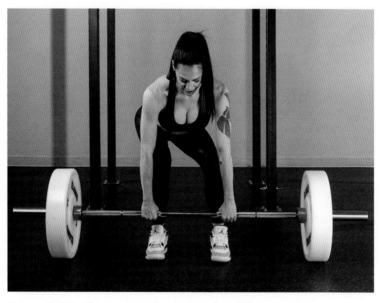

Figure 3.24 Knees cave in during deadlift.

The hips can create knee cave by not producing enough external rotation force to counter the internal rotation force of the adductor muscles during the lift. This is the prime responsibility of the glutes and can be stepped up by specifically cueing how to use the glutes more during the lift. Think of using the hips to actively push the knees wider. This will help prevent the knees from collapsing in. Imagining creating tension in the hips to cause the feet to spread the floor laterally can increase engagement as well.

Whether the feet are the problem or the hips are the problem, the solution is the same: create more tension to prevent the knees from caving in.

Issue: Lower-Back Discomfort at Lockout

The lockout typically requires the individual to stand as tall as possible, keeping the spine and shoulders vertically stacked over the hips. In some situations, the individual may lock out with more a lower-back extension and not let the hips get under the spine, effectively putting the spine into an extended and loaded position (figure 3.25). A simple fix is to flex the glutes hard at lockout and reduce the lower-back extension, plus maintain the bracing to help support the spine more effectively while under load.

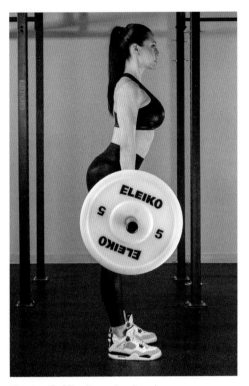

Figure 3.25 Poor lockout.

Conclusion

No matter your limb lengths and relative torso length, you can still benefit from squats and deadlifts, but you might find one easier than the other. Train them both anyway, and work on getting as strong as possible. These two movements, as well as their variations, are the prime strength training exercises we'll use for the lower body training for this program. Next, we'll dig into strength training movements for the upper body, namely pushing and pulling movements. Just as with the squat and deadlift, there are ways to customize the movements to your unique abilities, and some movements work better or not nearly as well for different people, so we'll look through the differences and figure out where you can get your best benefits for your upper body in the next chapter.

Pressing and Pulling Movements

The most common question asked of people who strength train is, "How much can you bench?" It's not that common to get a question about squats or deadlifts, but in terms of what the average person on the street is going to ask, bench seems to be the universally known movement. It doesn't matter if someone has no idea of what constitutes a good or not so good bench number, or whether they can tell relative to absolute amounts—if you bench, and it's more than their body weight, they're going to be impressed. Two hundred pounds (91 kg)? Three hundred (136 kg)? They don't know if that's good or not, but we all know that no matter what your real bench total is, just add 50 pounds (23 kg) to it, and whatever someone tells you their bench is, just subtract 50. Except on the internet, then it's 100. Maybe that's why Monday is International Bench Press Day every week in almost every gym, and no other exercise gets its own day. You gotta lead with what's important.

Because bench press is ubiquitous for anyone who lifts weights, knowing how to do it well and avoid common pitfalls is important. That being said, bench press is just a single exercise to develop the chest, delts, and triceps. There are many others, and in fact many that are better suited to training long term with fewer injury possibilities and better return on your training investment than bench press. Some people may have shoulders, elbows, or wrists that object to the restrictive orientations needed to push a strong bench press. Remember how we showed that there's some inherent asymmetry in hip structures for the squat and deadlift? Similarly, there can be asymmetric joint orientations in the upper body that make holding a straight bar and pushing through a fixed line of action less than ideal for some.

In the same way, overhead press is a challenging movement because the range of motion needed to do a true overhead press requires some serious thoracic extension, scapular upward movement, and shoulder joint mobility. The shoulder has a lot of moving parts to it, and a lot of muscles, tendons, and ligaments that all work in their own way. We have to approach the shoulder with a bit more thought toward technique, positioning, and orientation. I use the analogy that the shoulder is like a high-performance sports car, capable of a lot but very finicky and might need a lot of time in the shop—whereas the hip is like an old pickup truck that'll get the job done, even if things aren't that perfect. You can beat it up for a long time before it needs any sort of TLC.

Horizontal and Vertical Pressing

Because push and pull movements have a lot of moving parts, it's important to ensure they all do their jobs properly, or at least reasonably well enough to get the benefit you're looking for without the negative effects. Maintaining mobility through all the components of the shoulder—the glenohumeral joint (the clinical name for the shoulder joint), the shoulder blade around the ribs, and the thoracic spine to position the shoulder blade—is the key to successful training.

For a horizontal pressing movement, there's a different technique depending on whether you're lying on a bench or not. If you're lying on a bench, as in a barbell bench press or a dumbbell bench press, the bench acts as a stabilizer and force development platform. Because of this, your shoulder blades need to be pulled back and down to get the shoulder joint as close to that platform as possible and generate the most force possible. They stay tightly held in this position throughout the entire range of motion.

If the shoulder blades slide out and forward, it can be really hard to get them to slide back into place, especially since your body weight and the load you're lifting are pushing your ribs down into the bench and hindering that shoulder blade movement. A lot of high-level powerlifters consider bench press an upper-back exercise for this reason.

This "shoulder blade tucked" position also helps you use the bench as a stabilizer, reducing the demand on the rotator cuff muscles of the shoulder.[10] Anything that helps unload the cuff muscles to allow them to control the shoulder will reduce the chance of straining those muscles, and as a result reduce the possibility of overuse injuries or sudden trauma. This all adds up to longer-term lifting success.

For an exercise not performed lying on a bench, like a push-up, standing cable press, overhead press, or landmine press, the goal is to have the shoulder blades direct the movement as much as possible, sliding forward as you press and then returning to their starting position as you return the weight to the starting position. Because you're not using the bench as a force-generation platform, you have to use the shoulder blades and their connections to the rib cage to generate that push. Allowing the shoulder blades to wrap around the ribs in a horizontal press and to rotate upward during any overhead press can limit possible stress to the rotator cuff and reduce the likelihood of an impingement injury, all while maintaining more bone-on-bone loading to make force production more efficient. Plus, bringing more muscles to the party makes for easier work, so making the shoulder blades get their swag on can help you get more from your pressing movements than keeping them locked down.

Because exercises that don't use a bench have a smaller end range of motion and use a broader range of motion from all working joints, they are a better place to start, at least until range of motion is sufficient to press off a bench effectively. Pressing from a bench allows you to use maximum load, but if that's not a goal, there's no real reason to require pressing from a bench. It's important to note that an exercise or position that works the torso muscles can have a positive effect on rotator cuff muscle engagement,[1] so if you use a bench as your only form of pressing exercise you may be limiting your potential when it comes to balancing pressing strength with joint stability and resiliency.

For vertical pressing, there is a surprisingly large connection between thoracic extension and the ability of the shoulder blades to rotate upward to allow the overhead position to be as vertical as possible. Try this: sit up as tall as possible and bring your arms over your head, trying to get them vertical with your biceps touching your ears. Now try it again, except this time round your back and slouch. You'll probably find, as you flex the thoracic spine, that your shoulders roll forward and tilt, and when you try to raise your arms over your head you wind up shrugging and making your neck disappear as your shoulders become a part of your ears. You might even feel some notable discomfort in the shoulders and might not be able to get the arms vertical.

In this example, nothing has changed in terms of muscle strength, joint ranges of motion, or any common issue that would inhibit this range of motion. The only difference is the position of the thoracic spine, which affects how the shoulder blades move and where they wind up as a result. Aging tends to reduce thoracic mobility,[2] especially in extension, so the longer you've been around, the harder it can be to maintain this foundational postural expression and thus optimize your overhead pressing. A challenge in thoracic extension is that many people can't tell if they're extending from the thoracic spine or lumbar spine and might cheat by arching their lower back (i.e., lumbar spine) as far as they can in an attempt to compensate. Adjusting technique by feel goes only so far, so on occasion it might be worth taking a video of yourself trying to get a certain position or movement down, and then reviewing it to see what's actually happening when you think you're doing it correctly. And, of course, a good coach with a keen eye for this kind of detail is worth working with.

When you're pressing overhead, your shoulder blades should rotate out, away from the midline of the body, and elevate slightly. This movement is primarily driven by the upper trapezius, lower trapezius, and serratus anterior muscles, which each pull on a different side of the triangle of the shoulder blade and cause it to rotate against the ribs (figure 4.1). When this happens, the upper arm bone (humerus) socket begins to move. It changes from pointing horizontally to pointing vertically, which helps maintain bone-on-bone contact as you move into the overhead position. The more the humerus can stay centered in the cup of the shoulder blade (glenoid fossa), the easier it is to load without making the muscles of the rotator cuff work harder than normal to maintain control of the positioning, which means more successful pressing with less potential for injury.

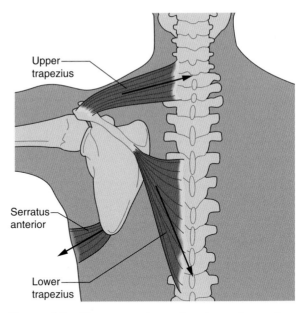

Figure 4.1 The upper trapezius, lower trapezius, and serratus anterior pull on the shoulder blade to cause rotation.

Getting overhead movement to come from the shoulder blade becomes even more important as an individual ages, because the shape of the shoulder itself can change over time.[3] The acromion process—the small, bony end that overhangs the shoulder joint and acts as an attachment point for the deltoid muscles—can change shape with time and get lower and lower over the shoulder, which reduces the space for the stuff that lives under it (supraspinatus muscle and subacromial bursa) to move around without problems. The supraspinatus muscle (top part of the rotator cuff) and subacromial bursa can get squeezed as the amount of space between the acromion and the humerus reduces, and in overhead movements, a shoulder blade that doesn't rotate up effectively will allow even less space for the arm to move vertically, intensifying that squeeze.

A smaller acromial angle and tighter subacromial space tend to correlate with a higher rate of rotator cuff tear injuries.[4] A 20-year-old may be able to press overhead without thinking twice or needing any mobility work and bounce back by tomorrow, but a lifter in their 40s or 60s might need more time to get their thoracic spine, shoulder blade, and shoulder joint into the right position to get the benefits from overhead pressing without waking up tomorrow unable to scratch the top of their head.

We'll dig into specific examples of how to improve mobility to get the best benefits from your upper-body pressing work in chapter 7.

Pressing Technique

Any horizontal pressing movement should be considered a full-body movement, not an isolation exercise. The torso, hips, and legs play a role in successful pressing, and ensuring they're involved in the process is one of the easiest fixes for a lot of common technical problems.

When preparing to do any pressing movement, start by taking a big breath, then bracing hard around that breath, similarly to how you brace with the deadlift and squat movement. With the brace, try to tense the glutes, quads, and calves to add tension through the lower body and develop maximum tension through the entire body. This summation of tension can actually make pressing movements easier and allow you to move more weight than just trying to isolate one group of muscles.

For a horizontal press (figure 4.2), as you lower into the movement or bring the weights toward your shoulders, let the shoulder blades retract and keep them low and away from your ears. As you begin to press, think of starting the push at the shoulder blades as they wrap around to the front of your ribs while the elbows extend. The elbows should form an arrow

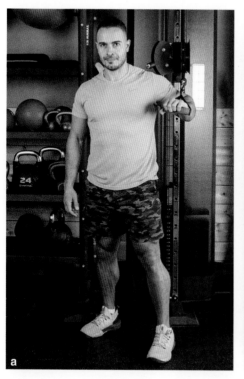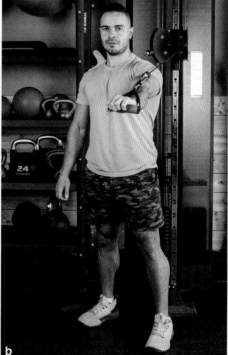

Figure 4.2 Cable horizontal press without a bench: *(a)* start position; *(b)* finish position.

with the body if viewed from the front or back, meaning they're not tight against the body and not flared out to 90 degrees in a T shape. As you press up, there will be a tendency to lose the arrow and move toward the T, so try to maintain the angle of the elbows throughout the movement. Exhale as you reach the fully extended position, without letting go of the core bracing as you breathe out. You don't relax the bracing until you've done the entire set.

COACHING CUES
FOR HORIZONTAL PRESSING WITHOUT A BENCH

Performing presses off a bench requires that the shoulders be set and stable against the bench so the bench can be used as a force generation platform. For pressing movements without a bench—think cable press, push-up, overhead press—the shoulder blades are a more integral and mobile part of the action. During these kinds of presses, focus on the following:

- Make the shoulder blades do the work. Retract as you lower, protract as you press.
- Maintain total body tension.
- Inhale to prepare, exhale on extension.

When pressing off a bench (figure 4.3), step one is to build the foundation from which the press will drive. Retracting the shoulder blades and trying

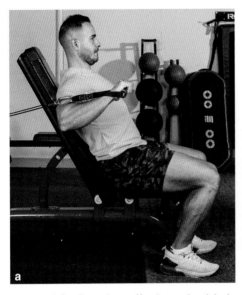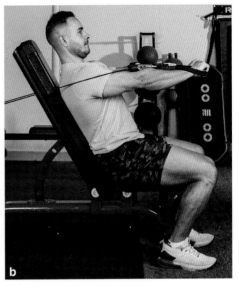

Figure 4.3 Pressing off a bench: *(a)* start position; *(b)* finish position.

to get them flat to the bench helps to reduce the stabilization requirement from the rotator cuff and increase the space that the supraspinatus can operate in, which can reduce the risk of impingement issues.[5] The heavier the loading, the greater the involvement of the latissimus dorsi and the less involvement from the pectoralis major.[6] This indicates that greater force is needed to stabilize the shoulders to the bench to successfully complete the lift.

Getting this retracted position is a stretch (pun absolutely intended!) for many of us, since it requires a large expansion of the pecs and ribs, plus some serious thoracic extension to make it happen, two ranges of motion that are commonly limited in many people. Whenever you feel like your shoulders are pulled back and down far enough, go another 2 or 3 inches (5-8 cm) and you'll likely be close.

Once you get the shoulders and upper back into position, it's important to make sure they stay there through the entire range of motion required in the rep. A common issue is to press the shoulders out as you get to the top of the movement. The downside to this is that, to get the shoulders back into the starting position, you now have to find a way to slide the shoulder blades between the ribs and bench while under loading.

COACHING CUES
FOR HORIZONTAL PRESSING OFF A BENCH

- Squeeze the bench with your shoulder blades.
- Get your upper arm bones as close to the bench as possible.
- Take a big inhale, brace, and drive. Push your feet into the floor, drive your shoulders into the bench, and straighten your elbows.
- Maintain the arrow elbow position. Avoid moving to the T elbow position.
- Don't let the shoulders shrug at the top of the press.

With an overhead press (figure 4.4), the movement of the shoulder blades is upward rotation instead of forward protraction. As you initiate the movement, think of the shoulder blades turning up and driving the arm into the higher position while extending the elbows. You must still consider the total body tension. Similar to the horizontal press, the best elbow line is slightly forward of the torso versus out to the sides. Throughout the movement, the elbows should be pointed slightly forward. Letting the elbows flare out as you press can result in the shoulder blades tilting forward versus rotating up, which puts the shoulder blade at an undesirable angle and can change the rotator cuff stress significantly. Another big benefit to keeping the elbows slightly forward is that it allows the forearms to stay

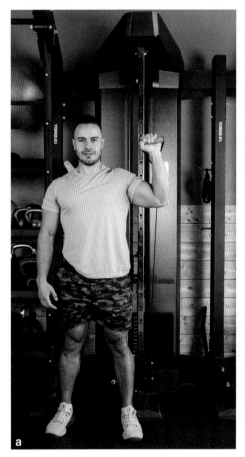 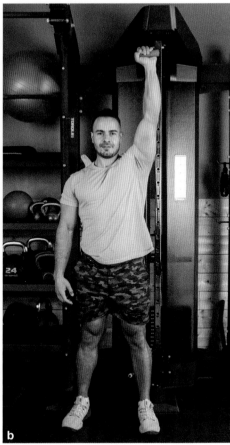

Figure 4.4 Overhead press: *(a)* start position; *(b)* finish position.

in a vertical line under the load. A vertical forearm allows for an easier press. If the elbow is behind the vertical line of the load being moved, the wrists and elbows have to work to maintain the weight in a vertical position versus falling forward.

COACHING CUES FOR OVERHEAD PRESSING

- Keep the chest up to support the weight.
- Drive through the shoulder blades. Think of scooping the shoulder blades forward and under the weight being lifted as the weight goes overhead.
- Keep the elbows pointed somewhat forward, not out to the sides and not back. Maintain vertical forearms under the wrists.
- Brace the abs and glutes when you press to avoid losing spine positioning or core tension.

Let's run through some examples of each pressing movement to give some context of how they should be performed, as well as the differences in cues and actions that are involved with each.

Horizontal Press Variations

There are a lot of ways to train the horizontal pressing movement that don't just require lying on a bench and pressing a weight toward the ceiling. Following are a few of the options to help build your pressing strength on and off the bench.

PUSH-UP

The push-up (figure 4.5) is essentially a full body moving plank. The goal is to make the movement come from the shoulders, shoulder blades, and elbows, and nothing else. Special focus should be given to bracing the core and glutes to prevent the lower back from sagging

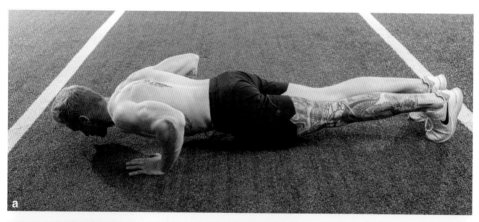

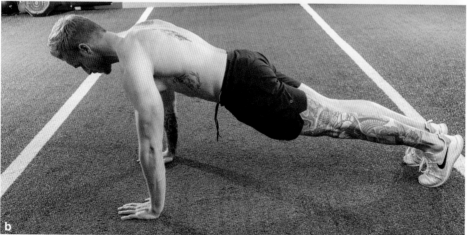

Figure 4.5 Push-up: *(a)* start position; *(b)* finish position.

and to ensure the head doesn't go lower than the chest during any portion of the movement.

During the lowering phase, lead with the chest, trying to make it touch the floor (or mat or whatever). Get as low as is comfortable, ensuring your forehead, abdomen, hips, and thighs are not touching the ground. As you lower, the shoulder blades will retract and come toward the spine, so try to avoid shrugging them toward your ears.

The raising phase is the reverse of this movement. Push your chest away from the floor or surface and drive the shoulder blades forward and around your ribs. Focus on ensuring your spine stays in the same orientation as during the lowering phase. Ideally, your body forms a relatively straight line from the crown of your head through the middle of your shoulders, middle of your hips, and down through your feet.

Foot position should be hip width or slightly wider, with tension through the quads and glutes to ensure the lower body is a solid lever from which to press off with the upper body. The hand position should be slightly greater than shoulder width and in line with your nipples at the point of contact to the floor. This will allow you to maintain an "arrow" alignment, with the elbows close to but not next to your body. Avoid flaring the elbows into a T position. Spread your fingers and think of gripping the ground. If using an elevated surface such as a barbell in a squat rack, wrap all your fingers around it and try to tighten your grip with all fingers. Think of gripping the floor and twisting it between your hands to increase tension in the upper body.

When preparing to lower into a push-up, inhale deeply and brace the core muscles around the breath. As you press into the raising phase, maintain the brace and exhale sharply as you get close to the top of the movement, ensuring you maintain tension through the core as you exhale.

To maintain the straight line through the entire body, think of tensing the quads, glutes, abs, eyeballs, toenails, and pretty much any other part of your body to prevent arching as you press up into the top of the movement. Muscle tension is your friend, so bring as many of your friends with you as possible.

A push-up typically will require pushing 97 percent of your body weight as a man and 80 percent of your body weight as a woman,[7] which can be a significant barrier to performing the reps effectively for beginners who may not have that much strength yet. You can adjust by putting your hands on an elevated surface such as a bench or bar in a squat rack (the higher the surface, the lower the pressing force requirements). You can adjust the height of your push-up surface to build the ability to do reps from the floor over time.

STANDING HORIZONTAL PRESS

The standing horizontal press (figure 4.6) can be done with a cable system set at or slightly higher than shoulder height or with bands attached to an anchor point (door, pole, squat rack, small child) that won't move or fall over as you do the exercise. (Small child results may vary.) Start in a split stance position with one foot in front of the other, ideally hip width or greater, although a narrower stance is more challenging Slightly bend the forward leg and lean forward slightly to load more weight on it than on the back foot; this will help you to maintain balance. Similar to the push-up, the goal of the exercise is to move from the shoulder blades, shoulders, and elbows without moving from other body parts. Brace the core and create total body tension from the feet up to maintain your positioning and create the best foundation from which to press.

Use a similar arrow elbow position as in the push-up and keep the elbows, forearms, and wrists in a straight line with the cable or band. Start with the arms fully extended and the hands in line with the chest. Lower the weight by letting the hands come toward the chest, thumbs coming close to your arm pits. As you press, push the shoulder blades forward around the ribs, ensuring you aren't rounding your upper back to get the shoulder blades to move. When returning the hands

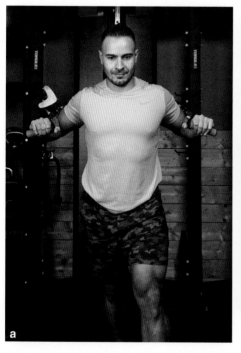
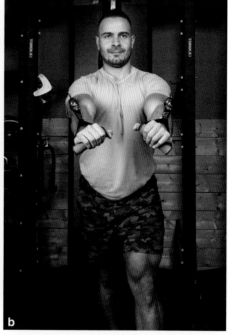

Figure 4.6 Standing horizontal press: *(a)* start position; *(b)* finish position.

to the start position, bring them in line with the lower portion of the chest, just under the armpits. The movement can be done one arm at a time, with alternating arms, or with both arms at the same time.

DUMBBELL BENCH PRESS

As discussed previously, the use of the bench requires a different technique and set up than a pressing exercise performed without a bench. A good idea is to practice the shoulder retraction needed prior to getting under weights, so try this: Standing with your back to a wall, move your shoulder blades as close to each other and as low on your ribs as possible (figure 4.7). Ideally, you should be able to get the shoulder blades flat to the wall. From there, do the pressing movement, ensuring you keep the shoulders stable on the wall without letting them slide out and forward as you extend your elbows. You can also try doing a bench press unloaded—that is, without weights—(figure 4.8) to get the feel of the movement before loading.

For the dumbbell bench press (figure 4.9), start by sitting on the edge of the bench with the weight on your thighs. As you lie back to get into position, tilt the dumbbells back to touch them to your chest. As you roll back and your back and head contact the bench, the weights will be in a good position to start the press.

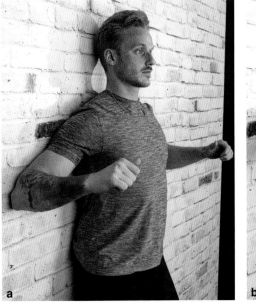
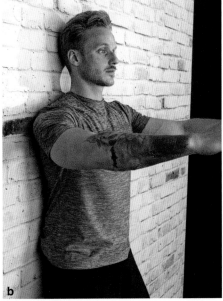

Figure 4.7 Wall press: *(a)* start position; *(b)* finish position.

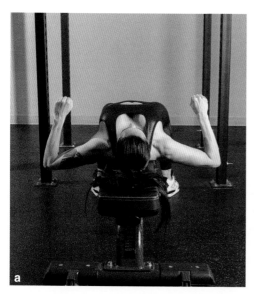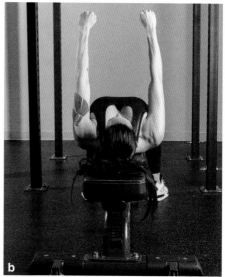

Figure 4.8 Unloaded bench press: *(a)* start position; *(b)* finish position.

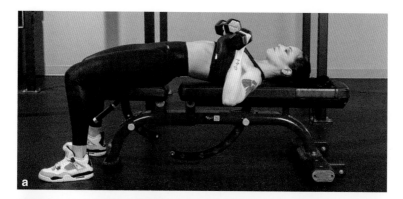

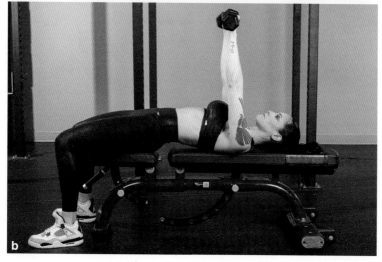

Figure 4.9 Dumbbell bench press: *(a)* start position; *(b)* finish position.

Using the arrow elbow position, hold the dumbbells so they make an arrow themselves (in other words, don't hold them in a linear or parallel position). This angled dumbbell position can reduce the rotation requirement from the wrist and elbow and make maintaining the arrow position easier overall, meaning an easier press with less potential for irritating some of the smaller joints in the arm.

Inhale as you lower the weight to your chest or as far as is comfortable. In preparation for the press, brace the abs hard, drive the feet into the floor, flex your glutes, and squeeze the bench with your shoulder blades to provide the strongest foundation possible. As you press, drive through the elbows, ensuring the shoulder blades stay tight to the bench. Exhale and move the weights from the vertical slightly outside of the shoulders to vertical over the shoulders in an inverted J shape. Try to avoid letting the elbows flare during the press and think of pressing your knuckles to the ceiling to maintain a strong wrist position.

BARBELL BENCH PRESS

Doing a bench press properly is how you get the training adaptations you want while minimizing the chances of developing shoulder discomfort in the rotator cuffs or AC joints. Here's how to do it.

Similar to a dumbbell bench press, for the barbell bench press (figure 4.10) you want to retract the shoulder blades and press them as tightly as possible into the bench. Set up so your eyes are directly under the bar. This shortens the distance between unracking the bar and bringing it forward over your chest while allowing room for the bar to move without hitting the hooks. The bar should be set at a height where you can set your shoulders in place and then only slightly extend the elbows to unrack the bar. If the hooks are too high, you'll have to push up through the shoulder blades to unrack the bar, and if the hooks are too low, you'll have to work really hard to lock out the elbows and bring the bar out of the rack.

When setting up to perform the reps, maintain the arrow elbow position and keep your knuckles square to the ceiling, with shoulders tensed and tight to the bench. Take a big inhale and brace your core around the breath, pushing your feet into the floor and tensing your glutes to build an arc of tension from the floor through the entire body and into the shoulders, squeezing the bench. Lower the bar in line with your nipples and avoid bouncing the bar off your chest unless you want to test the elasticity of your ribs. (Just kidding. Your ribs are not elastic and bouncing the bar off your chest will hurt.)

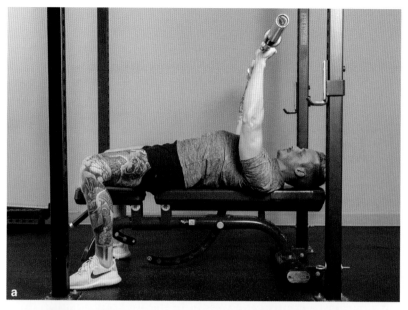

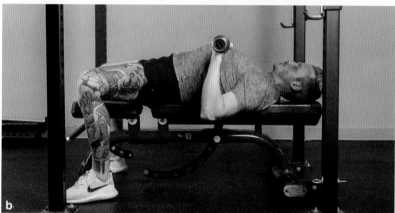

Figure 4.10 Barbell bench press: *(a)* start position; *(b)* finish position.

When you press up, keep the elbows from flaring out, drive through the feet into the floor, and straighten your elbows without letting the shoulder blades slide out from their tight, retracted, and depressed position. Exhale as the bar gets past the halfway point of the lift without letting go of your bracing.

A key feature of bench press success is developing and maintaining total body tension through the entirety of the exercise. At no point during the movement should you be "comfortable" or feel like the reps are easy; instead, you should feel like your soul is being ripped apart between the contrasting demands of moving the weight and maintaining your position. This duality of demands is one of the hardest features to master in a bench press but is one of the most important to achieving long-term success with the lift. Total body tension is one of the first things I check when someone says performing the exercise is painful or uncomfortable.

Overhead Press Variations

The movement for an overhead press involves a different set of muscles, different movement from the shoulder and shoulder blade, and a different stabilization requirement for the torso. Whereas a horizontal press involves movement of the scapula from retraction to protraction (except when pressing off a bench), the overhead press involves upward rotation of the scapula, a more complex and nuanced movement. The shoulder starts in greater external rotation during the overhead press than in the horizontal press, and the stabilization requirements at lockout are considerably higher. It's harder to control the weight in the lockout position during the overhead press than in a horizontal press.

When pressing overhead, you'll need to be in some degree of extension through the thoracic spine, but you have to get there without driving extension through the lower back. You can manage this by maintaining a hard abdominal brace and lifting your chest up high without relaxing the bracing. It's tough to do because the movement involves creating tension against tension, but it can help set the stage for the best movement from the shoulder blades. It can also help you maintain a vertical load over the shoulders and hips.

DUMBBELL OVERHEAD PRESS

When setting up for the dumbbell overhead press (figure 4.11), hold the weights at or slightly above shoulder height, with elbows pointing forward and the dumbbells in a similar arrow alignment as with the dumbbell bench press. You can press the handles in line with each other, but that orientation is considerably harder to maintain for the shoulder joint and doesn't as easily encourage activation of all the muscles that assist in upward rotation of the scapula. That said, you do you.

When preparing to press, take in a big breath, brace the core hard, and keep the chest up. Then push the weights by driving the shoulder blades forward and up under the weight, extending the elbows and pushing your knuckles to the ceiling. Try to keep your forearms vertical under the load throughout the entire movement. Exhale as

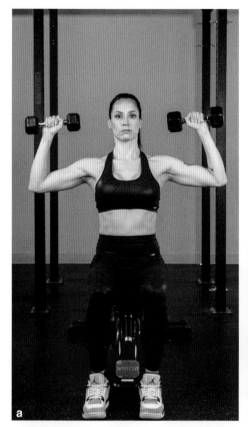 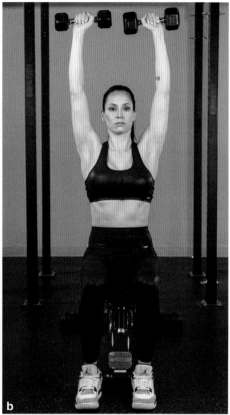

Figure 4.11 Dumbbell overhead press: *(a)* start position; *(b)* finish position.

you get close to the top of the movement, making sure you maintain your bracing and the weight is vertical over the shoulders and hips. Lower the weight back to your shoulders, ensuring you keep the chest up and core braced the entire time you're performing the exercise.

BARBELL OVERHEAD PRESS

As with the barbell bench press, for the barbell overhead press (figure 4.12) the hand positioning is locked and not easily adjustable, so there must be sufficient wrist and elbow mobility to accommodate the rotation needed. The technique for the barbell overhead press is the same as with the dumbbell overhead press; however, as you press into the lockout position, the elbows have to rotate back and point out to the sides to accommodate the hand positioning on the bar. The core bracing, thoracic extension, and scapular upward rotation driver are all the same, so it becomes a matter of personal preference, as well as whether you want maximal loading versus challenged stability. For max loading, a barbell is a better option; for challenged stability, choose the dumbbells.

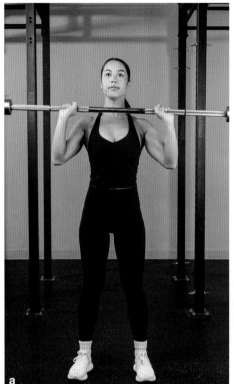 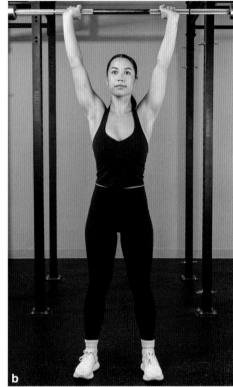

Figure 4.12 Barbell overhead press: *(a)* start position; *(b)* finish position.

NEAR OVERHEAD PRESSES

Sometimes the mobility to do a true overhead press just isn't there, but you can get some of the benefits of an overhead press by doing variations that go up above the shoulders but maybe don't go truly vertical over the shoulders and hips. These near-overhead presses allow users to get the most out of the mobility they do have and permits them to train toward an overhead press without pushing into a range of motion that might hurt their shoulders or their ability to maintain the desired alignment.

One option is to do an angled barbell press (figure 4.13) also commonly known as a landmine press. With one end of the barbell on the floor and the other in your hand, you can complete a pressing motion that's above shoulder height but not quite overhead. You can increase the angle of the press by moving from standing to half kneeling, and even include a forward lean at the top of the movement to coax more overhead range out of the press as available.

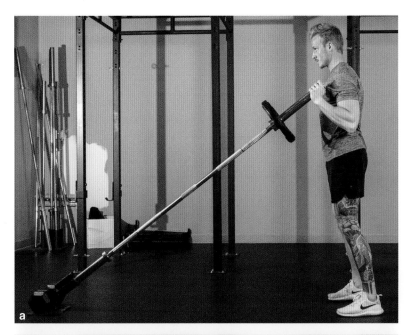

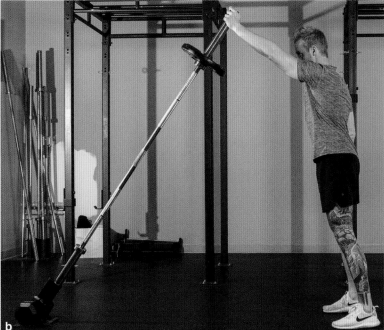

Figure 4.13 Angled barbell press: *(a)* start position; *(b)* finish position.

Another option is to do a Viking press (figure 4.14) in a squat rack. Remember *Rocky IV*? Training in a Russian barn, Rocky did a near overhead press using a cart with several people sitting in it. He pressed the handles up at an angle in front of his vertical overhead orientation, much to the amazement of the people in the cart. You can do the same in the gym without a cart but still amaze the people in the gym.

With the squat rack safeties set to about chest high or slightly lower, load one side and stand on that side to press. Ensure you have the barbell pulled far enough toward the pressing side so that you can put a plate on the anchored side to prevent it from sliding as you press. As you press the barbell up, the bar path will angle out in front of you, and the plate on the opposing side will press into the safety to prevent the bar from sliding out of the rack.

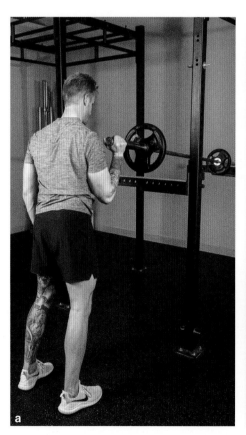 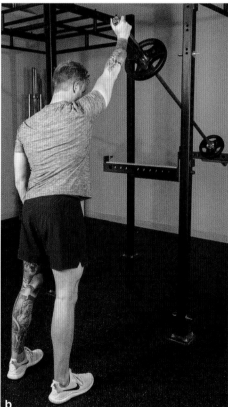

Figure 4.14 Viking press: *(a)* start position; *(b)* finish position.

A third option for the near overhead press is to use a high incline on a bench. This is known as a high-angled press (figure 4.15). Any angle between 45 degrees and 90 degrees works. You can use dumbbells, a barbell, or kettlebells for these, but again, go for the largest range of motion you can control through the vertical position.

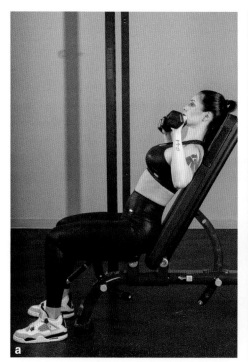 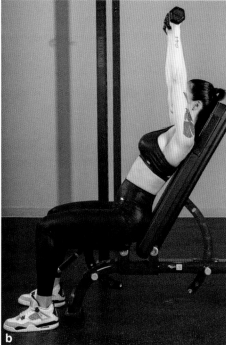

Figure 4.15 High-angled press: *(a)* start position; *(b)* finish position.

Troubleshooting Pressing Movements

Most common issues produced by pressing exercises come back to positioning and movement of the shoulder blades. Without enough scapular upward rotation, the rotator cuff has to work harder and thus gets pinched earlier in the range of motion than if the blade rotated more efficiently. With an anteriorly tilted shoulder blade that doesn't retract enough during horizontal press work, the front of the joint capsule, biceps tendon, and a few other structures get increased friction and loading, which can cause some discomfort. Without enough thoracic extension, your shoulder blades will have trouble rotating up and retracting back and down.

Let's say your shoulders are hating the idea of doing a vertical press. You could always adjust a few things, such as grip, equipment, angle, and volume, to make the movement easier:

- Switch from a barbell to dumbbells or kettlebells for a while.
- Make your grip width either narrower or wider on the barbell.
- Switch from a true vertical press to a near vertical press with the use of an angled barbell or Viking press that puts the weight in front of you and not over you.
- Complete fewer reps per set and increase the number of sets to reduce the potential of fatigue-related technical faults while maintaining volume.
- Spend more time getting shoulder blade motion down with some of the accessory exercises.

With horizontal presses, you could adjust the range of motion, type of pressing exercise, load and volume, or equipment, or add accessory exercises to train scapular and thoracic mobility:

- Switch from barbell to dumbbells or kettlebells.
- Change from a barbell to a football or Swiss bar with different grip positions, or another specialty bar, depending on what's available to you.
- Switch from bench-supported presses to unsupported presses and adjust range of motion (reduce the bottom position), hand positioning, and elbow angle.
- Reduce the number of reps per set and increase the number of sets to maintain volume but reduce fatigue-related changes in positioning.
- Spend more time working on accessory exercises to retrain shoulder blade positioning and movement and encourage thoracic spine mobility.

If any exercise creates pain or discomfort for any extended period of time, and if you feel that pain or discomfort even when you're not training, see a medical professional to get some further guidance on what's going on and how to proceed. It might mean you have to adjust your technique under the eye of someone who knows what they're doing, skip certain exercises altogether, or get some treatment to help the area recover more effectively.

Horizontal and Vertical Pulling

For pulling exercises, the same rules apply in terms of thoracic movement, scapular movement, and shoulder positioning. A horizontal row should involve the shoulder blades moving from a forward, protracted position to a retracted position where the shoulder blades almost touch or get as close as possible. For a vertical pull, the shoulder blades start in an upward rotated position and rotate down and in toward the midline of the body. Performing a row while concentrating on shoulder blade movement can help increase activity of the working back muscles and reduce the workload for the biceps or muscles that attach at the elbow, therefore reducing potential muscle strains and helping you to continue training hard without discomfort and with visible benefits.

With both horizontal and vertical pulling movements, the end position requires some thoracic extension, which is a hard position for many people to get to effectively, let alone with additional load. This is because the loading reduces the ability to access that thoracic extension. Starting off lighter than you think necessary and focusing on getting the movement of all segments down pat will produce better results than just crushing max weight by any means necessary.

A good rule of thumb with any pulling exercise is to use as much weight as possible while still successfully doing the full rep range of motion and feeling your target muscles squeeze at the peak contraction. If you can't feel your lats at the peak contraction of a row and instead feel your upper traps or elbows, you're not getting the shoulder blades to move to the right position and aren't getting the benefits from the exercise that you're trying to get. Reduce the weight and work on getting the movement from the shoulder blades and thoracic spine.

Horizontal Pulling Technique

Most horizontal row movements involve the same technique, regardless of whether you use a cable, band, dumbbell, or barbell. The only real difference is the direction of loading relative to gravity and your positioning relative to that loading to make the movement a horizontal row. For instance, using a cable or band at chest height requires a vertical torso orientation, whereas using a free weight requires a more horizontal torso orientation. The techniques are the same as the direction of movement relative to loading is the same, and the goal of the exercise in terms of muscles being used is the same.

We'll use a seated row as an initial example, knowing the same applies for a standing row, single-arm row, band row, and so forth.

SEATED ROW

For the seated row (figure 4.16), start with your torso vertical—avoid leaning back—and with a slight extension from the thoracic spine. Let the weight pull the shoulder blades forward to stretch the lats and rhomboids, making sure you allow slight thoracic flexion without any lower-back flexion. To start the row, extend the thoracic spine and retract the shoulder blades. Think of getting them to pinch in toward the spine and down to the bottom of your ribs. The combined movement of the shoulder blades and thoracic spine activates the targeted muscles. The hands pull the weight toward the ribs and beneath the pecs but above the belly button. The goal of the hands is simply to hold onto the weight, not direct where it goes. The movement of the shoulder blades and thoracic spine will dictate the end position of the weight. If max squeeze from the shoulder blades makes the hands wind up slightly in front of the ribs, don't try to use the hands or wrists to force the contact to the ribs, as this can alter the shoulder blade positioning and cause the shoulder joints to glide forward more than ideal to get that extra range of motion.

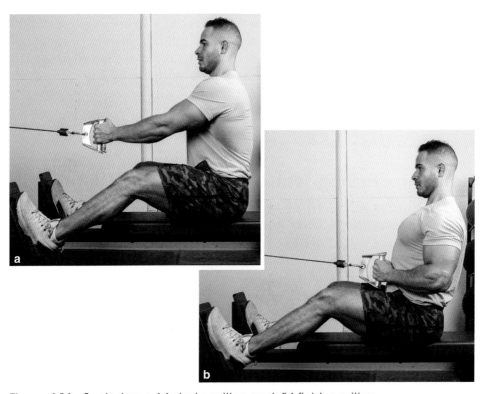

Figure 4.16 Seated row: *(a)* start position and *(b)* finish position.

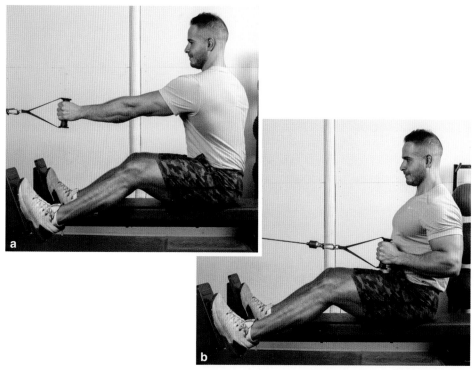

Figure 4.17 Single-arm cable row: *(a)* start position and *(b)* finish position.

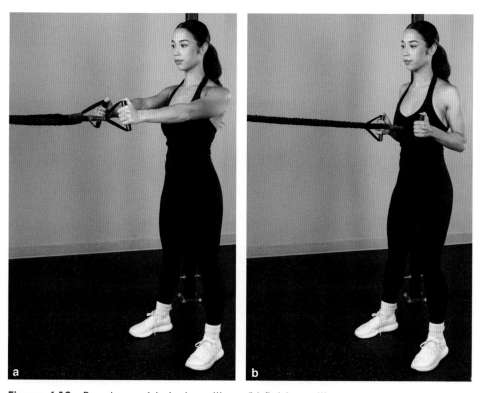

Figure 4.18 Band row: *(a)* start position; *(b)* finish position.

For a free-weight version, let's look at both a dumbbell row and a barbell row.

DUMBBELL ROW

For the dumbbell row (figure 4.19), use a bench or other supportive surface that your free hand can hold onto. Place your hand and the same side knee on the bench. Hold the dumbbell in the other hand and place the foot on that side on the ground and behind the hip. This foot positioning allows you to move the weight with less risk of bumping it into your leg during the reps.

Start with an extended spine, and chest up and out. Ideally, whenever you think you're extended enough, keep extending until it feels kind of comical how arched your back is and then you're probably pretty close. Imagine doing a cat-camel stretch, where you first round your back up to the ceiling and then arch to lower your back toward the floor as far as you can for the dumbbell row, you want to lower the back as far as possible, and then do the row from that position. With the weight vertical under your shoulder, let the shoulder blade slide forward toward the floor to stretch the lat and rhomboids. Avoid twisting the torso to get that reach.

When lifting the weight in the row, focus on pulling the shoulder blade back and down across the back toward the opposite pocket. Think of squeezing your armpit at the top of the movement without twisting or rotating the torso to get to that peak contraction. You should feel the muscle contract from your armpit all the way down to your hips.

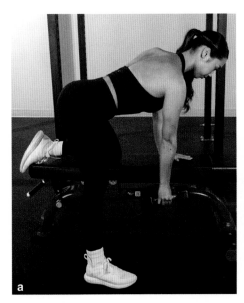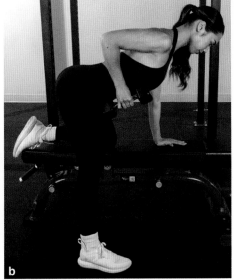

Figure 4.19 Dumbbell row: *(a)* start position; *(b)* finish position.

Try to keep your shoulders and hips square to the floor. Don't let the moving side lift higher than the stable side. Brace the abs to keep the spine movement controlled and stable. Similar to the cable row, the hand will wind up near the ribs, between the pecs and belly button, but don't force the hand to contact the ribs if it's not being moved by the shoulder blade. At the peak contraction, your shoulder should be retracted and tilted back on the ribs. If you look at your shoulder, the pec and collarbone should look stretched, not rolled forward.

A benefit of doing a single-arm dumbbell row on a bench is the ability to have three points of contact to provide stability to the exercise. Moving one arm at a time allows you to think about the movement of the shoulder and associated muscles more easily than if you were doing both at the same time.

BARBELL BENT-OVER ROW

A more challenging version of the free-weight row is the barbell bent-over row (figure 4.20). With only two points of contact to provide a foundation and no support for the upper body, you have to work harder just to set up and maintain posture during the exercise. Also, moving both arms at the same time makes it tricky to feel both sides working correctly. That being said, it's easier to add loading to this movement than to a dumbbell row, so if the goal is more weight and more challenge, this version will do the job.

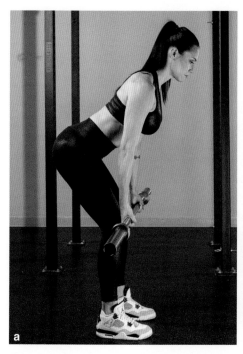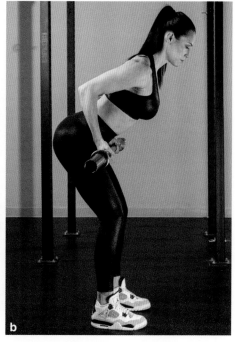

Figure 4.20 Barbell bent-over row: *(a)* start position; *(b)* finish position.

Start with the bar in a rack at about waist height. Grab the bar with hands slightly more than hip width in either a double overhand or double underhand grip. A double overhand grip makes it easier to hold on to the barbell, but for someone with limited wrist or elbow pronation, it might be harder to keep the elbows from flaring out. With a double underhand grip, it will be easier to get the elbows in tight and feel the shoulder blades move, but some people might find it harder to hold onto the barbell.

Once you are holding the bar, step away from the supports and hinge from the hips as in a deadlift, stopping when the bar gets to just below the kneecaps. Similar to the dumbbell row, ensure your spine is extended more than you think is necessary and then lock into this position for the entirety of the exercise. Think of a slightly extended spine position (though not as severe as the row described earlier) and then lock in place with the core bracing hard to prevent further movement from the spine. You will have a forward torso angle, but not quite parallel to the floor. From this position, let the shoulder blades stretch forward and reach the hands toward the floor without rounding the back. Retract the shoulders to pull the weight in toward the body at roughly the belly button. Squeeze the shoulder blades toward the spine and tilted down against the ribs, trying to avoid shrugging the shoulders up toward the ears. If the goal is to work your upper traps more, the shrug toward the ears is fine, but if the goal is to work the lats, it's the opposite of what you should be doing.

Vertical Pulling Technique

Vertical pulling movements are vertical pushing movements in reverse. The goal is to include scapular upward rotation at the top of the movement and downward rotation and a tight squeeze at the bottom position, whereas the horizontal row involves much more shoulder blade forward and back movement (protraction and retraction).

Vertical pull hand position tends to be easiest to perform and limits possible shoulder irritation when in a neutral position (palms facing each other), compared to a double overhand or double underhand grip. Double overhand is easy to hold but it can be more challenging to get the shoulder blades to fully move down (depress) at the peak contraction. With a double underhand grip, it's easier to get the shoulder blades to retract and depress properly at peak contraction but it's harder to hold at the full hang bottom position. Neutral hand position seems to be the Goldilocks grip for vertical pulls—not too much, not too little.

Regardless of the type of grip you use, the technique for a vertical pull remains fairly similar. Let's review a lat pulldown as well as a pull-up.

LAT PULLDOWN

For the lat pulldown (figure 4.21), set up with your preferred grip, letting the weight pull the shoulders up as far as they can comfortably go. As you initiate the pull, brace the abs and tense all your fingers on the handle, arch the thoracic spine slightly to lean back, and push your chest up and out. Think of pulling your shoulder blades down into the opposing pockets, squeezing the lat muscles right down to your hips. At the peak contraction, the shoulders should be behind the pecs and the shoulder blades tilted down. Think of pulling the handle into the collarbones, not lower to the chest. A lower pull will make it harder to keep the shoulder blades tilted back and down and will likely lead to the shoulders rolling forward to complete the range of motion.

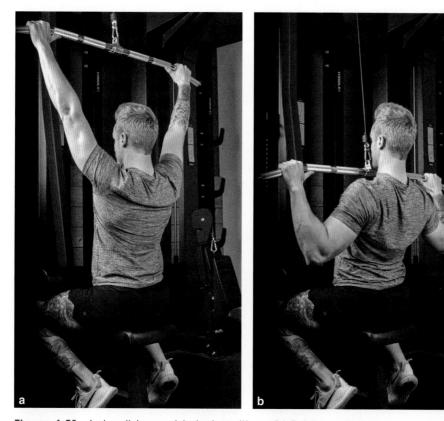

Figure 4.21 Lat pulldown: *(a)* start position; *(b)* finish position.

PULL-UP

For the pull-up (figure 4.22), using your preferred grip, grab the handle or bar, making sure you have a strong connection through all your fingers. Focus on generating maximal tension through the entire body, allowing the summation of force through the legs, hips, and core to assist in the force generation of the upper body. As you get set to initiate the first rep from the hang position, take a big breath and fill the lungs, then brace the core to squeeze that breath and generate as much pressure as possible, similar to when doing a squat or deadlift. When you initiate the pull, think of pulling the shoulder blades down and into the opposite pocket, lifting the chest to the handles. As you get to the top of the movement, continue lifting the chest and squeezing the shoulder blades while staying in constant tension. You can exhale at the top as long as you don't lose your bracing. Lower to the start position, with control coming from the shoulder blades sliding up and forward to their starting position in the full hang again. Throughout the movement, keep the knees straight and toes pulled up, with a strong emphasis on getting both glutes and your core to brace hard to add a layer of total body tension to the movement.

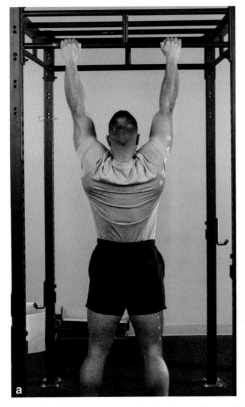 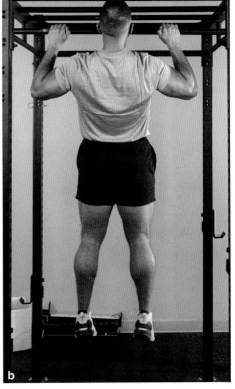

Figure 4.22 Pull-up: *(a)* start position; *(b)* finish position.

Because the pull-up starts with the expectation of being able to lift full body weight, this might be a more advanced version for some individuals. A lat pulldown allows for less than full body weight to train the movement, but you may also use some different options, such as a band assisted pull-up, to assist in completing the reps you're after. If you can bench press your body weight, you should absolutely be able to perform a few pull-ups as well.

Troubleshooting Pulling Movements

Poor row technique tends to fall into one of the following categories:

- Not enough thoracic spine extension
- Not enough shoulder blade retraction
- Forward rolled shoulder blade
- Too much wrist or elbow involvement
- Too much loading

For thoracic spine extension, rounding the upper back makes it considerably more difficult for the shoulder blade to retract and depress and get the lats to work effectively, and tends to crank up the upper trap instead. Think of proudly pushing the chest out and showing off the logo on the front of your shirt. You're a superhero striking a triumphant pose! If you're doing a dumbbell row, point your chest to the wall. If you're doing a vertical pulldown, like with a lat pulldown or chin up, angle the chest up toward the ceiling without leaning back.

A good cue I use with my clients is "Think chest up, not lean back." If you lean back, you might just wind up leaning back, not extending your thoracic spine. Lifting your chest up forces some degree of extension.

Getting enough shoulder blade retraction comes from gaining enough thoracic spine extension to allow that retraction to occur in the first place. Once you have the extension piece of the puzzle in play, you can focus on getting a tighter squeeze from the shoulder blades at the peak contraction. One of the most effective cues I've found is to simply tell people to squeeze their shoulders as hard as possible, then squeeze harder. Many people feel that they're doing their best, until you challenge them and then all of the sudden they find a little more movement from the shoulder blades.

When you get that extra squeeze, make sure you're trying to contract the muscles to pull the lower portions, not the upper portions, of the shoulder blades toward each other. If you shrug up, you're getting more upper traps involved and not letting the lats do their thing.

If your shoulders roll forward when you're trying to get the max shoulder blade squeeze, it's going to come down to a combination of subpar thoracic spine extension and not enough squeeze from the lower portions of the shoulder blades, or from trying to use a larger range of motion than the shoulder blades can achieve (bringing the hands too far into the body). What happens is that the shoulder blade tilts forward on the ribs versus sitting back and down flat against the ribs, which pushes the front of the shoulder forward. This is one of the most common technical flaws I see in rows of any kind. It usually doesn't hurt or feel off, and in the grand scheme of things it's a nuance, but it can make a big enough difference in your results that you have to address it properly.

Getting more posterior tilt from the shoulder blade typically means using less weight and focusing on the squeeze from the shoulder blades rather than on producing a larger range of motion in terms of where the hands wind up. You might also need a slightly wider hand position, with the caveat of keeping the elbows closer to the body. Using a mirror or even videoing yourself doing the exercise can provide valuable feedback about your position. It's tough to know what's going on back there without some form of feedback.

Wrist and elbow involvement typically comes in the form of forcing a range of motion that's not driven by the shoulder blades. Think of curling the hands or wrists to pull the handles closer to the body. If an individual feels their elbows on row movements more than they feel their back muscles, they're likely using the forearms and biceps to do most of the work versus using the shoulder blades and bigger back muscles to drive the pulls. The recipe for fixing this is again to focus on thoracic spine extension and shoulder blade movement. Imagine squeezing hard through the back muscles. Try to use only the range of motion you can get from that shoulder blade squeeze and concentrate on holding the handle with all your fingers engaged.

Loading can be tricky, since you might feel you can get through the reps without any discomfort or negative issues. But if the loading is too much and you aren't getting the right positioning and technique down, the muscles you're trying to work aren't feeling tired or may not feel like they're actually doing anything. Whether you're lifting 1 pound or adding plates to your body-weight exercises, you should be able to feel the target muscles contracting, regardless of the exercise. It can be tricky to get into the right positions to feel muscles like the lats or rhomboids contract, but it's important enough to spend time trying to find those suckers. If you feel your elbows, neck, the front of your shoulders, or other body parts working hard at the end of a set and don't feel anything in those target muscles, you're doing it wrong, and you need to step back the loading to find those muscles before adding any more weight.

As we said in the squat and deadlift section, a lot of the solutions to common problems come back to focusing on doing the exercise correctly, which means not focusing on just crushing max weight at all costs but sometimes stepping back, using less load, and working on the finite details of the movement. We'll go through some fixes for people who might have

PRESS TO PULL RATIO

There's a ton of content on the internet from excellent coaches talking about how many pull movements you should do relative to the number of push movements, and a general consensus is to do 2 pulls for every push movement to maintain shoulder health or reduce the likelihood of injuries as you train. However, there is no evidence to support this, nor is there any preferred ratio of pull to push exercises. This ratio is based on a few assumptions:

- Pressing hypertrophies and therefore tenses the anterior shoulder tissues, which causes them to roll forward. This posture can lead to a greater incidence of shoulder dysfunctions.[8]
- Pulling movements activate posterior shoulder and thoracic muscles that can adjust this scapular positioning, reducing the postural dysfunctions associated with an anterior roll.
- A relationship should exist between antagonistic muscle groups (hamstring and quad strength), meaning pull strength and press strength should be relatively close.[9]

Although it makes sense to maintain strength balance around associated joints, there isn't any specific evidence saying training more or less with push or pull will consistently maintain this balance or that it doesn't come without other issues such as elbow or biceps discomfort. The best way to maintain strong and resilient joints is to focus on effective technique, recovery, and variety of movements through all available ranges of motion within the training program versus max loading on a few movements all the time. A lot of muscles and directions of movement are available within the shoulder complex, so using a lot of options to train them all will in the long term give you better results than distilling your training down to only a few options done repeatedly.

What does tend to pop up more consistently is the idea that shoulder discomfort can be made more problematic with pressing movements versus pulling movements, so reducing the volume of press work and increasing the pull work tends to help in a short term to work around cranky shoulders. There isn't a ton of research to back this up, but it seems to be effective in a practical setting. I've worked with clients whom it has helped..

If you have uncomfortable shoulders, it would be worthwhile to adjust pressing work, range of motion, loading, or volume in a workout to find ways to train around or through discomfort, at least for a short cycle of training until your shoulders are feeling better, or work with someone for a second set of eyes on the problem. During this phase it might very well be worth using a 1:2 ratio of press to pull exercises, or even a 1:3 ratio for some people. Work on positioning and technique, adjust range of motion to what feels comfortable, and change the loading to find what will allow you to get your swole on without actual swelling.

lower thoracic spine mobility or shoulder blade control, and use those tools to help assist the development of these key movements in chapter 7.

Conclusion

Building a strong upper body and strong lower body are fantastic accomplishments, but we can't forget about the middle. In the next chapter, we'll work on some core training movements and exercises that help fill in the gaps that all the bracing and tension drills we've used in the previous sections may not get to sufficiently, and help you build a strong resilient body from top to bottom.

5

Core
Movements

Core training is sort of like cilantro: Some people absolutely love it and add it to everything, and others think it tastes like soap and do anything they can to avoid it. While core training may not taste like soap to them, it might as well. They figure they'll get their core strong with the Big Three of squat, bench, and deadlift and that's all they need.

Sure, most core training exercises may not be as exciting as moving a massive weight from point A to point B and back again, but there's something kinda cool about being able to walk for more than 5 minutes without your lower back cramping up. Being able to do stuff you want to do outside of the gym, like maybe turning, or bending down to tie your shoes, could be made easier with a few direct core exercises. Additionally, core exercises tend to have a direct impact on your ability to do the big exercises you're looking to hit up, so that should be enough reason to make them a part of your programming.

Direct core training can have a positive impact on performance in the gym, as well as performance in sport activities outside the gym.[1,2] The primary connection between core training and athletic or strength performance seems to be that core training increases the force production capability of the core muscles, improving their ability to increase force production in the working muscles of the extremities.[3,4] Essentially, a stronger core helps you to express strength from the rest of the body more effectively, so for this reason alone, you need to be doing some direct core work.

One fun benefit of doing core work is that it can actually be a useful tool to help reduce lower-back pain.[5] On top of this, regular lower-back and core strengthening can reduce the probability of future lower-back pain.[6]

In case you're not convinced yet, one more reason why working the core is great is that it helps your core resist motion during exercise. Your spine is constantly being bombarded with a combination of different forces when weight training (all good stuff, don't worry). The job of the muscles around the spine is both to promote motion and to stabilize all the structures within the spine. Adding core work to your routine will beef up your spine's ability to handle these stresses and stay healthier in the long haul.

Core training is more than just crunches and planks. The main functions of the core are to allow spinal movement into flexion, extension, lateral flexion, rotation, and any combination of these movements, but core muscles assist in breathing, development of intra-abdominal pressure, and accelerating force application from the lower body to the upper body and vice versa. Because the core has so many primary functions and operates on a continuum of force and velocity, you can't really train the core effectively with only a couple of exercises. You can use isometrics, concentric-eccentric activities, accelerative movements, and throws, and apply loading in various directions and with different implements.

As with most types of exercise, the details of how and why you're using specific methods of core training matter in terms of end result. If you want to be fast and explosive, doing lots of loaded carries and plank variations might not be the answer for you, but if you want to build a trunk of absolute steel, you'd be hard pressed to find better options. Using more throws or other rapid acceleration movements is great for building speed but might not be a good starting point for most people, especially if they have issues with lower motor control or a history of lower-back injuries. These exercises can still be worked in judiciously, but again, the devil is in the details of how, why, and where. Let's learn about some of those elements next.

Loaded Carries

One type of core training exercise that doesn't get the love it deserves is the loaded carry. This is a drill where you grab a weight and simply go for a short walk, trying to keep your spine stable and maintain the alignment of the ribs over the pelvis as you walk from one point to another. It sounds simple enough, and in terms of user experience it's not a very complex type of drill to execute. But in terms of challenge, it can be used therapeutically with post-surgical clients all the way up to max loading for competitive strongmen and strongwomen. The exercise can also be varied simply by where you have the loading, whether it's in one hand by your side, as in a suitcase carry, both hands by your side, as in a farmer carry; hands at your shoulders, as in a rack carry; or overhead, as in a waiter walk. You can use unstable loads, as in a slosh pipe carry or a keg carry, or use specific implements such as farmer walk handles or a super yoke, but the exercise simply comprises grabbing a weight and walking with it over a set distance.

The main challenge with loaded carries is the ability to maintain tension through the spine while shifting your balance from one foot to the other and back again, breathing, and not dropping the weight all at the same time. As the loading increases, the ability to maintain a brace and breathe becomes more challenging, and it becomes necessary to use more forceful breaths on both the inhale and the exhale to maintain that tension effectively.

A key feature for more loaded carries is grip strength and positioning of the weight in your hand to maximize your grip endurance. If it's a dumbbell, kettlebell, or similar implement with a handle, grab it so the handle is deeper in your hand than usual, and try to ensure that you have all your fingers actively engaged in holding the handle. Start with the pinkie finger and wrap it as far around the handle as possible, then work toward the index finger and thumb. Many people grab the handle to sit closer to the fingers than inside the palm, which is a more comfortable position but doesn't allow the same contact and friction to hold the handle. Additionally, many will focus on gripping predominantly with the index and middle fingers together with the thumb, limiting the involvement of the ring and pinkie fingers, which reduces possible strength and endurance for your grip. Five fingers work better than three, so make sure all digits show up.

Once you have a strong position and all your fingers are gripping the handle, actively engage the muscles of the shoulder and core to drive further neural flow to the hands and to increase grip strength and endurance. For any implement being held at your sides, think of crushing your armpits, trying to get your pecs and lats to tense and suck the upper arm into the socket as tight as possible, and then flex your abs all around as if you're about to go head to head with a heavyweight boxing champion who has a penchant for body blows. While tensing all these levels and regions, take measured steps that allow you to control the bracing and tension but move you forward. Try to breathe in short, hard inhales and exhales so you don't lose any of the tension you worked so hard to develop.

If the weight is in the rack position at your shoulder or overhead, you can still work on tension development, but it's going to be different since you won't be able to think of pulling the shoulders in and down as easily. Still, visualize getting all the muscles around the shoulder involved in the process, and work on ensuring you have total control over where the loading is and where you want it to go. No shaking, wobbling, or dumping the weight before the set is done.

Those new to loaded carries often have some basic questions. First, how far should I carry the load? This is a fair question, and one that doesn't have an easy answer. The best answer is "as far as possible," although that doesn't really help. I have people carry a load across the length of the gym.

In smaller spaces, they do a couple of laps depending on the size of the space. In the great outdoors, where they have literally no limit, we outline a distance based on landmarks, time, or goal-specific requirements. It might be "make it to that tree" or "complete as many laps in 60 seconds as you can," or "as a firefighter, you have to carry a charged hose over 300 feet, so let's set up that distance minimum and work on building endurance to surpass it." The key is to use your environment. Work on either carrying a load over a greater distance or a larger load over the same distance as you progressively overload the exercise based on your adaptation to it.

Second, how much weight should I use? This is also a fair question that doesn't have an easy answer. The best general answer is "as much as you can control" in the given position. This might be only 2 pounds (1 kg) for someone who is new to lifting to a 300 pounds (136 kg) per arm for someone who is looking to compete in strength sports, and everything in between. As with other exercises, decide on loading based on your competence to perform the exercise correctly for the duration required (given distance and time under tension).

Third, should I walk only over a flat surface when carrying the load? Not necessarily. Hills, whether you go up or down, are a different challenge. It can be a significant progression to go from a flat surface to a graded surface, so maybe start on a flat area and then once you're feeling spicy you can progress to something with a bit more of an angle to it.

Fourth, what if I keep dropping the weight? If this keeps happening, you likely have a stronger core than your grip or a weaker grip than needed for the implement or load being used. The benefit of training is that your grip will improve gradually as you consistently work it. The downside is that knowledge doesn't help you much in the moment if the weight doesn't want to stay in your hands. In a pinch, you can use straps to assist with grip, but be aware that loading heavier than your grip allows will put more strain on your spine and hips, which may be exactly what you're going for, but will bypass a specific limiting factor that would prevent you from overloading those regions until the grip strength improves.

If you notice any area of the body hurting or feeling more discomfort than ideal, reduce the loading and work on finding a way to brace that reduces the discomfort, or adjust where the loading is being held. Sometimes moving from a very heavy farmer carry to a lighter rack carry can present similar or greater challenges to stability but reduce the shear forces acting on the spine and thus reduce the discomfort you feel during the exercise. If you find your hands, elbows, or shoulders hurt during the loaded carries, adjust your grip positioning, change the implement being used or where you're holding the implement (to the sides, in front, slightly away from the body), and find an option that works more effectively for you.

Read on for some examples.

FARMER'S CARRY

The farmer's carry (figure 5.1) involves using two implements of roughly the same weight held at the sides, one in each hand. The balanced loading produces compressive loading and relatively balanced muscle activation on both sides of the spine.[7] This allows for a greater overall stabilization stimulus, and if the goal is producing stiffness through the spine muscles, this is a great exercise to incorporate.

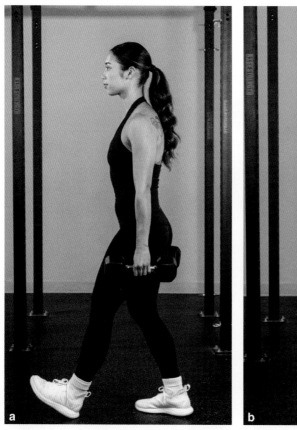 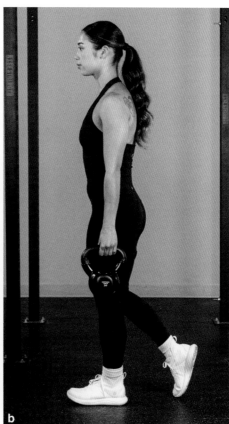

Figure 5.1 Farmer's carry with *(a)* dumbbells and *(b)* kettlebells.

SUITCASE CARRY

Similar to the farmer's carry, the suitcase carry (figure 5.2) involves using a load on only one side of the body. The unilateral loading produces greater lateral spine muscle activity as your body tries to balance out the unbalanced loading.[8] The unbalanced loading also requires more effort from the hips, especially on the side opposite the loading, to help maintain upright body positioning.[9] Because of the unbalanced loading, a suitcase carry can be significantly more challenging than a farmer's carry at the same single-arm load.

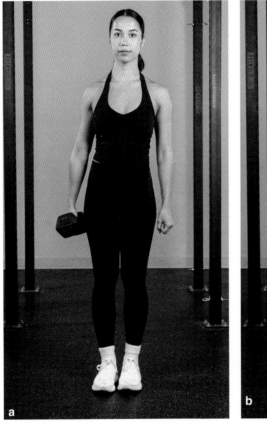
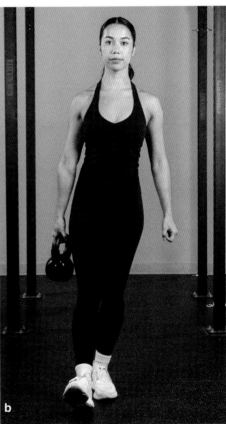

Figure 5.2 Suitcase carry with a *(a)* dumbbell and *(b)* kettlebell.

RACK CARRY

A rack carry (figure 5.3) involves holding the object, either a dumbbell or preferably a kettlebell, at the shoulder versus down to the side. You can do a rack carry on one side or both sides. The higher the load is relative to the floor, the harder it is to control and the greater the core stabilization requirements.

To hold the kettlebell, think of putting your thumb just below the collarbone, and keep the elbow in tight to the body (figure 5.4). The weight should slide to the front of your shoulder, resting in the angle between the upper arm and forearm. The shoulder muscles should be tensed, holding strong to keep the kettlebell centered and steady on the arm.

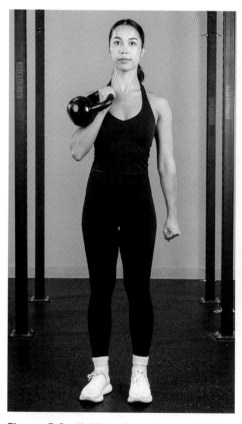

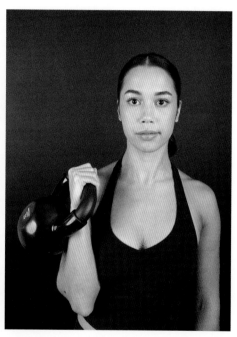

Figure 5.4 Position of the kettlebell at the shoulder during the rack carry.

Figure 5.3 Kettlebell rack carry.

For a dumbbell rack carry (figure 5.5), you should hold the weight with a part of the plates resting on the shoulder. Keep the elbow vertical under the hands and tense the muscles around the shoulders to maintain stability. Avoid draping the dumbbell over the shoulder and then just hanging on with your hand. Make sure your hand is supporting the weight.

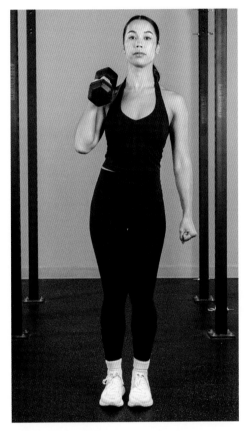

Figure 5.5   Dumbbell rack carry.

COACHING CUES FOR CARRIES

When doing any loaded carry exercise, make sure you get the most from the movement by maintaining a 360-degree brace throughout the exercise and breathing without letting that brace relax. You want to challenge your core endurance to maintain that brace but still find a way to breathe throughout the set. Think about bracing any time you're holding the weight. You should feel like you're maintaining your spine position and relative control without letting the weight affect that positioning or relaxing that brace until you're done with the set.

Rotational Training

While loaded carries are a fantastic way to train your core muscles to maintain stabilization around the spine, the core involves more than just stiffness. The core muscles exert a massive influence in producing movement of the ribs over the pelvis and vice versa, and an often overlooked training technique that directly affects this is rotational training. Rotation is often used in athletic events that involve throwing, running, kicking, skating, or hitting. The movements may involve rotation of the spine as driven by the core muscles, or it may involve a transfer of force from the upper to lower body or vice versa, with the core muscles tensing to provide a strong force transducer to ensure that power achieves the desired outcome.[10]

Much of this force transmission depends on the amount of load being moved or the velocity of the movements. Because spine rotation is a fairly small range of motion with relatively small moving muscles, exercises that involve spine rotation tend to be low in force production and move at slower speeds, whereas exercises that require more force and speed will be powered by the upper or lower limbs, with the core muscles working as stabilizers.

Rotational Training Exercises

We'll start off with the rotation movement exercises, and then move on to the ones that produce higher force and power.

BIRD DOG

Starting on hands and knees, reach the right arm and left leg out toward the far walls (figure 5.6). Think of pressing the heel and fist out as far as possible, bracing the abs so you aren't arching from the lower back or trying to raise the arm or leg higher. Then return the arm and leg under your body, trying to touch the hand to the knee, working to maintain balance and not fall over. Repeat the movement on the same side, then repeat on the other side.

The goal of this exercise is to control rotation while extending the opposing arm and leg. If you're not able to balance against this rotational challenge, you'll fall to either your extended hand or foot when performing the movement.

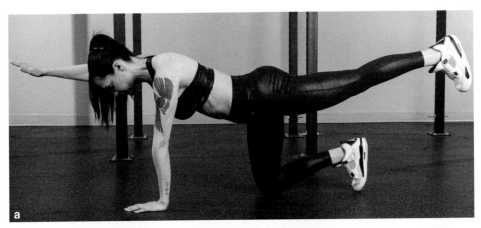

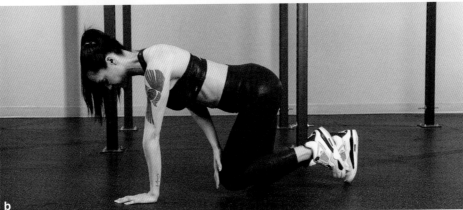

Figure 5.6 Bird dog: *(a)* start position and *(b)* finish position.

DEAD BUG SQUEEZE

Lying on your back with your hands vertical over your shoulders and knees bent and vertical over your hips, bring your left hand or elbow to your right knee and squeeze the two together as hard as possible (figure 5.7). This will take some rotation from the ribs and pelvis to bring the two together. Hold for a full inhale–exhale cycle, then try to maintain the core contraction and extend the right arm and left leg out away from the body as far as possible. Return to the starting position and repeat for the desired number of reps, then repeat on the opposite side. If you can't squeeze your elbow and knee together, you can regress the movement by pushing your hand and knee together.

   The goal here is to create maximal contraction from the core muscles while squeezing the elbow and knee together to create that rotation movement in a relative end range position.

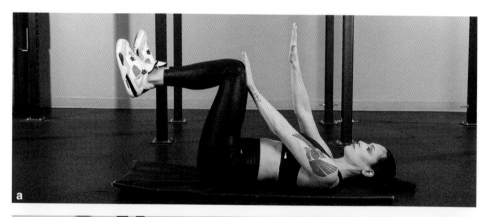

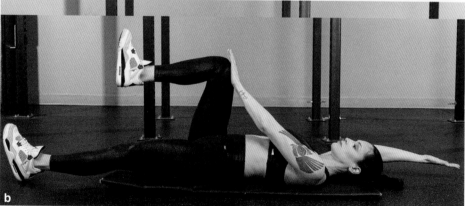

Figure 5.7   Dead bug squeeze: *(a)* left hand to right knee, and *(b)* extension.

PLANK ROTATION

Start in a plank position with your elbows and toes on the ground and the core braced hard. Pivot on the toes so that you raise one arm off the ground, turning your ribs and hips at the same time (figure 5.8). Turn roughly 90 degrees, or as far as you can maintain the locked ribs and pelvis, then return to the ground plank position. Make sure you're not shifting your ribs or pelvis first but keeping them moving together at the same time. Complete all of the reps on one side, then briefly reset and complete all the reps on the other side.

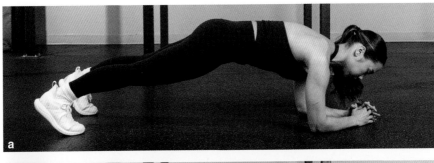

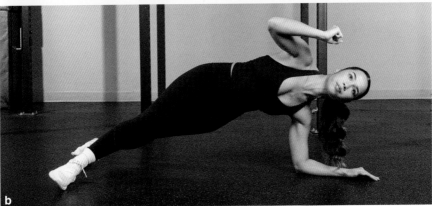

Figure 5.8 Plank rotation: *(a)* start position and *(b)* rotation.

If the exercise is too difficult to do from the floor, start with your elbows on a bench (figure 5.9) or other elevated surface instead. For a further regression, you could start with your elbows on a wall with a slight forward lean.

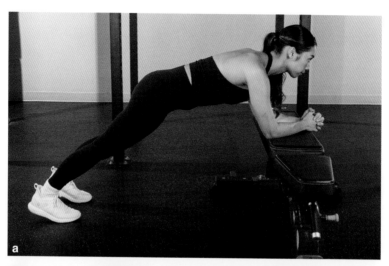

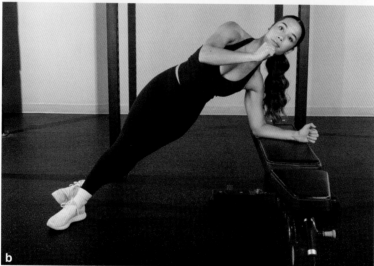

Figure 5.9 Bench plank rotation: *(a)* start position and *(b)* rotation.

Antirotational Training Exercises

The exercises so far teach control against intended rotation of the torso. While we're working on rotational exercises, we should also work on exercises that control against undesired rotation. Similar to how a deadlift trains extension of the hips but involves contraction of the spine muscles to resist against flexion, we can train the core muscles to resist rotation, building those muscles to create stiffness on demand.

PALLOF PRESS

Let's start with an anti-rotation exercise called the Pallof press. You begin the Pallof press by holding a cable at chest height, standing at a 90-degree angle relative to the direction of pull, bracing the core to hold the ribs and pelvis together, and pressing the cable out away from the body (figure 5.10). As you press the cable out, the lever arm of the resistance, which is trying to pull the torso and cause rotation, increases. This increases the force required to resist the rotation. For added points, raise your arms once the arms are fully extended; keep

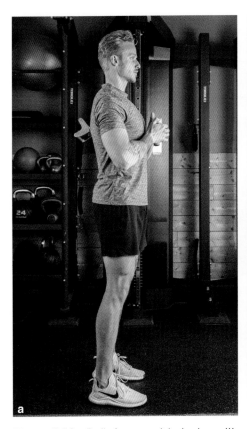
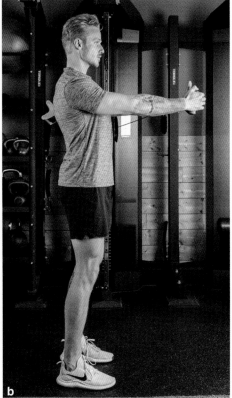

Figure 5.10 Pallof press: *(a)* start position and *(b)* press.

them straight and try to avoid torso rotation. Return the hands to the chest and repeat for the number of reps given, then do the same facing the other way with the cable pulling in the opposite direction.

You can do this drill with a variety of different stances, with feet shoulder width apart or wider than shoulder width, a split stance, a half-kneeling (figure 5.11) position with one knee down and one leg

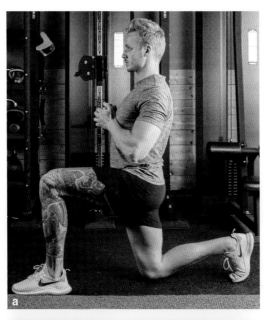

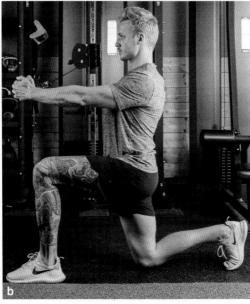

Figure 5.11 Half-kneeling Pallof press: *(a)* start position and *(b)* finish position.

forward, or a tall kneeling position on both knees (figure 5.12). The big difference in the various stances comes down to altered base of support and balance requirements. The narrower the stance or foot position, the harder it is to balance in the movement. Ideally, you should use a position that challenges you but allows you to maintain your balance and use the core to stabilize during the movement without flailing around.

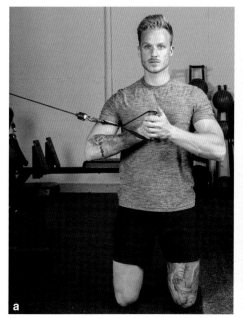 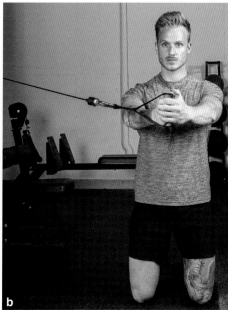

Figure 5.12 Tall kneeling Pallof press: *(a)* start position and *(b)* finish position.

MEDICINE BALL SEATED ROTATION

Sit on the ground holding a medicine ball. Lean back slightly to start the abs contracting. Focus on keeping a long, tall torso without rounding or flexing your spine. For additional difficulty, you can raise your feet off the ground. Start with the medicine ball held out in front of your chest. Turn to one side, trying to touch the ball to the floor beside your hips (figure 5.13). Return to the middle, then turn to the opposite side, trying to maintain that upright, straight torso position. Focus on maintaining a core contraction and trying to breathe thoroughly throughout the entire set. To heighten the challenge, increase the movement speed, hold the arms in a straighter position, or use a heavier ball.

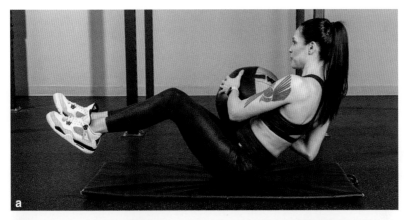

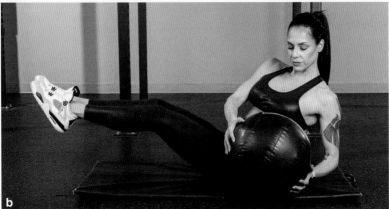

Figure 5.13 Medicine ball seated rotation: *(a)* start position and *(b)* finish position.

High-Force Production Rotational Exercises

There are many more rotational core training exercises that work on controlled force production into rotation as well as maintaining core position against rotational forces. Learning the basics of the exercises described in this chapter will allow you to get more from any other exercise that has a similar goal.

Now let's look at some higher force production rotational movements. For many of these movements, you will need to move a weight very quickly or move a larger weight as fast as possible. The very quick movements typically involve either throwing a ball for distance or against a wall. The heavier, fast movements involve moving as quickly as possible but not letting go of the weight, which means a greater emphasis on decelerating the weight compared to a throw or slam. With a throw or slam, you let go of the weight and don't have to slow it down, meaning all that momentum makes it sail away from you. If you hold on to the object, you have to fight against that momentum to slow it down.

Both types of exercises can be used effectively across a wide range of goals and abilities. The key is simply to scale the work to what you can manage effectively, and ramp up intensity gradually over successive workouts.

ANGLED BARBELL STRAIGHT-ARM ROTATION

Begin with one end of a barbell on the floor and against a wall, preferably either in a corner or landmine attachment or apparatus. Hold the other end of the barbell at roughly eye height with straight arms. With your weight on the balls of your feet, turn your hips and pivot on your toes to turn the barbell to your side (figure 5.14). Lower the end of the bar toward your thigh, trying to maintain a tall torso. Next drive through the feet and hips. Rotate the barbell away from your thigh and in an arc back to the start position at eye height, then over to the opposite thigh. Gradually increase the speed of the movement as much as possible with good core control and a vertical torso while controlling the weight.

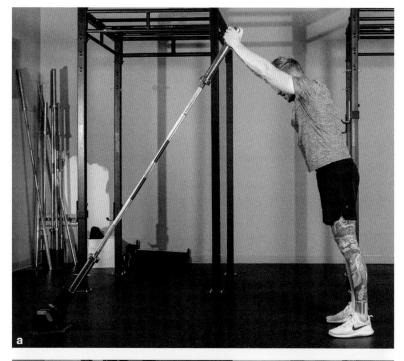

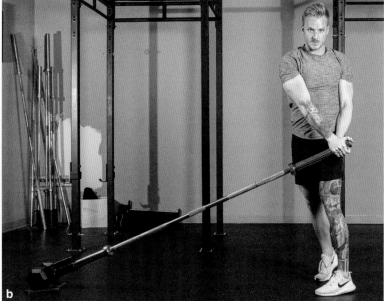

Figure 5.14 Angled barbell straight-arm rotation: *(a)* start position and *(b)* finish position.

CABLE LUNGE AND PRESS

This movement is similar to taking a step in to swing a baseball bat. The lower body drives movement into the core and through the upper body for the finishing extension. Start with a cable and handle set at roughly shoulder height. Hold the handle in the hand closest to the cable unit while standing at a 90-degree angle to the direction of cable pull. Step away from the cable unit with the outside leg. When your foot contacts the ground, pivot through the hips and feet to turn in line with the direction of cable pull, then extend the arm in a pressing movement along the same direction. As you extend the arm, bend your knees into a lunge position (figure 5.15). Return to standing, facing the same starting direction. Try to make one smooth, fluid movement. Complete reps on one side, then repeat on the other side.

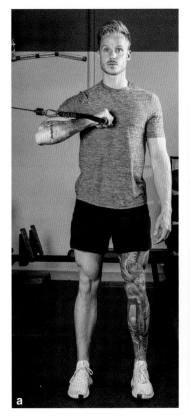
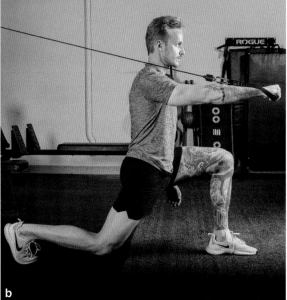

Figure 5.15 Cable lunge and press: *(a)* start position, *(b)* lunge and press.

CABLE SPLIT STANCE CHOP

Use a cable system with the attachment as high as possible. You can use a handle, rope, or stick attachment. Stand at a 90-degree angle to the direction of the cable pull in a split stance, with the foot farthest from the cable unit forward and the foot closest to the unit behind. Hold the cable attachment with both hands. Pull the cable from the high position across the body and down to the side of your outside hip or thigh in one smooth movement with straight arms (figure 5.16). Exhale as you get close to the finish position. Try to drive the movement from the hips and core rotation. Return to the start position and complete the outlined number of reps on that side. Switch to the other side and repeat.

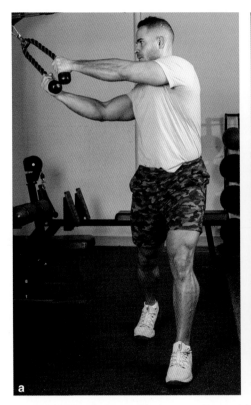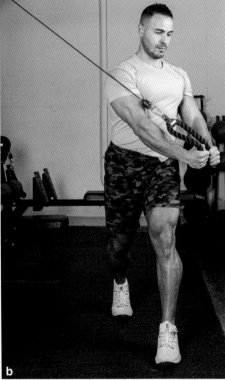

Figure 5.16 Cable split stance chop: *(a)* start position and *(b)* finish position.

MEDICINE BALL HALF-KNEELING ROTATIONAL THROW

Using a medicine ball and a wall sturdy enough to throw the ball against, set up in a half-kneeing position with your leg closest to the wall forward and the leg farthest from the wall down. With a strong grip on the ball, rotate through the core and shoulders, opening the chest and torso away from the wall to load the muscles and prepare to throw (figure 5.17). Rotate toward the wall and release the ball at the wall with as much speed and force as possible. Exhale as you release the ball. Try to avoid falling over. You should throw hard enough for the ball to bounce off the wall and come back to you. If you use a sand-loaded ball, the rebound will be nearly nonexistent. If you use a very bouncy ball, have your hands ready to catch the ball very quickly after it hits the wall. The half-kneeling position reduces the movement available from the lower body and requires more of the movement and force development to come from the torso and shoulders. If you want to increase arm and torso involvement without letting the lower body do all the work, a half-kneeling position can divide the work between the upper body and the lower body.

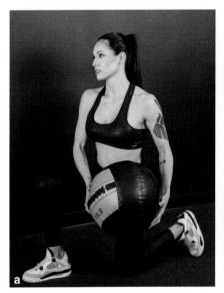 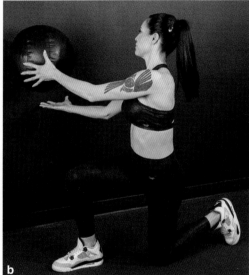

Figure 5.17 Medicine ball half-kneeling rotational throw: *(a)* start position and *(b)* finish position.

MEDICINE BALL STANDING ROTATIONAL THROW

The half-kneeling version of this exercise limits how much drive and pivoting you can get from the feet and lower legs, which in turn limits the total power and range of motion of the throw. The standing version allows greater involvement of a wider volume of muscles and joints, which means a larger force production and range of motion come together to let you cause some chaos with a medicine ball and a wall.

Start with your feet in a square stance: feet in line with each other, about hip or shoulder width apart, at a 90-degree angle to the wall. Rotate the ball away from the wall to load the throw, ensuring your core is braced and strong but elastic, not under maximum stiffness as with a deadlift. Rapidly accelerate the ball to the wall by driving off your hips, pivoting on the feet, and directing the ball toward the wall with violent intent (figure 5.18). Exhale as you release the ball, then complete the number of reps outlined on the same side. Repeat on the opposite side.

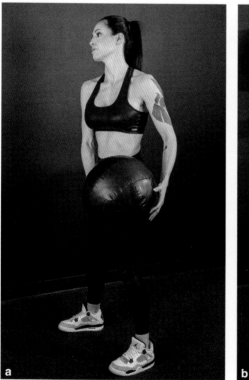
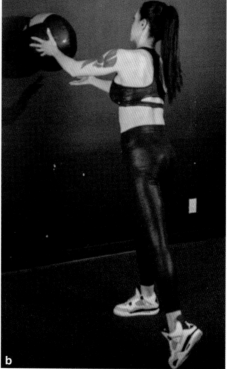

Figure 5.18 Medicine ball standing rotational throw: (a) start position and (b) finish position.

MEDICINE BALL SLAM

A medicine ball slam is a great way to get out any stress or rage you might have and direct it toward an unsuspecting ball that simply smiles and takes all that you can give it. Ideally any medicine ball you use for slams will have minimal bounce, like a sand-filled ball. A ball with too much bounce earns your dentist another boat payment while also crushing your dreams of posting your smiling post-workout selfie with all your teeth in their original places. For this reason, perform a test bounce to gauge the bounciness of the ball you're planning to use before you have an up close and personal meeting with it and your gum line. Hold the ball out at about shoulder height and just let it fall to the ground. If it hits and just stops dead, you've found a winner. If it bounces back up to any appreciable height, like over your knee or up to your waist like a properly inflated basketball, I'd avoid slamming it into the floor with reckless abandon.

Start in a square stance, holding the ball with both hands. Reach overhead with the ball as high as possible and slightly behind your head. Stand as tall as possible, pushing your hips forward, and even getting up onto the balls of your feet. As you prepare to slam the ball, take a big breath in and squeeze the breath. In one smooth and explosive movement, drive the hips back, drop your heels to the floor, and swing your arms down to smash the ball into the floor between your feet and about a foot in front of them (figure 5.19). Exhale rapidly and tense the abs even more as you accelerate the ball toward the ground. Try to catch the ball as it comes off the floor, ideally with your hands and not with your face.

Avoid rounding your back as you slam the ball. Instead, focus on flexing from the hips and the abs to create the acceleration. There will be some spine flexion, but make sure the movement is coming from every segment of the body simultaneously and not just exclusively from the spine.

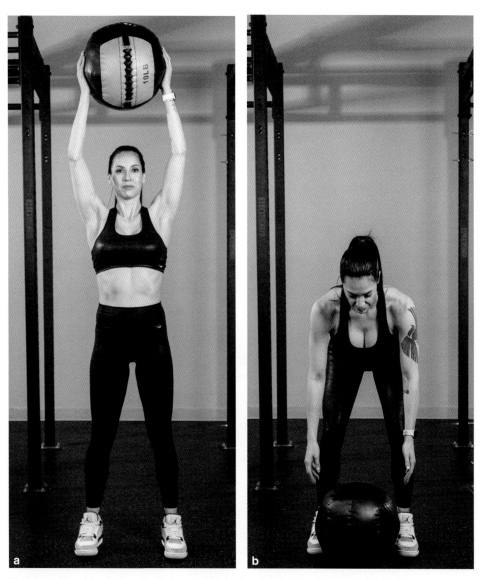

Figure 5.19 Medicine ball slam: *(a)* start position and *(b)* finish position.

Key Core Exercises

Some core exercises don't fit into the outline of resisting movement or moving explosively, but still add a ton of value to the mix. This next section covers key core exercises that help fill in the gaps and expand your movement capacity with regard to spine and core training.

HANGING KNEE RAISE

A major benefit of this movement is the involvement of the upper body with respect to how you engage core muscles. The hang itself has to be a fairly active process; you can't just dangle. The grip has to be strong enough to keep you on whatever you're hanging from. Your arms and shoulders have to be engaged to keep tension through the shoulder blades as they attach to the torso, which can create a deeper involvement of the core muscles being used to lift your legs. Ideally, the movement is like the beginning phase of a pull-up that morphs into a raise of the legs before your elbows have a chance to bend. Controlling how the spine produces movement of the hips and ribs can help improve motor control through the region, which itself can help reduce the potential for muscle or joint strains when the spine moves in other exercises or activities.

Hang from a straight bar, chin-up multigrip bar, or whatever you have available. Make sure all your fingers are wrapped tight to the bar and tense the shoulder muscles around the ribs. Inhale, then drive the knees up toward your chest (figure 5.20). Think of pulling your torso from a vertical position to slightly more horizontal from the shoulders. The movement at the top should feel like you're getting some spine flexion; you are not just raising the knees but performing more of a crunch movement. Exhale at the top of the rep, and lower under control.

If you start swinging from the bar, adjust your tempo. Spend a little extra time lowering your legs compared to the time spent raising them. If you find your grip is failing before your abs, spending more time in a hang like this will help build up your grip endurance, but you could also use straps to reduce the demand on the hands (which would also reduce the benefit from the movement itself, but you do you). If you find you can't hang at all, you could use an elbow-supported Roman chair to perform the movement, or switch the exercise for a bench leg lift, which is described next.

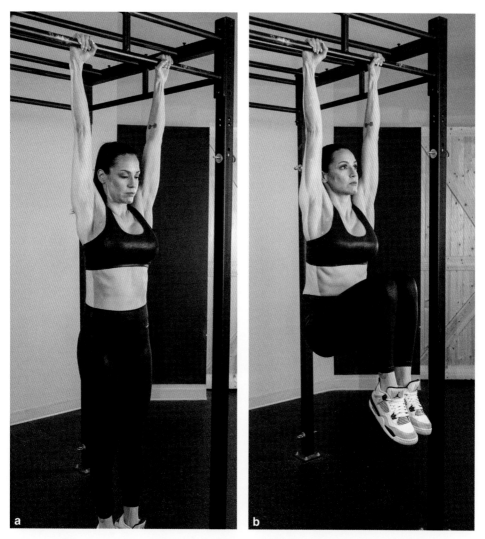

Figure 5.20 Hanging knee raise: *(a)* start position and *(b)* finish position.

BENCH LEG LIFT

Lie on a bench and grab the bench beside your ears with both hands. Raise both legs up with knees relatively straight. Curl the hips off the bench as your legs reach the top to get an extra crunch out of the abs (figure 5.21). Bonus points if you raise the legs, then push your feet toward the ceiling, raising your hips and back off the bench as high as possible. Lower your hips and legs to the starting position and repeat. Training the spine to flex and lower in different ways and different directions relative to gravity can help build the muscles of the core and spine to improve stress tolerance from other exercises or activities that the spine might be exposed to in daily life.

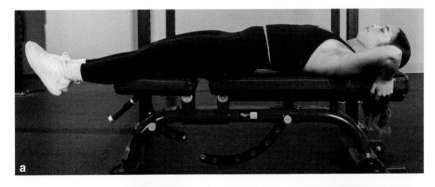

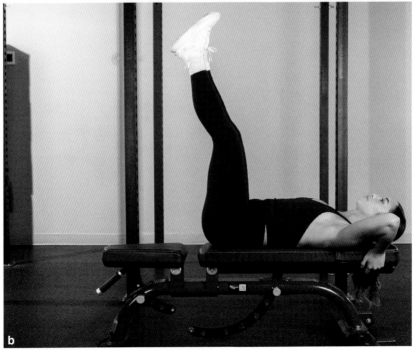

Figure 5.21   Bench leg lift: *(a)* start position and *(b)* finish position.

AB WHEEL ROLLOUT

The ab wheel is likely the most economical and beneficial piece of exercise equipment you could have in your arsenal, but also the one piece of equipment most commonly used incorrectly. An ab wheel rollout is essentially a moving plank; you start with the hips over the knees and the hands under the shoulders then roll forward as far as possible without changing the spine's position. Many people lose core control and wind up hanging off their hip flexors and spinal ligaments versus using their ab muscles to keep the ship steering straight and strong. The core should be in a slightly flexed position but stay rigid throughout the entire movement. Ideally the lower back shouldn't drop into any extension or shift as you move from stretching out to coming back to the start position. Often this means going only about 80 percent as far as you think you could go.

Begin on your hands and knees, holding the ab wheel under your shoulders. Brace the abs so that you feel a strong controlled contraction throughout the abdomen. Take a big breath in and lock it down, then start pushing the wheel forward by pushing your hips forward and slowly moving your hands forward from under the shoulders (figure 5.22).

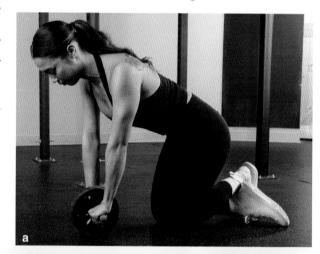

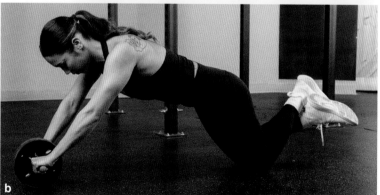

Figure 5.22 Ab wheel rollout: *(a)* start position and *(b)* finish position.

Make sure you are able to maintain the core contraction. Stop forward movement at any point at which you feel you are not able to maintain that tight core position or if you feel your lower back drop into extension. Use the abs to pull the wheel back toward your knees and return to the start position, exhaling as you get to the finish. This is one of the more challenging and self-limiting core exercises you can do, especially if done with a high level of intent and focus on maintaining position and challenging your range of motion without losing your brace or spine position.

HARDSTYLE PLANK

A plank is a fairly basic exercise, but with the right focus on developing total body tension and maximizing intensity you can make this simple exercise one that leaves you completely wasted in a short order of time. Generating total body tension to build torso endurance is a fundamental requirement for a lot of athletic events and strength movements, so this plank variation is fantastic for building that endurance.

Starting on your abdomen, set your elbows under your shoulders and press up so that your torso is off the ground and you're supported on your forearms and toes with your body and legs in a straight line (figure 5.23). With your feet about hip-width apart, tense your quads, glutes, abs, and pecs, and think of trying to drag your elbows back toward your toes without losing that straight line torso position. Essentially, make every muscle in your body tense. From there, ramp up the intensity more and more until you're almost able to see through time and smell colors, and don't forget to breathe forcefully, much like the Big Bad Wolf trying to blow over some houses. Ideally you should be completely spent within about 20 seconds if you're doing this properly.

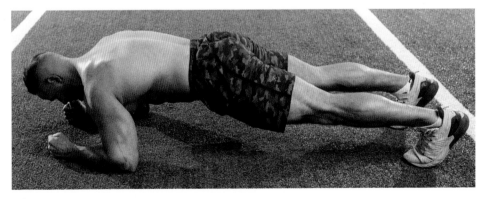

Figure 5.23 Hardstyle plank.

Breathing, Bracing, and Core Training Beyond Crunches

Breathing and bracing operate at opposite ends of a continuum. Easy breathing typically involves little to no core bracing, whereas maximal bracing makes breathing next to impossible. Because of this, bracing has to be used on a dial—it's not an "all or nothing" concept. For maximum-intensity lifts, a maximum-intensity brace is needed, but for that breathing has to be paused or limited significantly. For activities that involve more endurance to maintain a brace, there has to be a slightly submaximal intensity with the brace and more effort given to being able to actively and forcefully breathe so that you aren't negatively affecting your bracing.

A loaded carry is a great example of a bracing endurance type of activity. Your brace has to be strong enough to maintain control of the spine under load but still allow you to breathe for the duration of the activity. If you locked down your bracing so hard you couldn't squeak any air in or out, you'd be stable but likely pass out after a few seconds or have to drop the weight to release your brace and take in some air again. Neither outcome is desirable.

For speed-based exercises, the bracing has to be maximized at the moment of peak force. Think of a boxer; when their hand hits the target, they want to stiffen their core and brace as hard as possible to transfer as much force as possible from their lower body to their upper body. Similarly, when throwing, the core will stiffen as hard as possible at the moment when the lower body drives forward and starts to require the upper body to lock and rotate with the hips. These activities require a rapid increase in muscle tone and a pulsed exhale rather than a forceful or drawn-out exhale. It's more of a puff through pursed lips versus a fire-breathing dragon or gentle breeze.

As discussed in chapter 2, bracing ideally involves all the torso muscles supporting the spine. The degree of bracing tension is directly proportional to the amount of loading in relation to an individual's maximum capability. As the loading goes up, it's next to impossible to isolate any specific core muscle, so focus on bringing the whole team to the party, rather than any one muscle or group of muscles. As loading decreases, it's easier to think of working individual muscles, which can be beneficial for training specific movements, building localized strength and endurance, or recovering from injury. Sometimes you also just want to get an extra pump from the obliques or make your six-pack pop more, so targeting muscles with less than maximal loading can be worthwhile and will require more of a steady tension with more consistent breathing than locking down and performing a Valsalva maneuver.

A good question to ask is: why is breathing so important to core training, specifically intensity? That's a fine question, and I'm so very glad you asked it. During inhale, the lungs expand to allow more air volume, raising the ribs. The diaphragm, a large parachute-like muscle underneath the lungs, contracts, going from a dome shape to a flatter shape and pushing down into the abdominal cavity. When the diaphragm contracts and pushes down, the contents of the abdominal cavity become more pressurized and need to go somewhere to avoid being squished. This typically results in the abdomen pushing forward slightly.

Now you can imagine that bracing the ab muscles hard limits your ability to push the abdomen out and accommodate the diaphragm depressing and pushing your guts forward. A hard brace also tends to lock down the ribs, which makes it difficult for them to expand and rise as well. So the ability to fully inhale requires the core muscles to let the ribs elevate and the diaphragm push down as the abdominal cavity pushes down and forward. To get that breath, you have to relax the abs and not brace very much.

You can still breathe without letting your bracing go, but your breathing will be shallower, with a smaller volume per breath, and require more work from the muscles of the ribs and shoulders, plus you have to push against the resistance of the core muscles trying to brace and hold the spinal position, which makes the relative effort of the process much higher and more uncomfortable.

Similarly to the inhale, the exhale involves the movement of the ribs and diaphragm but in the opposite direction of the inhale, as the volume of the lungs is reduced to push air out. At relatively low intensity or at rest, exhalation is often a passive event, where you just reduce the involvement of the inhaling muscles and let the expanded volume reduce. While under tension, you don't really want the exhale to be passive; rather, you want to use those core muscles to contract and squeeze the air out of the lungs. This increased force of exhalation tends to ramp up the intensity of the intercostal and abdominal muscles, which can help increase the bracing strength through the core and pull the ribs down to restore the canister position we've used with more of the strength-based movements.

Pretty much any time you're lifting a weight or putting your spine under loading from exercise, you should be using a brace in some form or another, the intensity determined by the amount of load or how fast you're planning to move it. As the intensity goes up, the bracing increases, and your breathing will go from free and easy to labored and restricted, and eventually to not more than a big inhale to prepare and an exhale when the work is done for near max intensity.

Matching the manner in which you breathe to the task and intensity at hand can often be the secret weapon to getting the most out of the exercise. Focus on working with the highest intensity you can manage to perform the exercise properly, breathing as outlined earlier. Maintaining control of the torso helps to produce the best results from your core training program. Crunches are cool and all, but so is carrying a heavy weight across the gym floor, throwing a medicine ball into the wall, and rocking out with some of the other cool stuff we've outlined in this chapter.

Conclusion

Now that we've reviewed the basic strength exercises we'd like to use during the training programs, we have to learn how to use them. To use a delicious metaphor, the exercises are the ingredients to our meal, and now we have to figure out how much of each to use to make it tasty. The next chapter outlines how much volume and intensity to use with each, and considers the different ways to manipulate these variables to produce different outcomes depending on the goal of the exercise, the training program, and the stage of training that you're in at the moment.

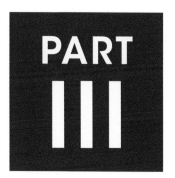

PART III

Programming Considerations

6

Volume and Load

To continue our food metaphor from chapter 5, the exercises we've outlined so far are the main ingredients in any kind of training program, but the recipe you use matters just as much. That's why we're going to spend this chapter talking about how to play with all the ingredients (important variables) to get the desired outcome (meal) you're looking for.

All exercise is stress applied to the body. The body adapts to the amount and type of stress in order to manage it more effectively in the future. That's training. The challenge is to find the amount of stress necessary to see these adaptations without causing so much stress that the body breaks down, gets injured, or succumbs to overtraining, where the continued application of stress actually causes negative adaptations instead of positive ones.

While it's nice to go full beast mode and YOLO yourself in the gym all day every day, there's actually compelling research that always expending maximum effort may not provide as much longevity benefit as blending high-intensity exercise with moderate-intensity exercise.[1] When viewed in the context of the gym, making every exercise as stressful as possible isn't really necessary for everyone, and very few benefits result from this approach. In essence, there's nothing wrong with exercise you can tolerate and recover from more easily. Sure, there are genetic fortunates who can manage continuous high-intensity workouts really well, as well as people on all types of pharmaceuticals that help them produce higher intensity and bounce back faster, but they have their own problems and we won't address that in this book.

Developing Muscle Mass

Does lifting heavier weights for fewer reps produce more muscle mass than lifting lighter weights for more reps? The answer is long, but to boil it down, the short answer is: kinda. If you match the total workload between heavier weights and lower weights by assigning a lot more reps and sets to the lighter-load workouts, the results are pretty similar.[2] If you've been working out for a while, you can actually still see some muscle growth by using lighter loads and higher volume.[3] Plus, lighter weights won't beat up your joints as much as heavier weights, although the fact is that the only way to really increase your maximum strength is through heavier loads.[4]

So what are the necessary ingredients to getting bigger muscles? Dr. Brad Schoenfeld has researched this very question, and he came up with three main ingredients to get more jacked:

- Mechanical tension
- Intramuscular damage
- Metabolic stress[5]

You have to stress the tissue enough (in our case, by lifting heavy) so that it incurs mild damage from which it can recover and synthesize new protein to build new muscle tissue. You have to work hard enough to make the muscle suck up enough oxygen and carbs and push out enough carbon dioxide and water to make the tissue adapt effectively. Once those conditions are met, you can either use lighter weights for more reps or heavier weights for fewer reps to meet your goal of being an absolute jacked unit.

Is there a specific load or number of reps that helps you adapt best—makes you stronger, bigger, or more resilient? Not really. Most of the research shows that you can see these adaptations with a wide variety of loads (based on percentage of maximum being lifted) as well as across a wide range of reps completed per set, and number of sets within a workout.[6] Some people respond really well to doing just a few very heavy reps per workout, whereas others might need 20 sets of work to feel like they're getting into the groove with no set of fewer than 20 reps. Both are valid, as is any option in between.

One consideration in the discussion of heavy versus light is the tempo, or time it takes to complete a rep. Often this can be written as "lowering-pause-raising time," in seconds, so a 3-2-1 tempo would involve lowering the weight for 3 seconds, pausing at the bottom of the range of motion for 2 seconds, and then returning to the top position in 1 second. If you have a device that can measure bar speed, it usually comes out in meters per second, 0.7 m/s, for example.

Speed can play a role in training through two main factors: time under tension (TUT) and power production. TUT is typically used when force production doesn't have to be at or near max, and where loading is light enough for you to control the tempo effectively. By increasing the TUT during a set with slower reps, you can increase the muscular damage and metabolic stress even with a sub-maximum load. Conversely, moving a weight fast requires a greater power production from the muscle. The mathematical formula for power is

$$P = M \times D/t$$

where P is power (also commonly shown as W for work), M is mass, D is distance, and t is time. Moving the same mass over the same distance in a shorter amount of time requires greater power from the working muscles. This can create greater mechanical tension and also be helpful in developing more strength compared to lifting lighter weights more slowly.

Developing Strength

Similarly to hypertrophy, there seems to be a benefit to using a variety of tempos when trying to get stronger.[7] Using a combination of near-maximum slow, grinding reps as well as lighter load but maximum-velocity reps can be a great way to use multiple influences to develop strength. Both techniques involve a massive spike in neural drive (the strength of the impulse from the nerve, like the current in an electrical wire) into the working muscles, just in different ways, but the end result is you get stronger.

As the amount of loading goes up, there's always an increasing risk of injury. While it's possible to train and use heavier weights, if you're not specifically training for a powerlifting competition or other sport that requires max or near max loading, the risks tend to outweigh the benefits. In many cases, you can still see improvements in muscle size and strength by training through a variety of intensities, volumes, and speeds of movement, so limiting injury risk and getting similar benefits is always a smart strategy. The heavier the weight becomes, the smaller the margin of error becomes, which means a small shift in where the weight is or how you're standing could mean a trip to the surgeon's office.

This isn't meant to scare you off from lifting heavier, especially if that's something you really love doing, but just to say you can actually get what you want in terms of the specific benefits from the heavier weight *at a lower-risk level of loading*. If heavy lifting is something that sparks joy, go heavy and hard, but if it doesn't, you can skip it in favor of slightly lighter weight with a few more reps and still become a dieseled-out monster, if that's what you're after.

In many cases, occasional heavier lifting can produce some significant strength improvements, and it can be done safely when included in a long-term training program. While a 20-year-old may be able to hit the gym four days a week and push max effort on every single workout for a long time, someone in their 40s or 60s may only be able to do max effort lifts for two or three phases each calendar year, and likely build up to max effort for only a short period of time in each of those phases. The longer you've been training, the longer it's likely to take to work up to a true max effort lift in terms of both in-workout warmups and programming weeks leading into the heavier or peak phase of lifting, and to do so safely with relatively good recovery afterward. Max effort when you're not ready for max effort can really mess up some people, and it occasionally causes flu-like symptoms for a few days while your body tries to figure out what the heck just happened and recovers from the stress. You might feel like you're jet-lagged, wearing a weighted vest, undercaffeinated, and kind of sobby—all at the same time. Not a fun place to be, but still cool if you posted a personal best.

For most of the training calendar, the lifts will be best in a relatively sub-maximum intensity, working toward mechanical failure at 3 to 10 reps per set, depending on the amount of loading and volume of sets, other life stuff going on, and so forth. Most average gym-goers don't really need to attempt max-effort lifts, but for those who want to, it makes sense to try them about every 4 to 6 months, meaning two or three phases per year of building toward heavier lifts, with appropriate amounts of time to build up and recover from those efforts. Ideally, a build-up toward max effort shouldn't be less than 4 weeks or more than 8 weeks, as adding intensity over a long time frame will likely lead to some extra soreness and cranky tissues.

So how do you do a build-up? By simply adding a little more weight and reducing a couple of reps each week over the span of the build phase. For instance, let's say you want to test your bench maximum next month. This month, you would start with 4 working sets of 5 reps with a weight that allows for a roughly 8 or 9 out of 10 rating of perceived exertion (RPE) or 1 or 2 reps in reserve (RIR) per set, meaning at the end of the set you still feel like you could do another 1 or 2 quality reps. Let's assume for example, that this is 185 pounds (84 kg). You finish the workout, everything's great, you can move your arms the day after, great success.

In week 2, you'd up the loading to 195 (88 kg) or possibly even 205 pounds (93 kg), and aim for 5 sets of 3 reps, with again the aim of 8 or 9 RPE and at least 1 RIR at the end of each set. After you complete the first 2 sets at 195 (88), you feel super strong, and bump to 205 (93). You grind out that set and think you probably didn't have any reps in reserve, so you drop back to 195 (88) for the next 2 sets. Solid choice, since you finish the remaining sets within the above targets.

In week 3, you up the weight to 205 pounds (93 kg), and aim for 5 sets of 2, still 8 or 9 RPE and 1 RIR. You go through the sets, feeling good until set 4 is a grind, and then you drop down to 195 (88) for the final set. You're still adding weight to your workouts, and managed 4 sets of 2 at 205 (93), when last week you finished only 2 sets of 3 at 205 (93), meaning you went from 6 reps up to 8 reps at that loading. Solid progress!

In week 4, you're ready to push and try 3 singles, working at 205 (93) to get the groove, then 215 (98 kg), and attempt 225 (102 kg) for the final rep. Your targets are 10 RPE and 0 RIR for the final rep. You manage to finish the rep with a little grind through the sticking point, but it's still up and done. You added 40 pounds (18 kg) to your loading, while dropping the total volume from 20 working reps in week 1 to 3 in the final rep, gradually adding to the load and getting closer to a max effort RPE while leaving nothing in the tank. After your workout, you're on cloud 9, light as a feather, but wind up crashing hard. You need a nap about 3 hours after the workout, and feel a bit foggy for half the day afterward, but you wind up recovering well after that.

Here's the outline of the progression to this effort over 4 weeks for just bench:

Week 1: 4 × 5 reps, 185 lb (84 kg), 8-9 RPE, 1-2 RIR; volume = 20 reps; loading = 3,700 lb (1,678 kg); load/rep = 185 lb (84 kg)

Week 2: 5 × 3 reps, 195-205 lb (88-93 kg), 8-9 RPE, 1 RIR; volume = 15 reps; loading = 2,985 lb (1,354 kg); load/rep = 199 lb (90 kg)

Week 3: 5 × 2 reps, 195-205 lb (88-93 kg), 8-9 RPE, 1 RIR; volume = 10 reps; loading = 2,030 lb (921 kg); load/rep = 203 lb (92 kg)

Week 4: 3 × 1 reps, 205-225 lb (93-102 kg), 10 RPE, 0 RIR; volume = 3 reps; loading = 645 lb (293 kg); load/rep = 215 lb (98 kg)

For this example, volume went down in successive weeks by 25 to 33 percent, and load/rep increased by 4 to 6 percent per week. The max effort of 225 pounds (102 kg) means the loading used in the first week was only 82 percent of the max. While we could write a doctoral thesis on these kinds of percentages, for the most part they need an explanation of the amount of effort used to get them. Because in week 1 the RPE was only 8 or 9 out of 10, and there was ideally still 2 RIR, this wasn't a true max effort. Most charts and tables on predicting 1 rep max (1RM) and number of reps at percentages of 1RM are assuming the work being done is taken to failure, not stopping with one or two reps left in the tank, so they don't truly apply with work being done at submax intensity.

It's also tough to predict a max from a submax loading not done to failure, so testing it on occasion is fine, but because most of the work being done within the framework of this program doesn't require knowing your max, it's more of a novelty and indicator of progress than a requirement. Don't put too much value on testing it, using it, or getting into the calculus of what it means relative to the other stuff you're doing and how that number determines everything else you'll be doing going forward. As we've discussed, we'll use some different methods that are a bit more forgiving, easier to adjust as you go along, and give some more leniency for good and bad days in the gym versus hard percentages. Its main benefit is having a ready answer to the question "How much can you lift?"

Measuring and Adjusting Loading for Max Benefits

Most training programs are based on the concept of progressive overload, where you gradually add more and more stress through the course of a training plan with workouts that have you lifting more weight or where you do more work during a given workout through either completing more reps or more sets at the same load. The challenge with this is that eventually, you'll max out how much stress you can handle while seeing good adaptations—in other words, you'll stop making progress.

How can you tell how much stress you're applying to your body with exercise? The best way is to simply keep a log and refer to it on occasion. Do some accounting in terms of how many sets, reps, and pounds you're lifting in each workout, and see if it's changed much over time or if there have been any sudden spikes or drops. Once you see what kind of volume and load you're used to working with consistently, try varying a few things every now and then. Try using a lighter weight for a few more reps or a heavier weight for only a couple of reps, add a set in a few exercises, take one or two out of others, and see what these variations do for you. Later we'll look at these variables and how to manage them in a training program. We'll also explain what to expect if you switch things up, as well as how much to change so you don't wind up demolishing yourself by trying something "fun."

As loading goes up, the volume of work you can do per set will go down, and the total volume of good reps you can get into a workout will diminish pretty significantly. There's a saying among sprinters and track cyclists that you get only so many matches, which means you can do high-intensity work only so many times in a workout before you don't have anything left to produce at that intensity. Once that match is burned, you can't unburn it in that workout. If you're doing max efforts in the gym, you'll get only a few good reps before those matches are burned. Consistent training can help you gradually increase the number of higher-effort sets you can complete, but even very skilled athletes will be able to attain only 2 or 3 true max efforts in a single training session—and sometimes only one.

For the average nonprofessional or individual who wouldn't classify themselves as a genetic fortunate, they might be able to get about 10 reps of near max effort throughout a workout. This might mean 3 sets of 3, 5 sets of 2, or some similar iteration. At maximum, they might get only 2 or 3 reps. The main reason why you can't do more is that you can't come back from the relative fatigue of the heavier efforts with cardio recovery, refueling with carbs, or boosting your caffeine intake through the roof.[9] Your brain and nervous system can send a supercharged impulse to the muscle to contract as hard as needed to lift the max weight, but the higher the demand, the longer it takes to recover. Most strength athletes might feel like they're in a movement fog or muscle haze following very heavy training, where the body just doesn't respond the same way as before the training. For many who get to this level of fatigue, it might take a full day or more to be able to produce similar force outputs again, so maxing out every day isn't the best option for most. (Side note: Movement Fog and Muscle Haze would make fantastic band names.)

For non-max-effort lifts, there are two main types of fatigue to be aware of:

- Technical fatigue
- Muscular fatigue

Technical fatigue is where you're not able to do the exercise with the required technique due to movement patterns starting to break down. Imagine doing a squat and the first few reps go really well, but then your knees are caving in, your back is rounding, you're shooting your hips back and up too early, or you're seeing any element of poor technique that you're not able to correct. Fatigue is limiting your ability to perform the exercise properly, even though you can still grind through some more reps if needed. You've hit technical fatigue, even though the muscles are still powering through (poorly).

Muscular fatigue is when the working muscles can't complete the rep against the given resistance. Imagine doing a biceps curl with a dumbbell, and you get up to the eighth rep, then the weight starts to slow down, rep nine is an absolute grind, and rep 10 gets halfway up, stalls, and no matter how much you will that dumbbell to move or how many Jedi mind tricks you employ, it's just not happening, so you can't complete that tenth rep. You just hit muscular fatigue.

For exercises that require more skill or technique, like heavier compound lifts, technical failure is the place to stop. For accessory work or isolation exercises, you can push to muscular fatigue since the technique is rarely affected enough to warrant stopping prior to the muscle's inability to complete a rep. Skilled movements require learning to do the task properly, so pushing past technical failure doesn't reinforce how to do the movement correctly and winds up creating poor movements that aren't going to give you what you're looking for from the exercise. Maintaining proper technique for as many quality reps as possible is a better goal than grinding for the sake of grinding.

You can increase your strength in most of your training reps at less than maximal loading while only occasionally dipping into more challenging or near-max-effort work. Most powerlifters and Olympic lifters see a lot of progress year over year by keeping most of their work at 70 to 80 percent of their max and focusing on technique while building a base of reps, and pushing toward max efforts only a few times a year to gear up for competitions. Trying to max out every day is a good recipe for frustration when you miss reps, feel overtrained, and possibly get injured along the way, so focusing on quality technique and submax work can go a long way to producing the benefits you're looking for. What's more, this give you a better chance of actually walking out of the gym and enjoying your life later on that day.

For most non-max efforts, you shouldn't be taking the set right to the limit, especially if that exercise has a higher skill requirement and where fatigue could make the quality of the reps less than beneficial. This could be true of your compound strength exercises, as well as any higher skill-based movements such as throwing or Olympic lifts. Keeping a non-max loaded set feeling like it's challenging but still doable is a challenge to figure out, but there are some methods to make it possible.

One method is to use a scale called rating of perceived exertion, or RPE, which we touched on previously. This is classically something that's been used with cardio testing or programming to determine whether the intensity matches the individual's experience. If you're working at 80 percent of your heart rate max, your RPE will likely be around 7 or 8 out of 10, where 1 would be simply existing and 10 would be running away from a bear while you're on fire, and the bear is on fire, and everything is on fire.

With strength training, you could use the same scale as a measure of intensity during the set. Say the set called for 5 reps, and at the end of the fifth rep, you returned the weight and felt it was roughly a 7 out of 10 RPE. That means you're likely working at around 80 percent of the weight you could manage for that set for 5 reps if it was a true max effort. A challenge with RPE is it's entirely based on the individual's ability to accurately determine how hard they were working on that set relative to the max they would likely be able to handle. This is often wildly inaccurate, but it's at least a place to start. A major issue with defining effort is whether the individual has ever actually experienced maximum effort, as well as whether that maximum effort translates to different exercises or specific body parts,[10] If someone doesn't actually know what maximum effort feels like, they can't accurately compare what they're doing against it.

Another option would be to try to determine if you could do any more reps at the end of your set, and make a game plan for a load that would allow you to finish the set with that many reps still possible. This is called reps in reserve, or RIR, also introduced in the last segment's example. Essentially, if you did the same set of 5 reps and at the end feel like you could do another 2 reps with reasonably good form, you would have 2 RIR. This is something I first heard from Dr. Mike Israetel of Renaissance Periodization, and it seems to be a reasonable metric for many people to understand. However, similar to RPE, it relies on the individual's ability to determine how many reps they could do at the end of the set, which is often inaccurate.

Most experienced lifters tend to slightly underestimate their RIR,[11] under-predicting by almost one full rep, with the greatest accuracy as the individual got closer to failure, and where the total number of reps in the set was less than 12.[12] So for lower-volume stuff, most people will be able to accurately squeak out one more rep than they think they can, even if they have a pretty good understanding of their lifting capability.

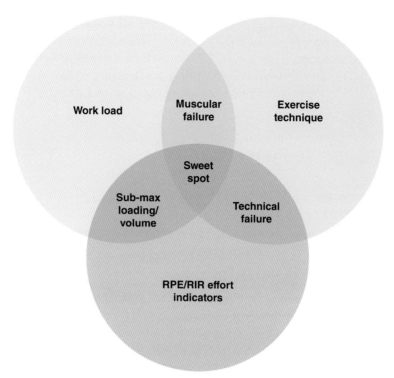

Figure 6.1 Venn diagram of relation between workload, exercise technique, and effort indicators in developing your best exercise response.

There's a sweet spot where the main factors of workload, technique, and effort all create the ideal situation for lifting, but where an imbalance on any of these elements might not give you what you're looking for. The Venn diagram in figure 6.1 outlines some of those considerations.

If you really want accuracy, you could use a device that measures the velocity of the bar being moved to track the speed of each rep. If you're moving at, say, 0.7 meters per second for most of the set, and then the bar slows down to 0.6 meters per second and then 0.5 meters per second, you would stop the set there versus trying to keep going. Any drop in speed of 10 to 20 percent typically means you're getting close to the limit of how many reps you can do at that weight.[8] There are some really cool velocity-based training (VBT) toys out there to help get more data from your training approach, and we'll talk a bit more about that in later chapters.

No matter how you choose to measure your intensity, the key features should be the ability to do the exercise correctly (within technical failure parameters) and to feel like completing the set is a challenge. If you know you can squat 200 pounds (91 kg), lifting 50 pounds (23 kg) will let you finish the set with good technique, but won't be much of a challenge. For most heavy exercises, it's worthwhile to do a few build sets before your working set. A build set is essentially a warm-up set with weight that gradually increases from one set to the next, up to the weight you're planning to use for the working sets. These build sets allow you to rehearse the technical components of the lift, refine your movement pattern, and warm up the working muscles and joints before starting the heavier sets.

For example, let's say you're planning to deadlift today, and want to work up to 315 pounds (143 kg) for your main working sets. Your build sets would be:

Set 1: 10 reps with the empty bar

Set 2: 10 reps with a 45 lb (20 kg) plate on either side (135 total lb or 61 kg)

Set 3: 5 reps with a 45 lb (20 kg) and 25 lb (11 kg) plate on either side (185 total lb or 84 kg)

Set 4: 5 reps with two 45 lb (20 kg) plates on either side (225 lb or 102 kg)

Set 5: 3 reps with two 45 lb (20 kg) plates and a 25 lb (11 kg) plate on either side (275 lb or 125 kg)

Following these build sets, you could start your main working sets with 315 pounds (143 kg), assuming everything felt fine and ready during the build sets. The build sets should gradually add challenge with loading but not use so much volume that you feel tired after completing them. That's the job of the working sets. The build sets are meant to prepare you for the working sets, not destroy you on the way there, when you're supposed to be gauging how you're feeling as you move toward the working sets. This isn't Frodo walking to Mordor here, so don't make the build sets a perilous journey.

The build sets also work as a self-audit to see how you're feeling and if the working sets are going to go as planned. Maybe you just got back from international travel, slept poorly, had a fight with your partner, cut your calories way back, or have a ton of work stress, so the conditions to work out hard aren't great. As a result, maybe the build sets are feeling extra heavy and hard today, so you decide to adjust the working sets a little, either dropping the weight a tick or dropping a rep or two from the end of each set. We'll talk about autoregulation and how to adjust your training based on how you're feeling in chapter 9, but in summary, some days you're just not feeling it and need to call an audible once you're under center and make a few adjustments to the plan.

Without those build sets, you would have jumped right into the working sets, for better or worse. With lightweight or accessory stuff, it's no problem, but with bigger weights, you have to dial it in a little more with a smaller margin of error, so working through some gradually increasing loads can have a big impact on your ability to complete the desired workload, while also determining if today's a good day or a day to just punch the clock and get through the basics.

Let's use those build sets as an example of how you would adjust your working sets based on two possibilities. For option 1, you feel absolutely terrible during the build sets and going through them doesn't get you feeling better and ready to lift more when they're done. In option 2, you're actually feeling like each build set gets better and better and like you're ready to smash everything in sight by the time you get to your working sets.

Option 1

Set 1: 10 reps with the empty bar. Felt cranky and way heavier than it should.

Set 2: 10 reps with a 45 lb (20 kg) plate on either side (135 lb total or 61 kg). Felt like positioning was off, like you couldn't get your bracing effectively, and like your hamstrings were immobile steel cords not willing to participate in these shenanigans. As a result, you got a lower-back pump from that set, meaning you were likely just bending your spine to lower and raise the weight. Not a good sign.

Set 3: 5 reps with a 45 lb (20 kg) and a 25 lb (11 kg) plate on either side (185 lb total or 84 kg). Felt like an 8 RPE for only 60 percent of what you would be using on your working sets. But today it was way too heavy and hard, and you want to curl into the fetal position in the corner and have someone pat your head and tell you you'll be okay.

Set 4: 5 reps with two 45 lb (20 kg) plates on either side (225 lb total or 102 kg). Hot buttered death, but with more chalk. You start reexamining all your life choices that led you to this moment and figure that it's likely going to be a terrible workout because everything sucks, you suck, everyone else sucks, and deadlifting today sucks the most of all.

Set 5: 3 reps with two 45 lb (20 kg) plates and a 25 lb (11 kg) plate on either side (275 lb total or 125 kg). You grind through the first rep, then the bar is welded to the floor on the final two efforts, doesn't even budge. You throw your hands in the air, swear a little, maybe weep softly, and think about how you can hide under a blanket on the couch and avoid the world for the rest of the day.

In this example, you're just not feeling up to using the working weight prescribed, so we have a couple of possibilities here. First, you could suck it up and try the working weight, knowing it's likely not going to give you the best workout and could increase the risk of injury or just massively frustrate you. Second, you drop weight off the bar and work within the RPE and RIR guidelines you planned for the working sets. You're still doing some work and honing your technique, even though it's less loading than you ideally would have worked with. You might not get the benefits from the workout you had originally planned, but it's still been productive. Third, you ditch the barbell and switch to a different deadlift exercise, add in a couple of accessory lifts if needed for some different training stress, or just skip that barbell exercise and make it more of a general fitness-type workout where you just do stuff without worrying about the specifics.

Sometimes your head and body aren't in it to push hard, but some movement and trying to find some level of enjoyment from the process is better than grinding or giving up altogether.

Let's look at the other possibility: You show up and feel like a god ready to tackle all the weights.

Option 2

Set 1: 10 reps with the empty bar. Felt like a waste of time, it's so stupidly easy.

Set 2: 10 reps with a 45 lb (20 kg) plate on either side (135 lb total or 61 kg). Felt like absolute butter. The core was working, hamstrings felt stretchy, back was lit up like a chandelier, and nothing felt like it was working too hard or doing all the lifting.

Set 3: 5 reps with a 45 lb (20 kg) and 25 lb (11 kg) plate on either side (185 lb total or 84 kg). Felt like a 2 RPE, which means 315 lb (143 kg) will likely feel like a 5 at this rate. Time to get serious and see what's possible today. It was so easy that your heart rate didn't even go up and you could hold a conversation with your gym crush through all the reps.

Set 4: 5 reps with two 45 lb (20 kg) plates on either side (225 lb total or 102 kg). You start getting excited and turn this into a speed set, trying to demolish the bar with your hips on every rep. Other gym members start to stare in awe, which is weird because you work out at home, alone. Who let them in? This could be fun.

Set 5: 3 reps with two 45 lb (20 kg) plates and a 25 lb (11 kg) plate on either side (275 lb total or 125 kg). You're still not even registering anything other than a warm-up level of effort. Everything feels great, the weight is moving super fast, and the last reps felt like you were about to clean the bar to your shoulders.

In this example, you're feeling like everything is just clicking for you. Similar to the first example, there are a few things you could do. First, you use the loading you set out to work with, in this case 315 pounds (143 kg), but you keep in mind the effort parameters you'd established with RPE and RIR and adjust weight on subsequent sets based on how the first few sets go.

For this case, let's say hypothetically 315 pounds (143 kg) moved super easily and you felt your RPE was 6 when you had expected it to be 8, and the RIR was easily 4 or 5, when it was supposed to be 2. You could add another 20 pounds (9 kg) to the bar and see how it feels, to possibly get the working set within your preset parameters for effort. On the second set, 335 pounds (152 kg) moved really well, and the effort and reserve were both around where you would have expected it to be for the 315 lb (143 kg) set, which means this loading is appropriate for how you're feeling today.

Second, you could jump up the weight right out the door to what you think would be appropriate for the effort parameters, given how you felt on the build-ups. For this example, you jump into your first working set with 335 lb (152 kg) instead of 315 lb (143 kg). This could go really well or it could be a case where you bite off more than you can chew. If you overshoot how you feel on set 1 and it winds up causing you to miss reps, hit technical failure too soon, or exceed your effort parameters, you'll either have to dial the weight back on the subsequent sets or try to appease your ego by keeping the heavier weight and working way harder than you thought you would or risk some damage from a weight and volume you can't properly control.

The third option is a pretty simple one. You do the working sets as outlined. Maybe, as you finish the second-to-last set, you gauge how you're feeling. If you felt good and didn't expend much effort on the previous sets, you add a bit more weight just for the sake of adding on the last set. It's sort of like option 1, but slightly more conservative because you have an element of change only on the final set versus possibly pushing the weight up earlier. In each of these scenarios, you're using the build sets as an indicator that you'll likely be able to add more weight today and adjust based on how you're feeling during the working sets and whether you're able to maintain the effort parameters and technical capability of the exercise.

In both options, the key considerations were how the build sets felt, whether they allowed you to feel like you were adequately prepared for the working sets, and whether you felt you could continue at the desired loading or needed to adjust for that day. These real-time considerations of increasing weight, technical capabilities, and physical readiness all contribute to your performance, so it's valuable information that can help you see the best benefits for your workout at that point in time. Similarly, it helps you fine-tune your effort parameters, allowing you the confidence to work hard enough to see the benefits you want, while also not pushing so hard that you have to expand effective recovery time frames between workouts. It's not meant to be precise or entirely prescriptive but allows the flexibility to adjust the plan as needed to accommodate normally occurring fluctuations in readiness.

If we were cyborgs who responded perfectly to everything as written, we'd have no bad days or peaks or valleys in energy. However, humans are consistently variable, so a training program that is too rigid in how loading is used or progressed may not be beneficial, tolerable, or even doable. A little flexibility in loading and willingness to adjust as needed makes it easier to get through the workouts and can increase the willingness of the person doing the programming—you—compared to programming that doesn't offer enough leeway for personal adjustments.

Varying High-Volume and Low-Volume Days in Training Programs

The volume in a workout or in a specific exercise is the amount of work being done during that particular interval. You could express it as the number of sets and reps within an exercise, the total amount of sets and reps being done within a specific body part, or the total number of sets performed throughout the week. Let's say that for upper-body push work, we do a bench press for 5 sets of 3 reps, which works out to 15 total reps for that exercise. We also do other pressing exercises, and the total volume of sets for that specific workout winds up being around 18 sets. We repeat that workout later in the week, and complete 36 total working sets for press work that week.

The total sets within a week gives a good bird's-eye view of the programming, including frequency of application. The volume within the workout gives a more detailed view of what's going on, and the volume within a specific exercise is a zoomed-in view of how the workouts are progressing. As with any form of accounting, knowing the details matters, but having a relatively concise overview can speed the review process up a lot. The details of a given exercise can outline how hard each rep is and how much weight is being lifted, whereas the total weekly volume can give an idea of how the structure of the program is built and whether there are any fluctuations from week to week or things that may need to be adjusted to allow for better results or improve recovery.

It can be pretty tough to just keep slapping more weight on the bar and do more work within a given exercise, as you'll eventually max out what you can lift effectively. However, it can be possible to use the same weight, and either add in an additional set, or maybe add another rep on a few sets, or even drop a rep from each set and make up the difference with more sets within that exercise. If I'm used to doing 4 sets of 5, and today I decide to do 5 sets of 5, I've added 25 percent more volume. If I decide to do 6 sets of 4 reps, the total work volume went from 20 reps up to 24 reps, even though I'm doing 1 less rep per set.

Adding volume adds stress, which allows for greater possible adaptation to the work being done, while also challenging the recovery from the work itself. Increasing volume can be a fantastic way to see progress, but as with adding weight to the bar, there's usually a limit to how much volume you can add before you hit a ceiling, either in terms of time spent in the gym, how well you can maintain intensity in the workout, or your ability to recover from the workouts. A small weekly increase in total volume can boost the workout stress but should also include a point where the volume is reduced to give the body a break, allow for some deeper recovery, and potentially recover from any mild aches and discomforts that may have popped up as the volume increased.

Let's say we have someone doing 10 sets of work each workout, and they train for 4 workouts each week. That's 40 total sets each week. We could do a few things to increase the total volume gradually. First, we could pick one exercise on each day and add in one additional set. This would bump the total work from 10 sets each workout up to 11 and move the total weekly volume up from 40 sets to 44 sets. This would represent a 10 percent increase in volume from week 1 to week 2, which would be significant, but hopefully not too much of a challenge in terms of post-workout soreness, sleep, or other metrics of recovery. The following week, we could add another set to another exercise for another bump from 11 sets to 12 sets within the workout, moving from 44 to 48 total sets within the week. This would be a 20 percent increase in work over 2 weeks, which for most people would also be relatively doable on occasion.

If we did this again in weeks 3 and 4, we'd be up to 13 sets per workout and 52 sets each week, or about a 30 percent increase over week 1 volume. That's pretty significant and would cause the individual to feel a bit tired and maybe a little beat up. Another option could be to bump volume in each workout for a few weeks, then add in an additional workout each week, which would also add volume to the week's total. Could we keep progressing like this? Probably for a little while, but as the person doing the work gets tired, feels like they don't have time to spend at the gym, or begins to show signs they aren't recovering effectively, they may need to take a bit of a volume vacation, or a deload.

Similar to how you need to have some time off from your job or from school every now and then, a deload allows you to recover more deeply than you can by just getting a good night's sleep. Many of the connective tissues in the body adapt at a slower rate than muscle tissue, so including a time frame of reduced volume and intensity can have a beneficial effect: it lets those tissues adapt more effectively instead of requiring them to keep up with the muscles. A deload is a significant drop in either volume or intensity, or both, for a short period, usually a week or two, depending on how built up the training program was and whether the individual was pushing to compete or just complete a training block.

The build weeks typically involve increasing volume and/or loading for 4 to 16 weeks, so the longer the build phase, the longer the deload will need to be to permit recovery from the training stress. Often these deloads involve cutting volume in half while trying to maintain some element of intensity, although for very high-intensity training blocks, such as max effort lifts, jumps, sprints, or similar drills, reducing intensity might be required with a shift to other drills that can help maintain specific training qualities without stressing the body excessively.

An example of building and deloading weeks, based on the hypothetical given earlier, would look like this:

Build week 1: 4 workouts, 10 sets each workout, 40 total sets

Build week 2: 4 workouts, 11 sets each workout, 44 total sets

Build week 3: 4 workouts, 12 sets each workout, 48 total sets

Build week 4: 4 workouts, 13 sets each workout, 52 total sets

Deload week: 4 workouts, 7 sets each workout, 28 total sets

A longer calendar might involve something like this:

Build week 1: 4 workouts, 10 sets each workout, 40 total sets

Build week 2: 4 workouts, 11 sets each workout, 44 total sets

Build week 3: 4 workouts, 12 sets each workout, 48 total sets

Build week 4: 4 workouts, 13 sets each workout, 52 total sets

Deload week: 4 workouts, 7 sets each workout, 28 total sets

Build week 1: 4 workouts, 12 sets each workout, 48 total sets

Build week 2: 4 workouts, 13 sets each workout, 52 total sets

Build week 3: 4 workouts, 14 sets each workout, 56 total sets

Build week 4: 4 workouts, 15 sets each workout, 60 total sets

Deload week: 4 workouts, 8 sets each workout, 32 total sets

You can see the second month started at a higher volume than the first month, but not at the same volume with which the first month ended. It was a step down from the peak, but not all the way down to the volume being used at the very beginning. The deload week even had a small bump in volume to reflect the increase in volume used during this phase, but the key is that it was a small increase to reflect a greater ability to handle stress effectively.

The point of the deload week is to still get some stress, but only enough to prevent the body from detraining and losing a step against what you've worked to build. By the end of this week, you should be feeling like you can get back into the greater volumes again without problem—maybe you even crave the bigger workouts—but the point is to feel recovered and ready. This phase can make it easy for the lifter to say, "That's it? I think I should add in some more heavy back squats or test my overhead press max. I'm feeling good and want to throw in some extra stuff to make it a full session." Try to avoid doing this as it defeats the entire purpose of the deload in the first place. Don't substitute other workouts, additional runs, or conditioning work, or do other challenging activities like building a stone patio or climbing a mountain peak or other stuff that would ramp up your physical stress.

When going through your build phases, your performance, readiness, and overall physical well-being should dip as the volume and workload goes up. You're causing more and more stress to accumulate through each week, pushing your body to adapt, which is the point. If it was easy, it wouldn't cause adaptation. The deload allows recovery so that your performance capabilities come back up to a supercharged level compared to where they were before. The manipulation of these types of variables and timing is what allows elite athletes to hit their peak for competitions and smash world records, and you can take advantage of the same concepts with your training.

There are a few ways to view total volume. You could consider only the working sets of all the exercises done after the warm-up, all of the sets including build sets and warm-ups, or categorize volume by intensity, such as low, moderate, or intense. This third option gives more detail and can allow you to tailor each element of your workout more effectively than by relying on total volume, but it does require a bit more work to break exercises and work into these different intensities.

Let's say that in the original example of working out four days a week with 10 sets per workout, three of those sets were considered light activation exercises, four were heavier strength work, and three were medium-intensity accessory exercises. Adding one extra set of the warm-up would have a very different effect compared to adding one extra set of the heavy strength work in terms of the stress on the system. Using intensity blocks to describe the volume makes this a more effective method of tracking volume throughout the week and through a training phase.

If we started with three light, three medium, and four heavy sets in week 1, then increased to three light, three medium, and five heavy sets in week 2, then three light, four medium, and five heavy sets in week 3, and so on, we would see more detail *and* get an overview of how the programming is progressing from start to finish. If you just consistently add in more heavy sets each week, you will likely burn out as your body recoils against more and more intensity. You'll burn through all your matches pretty quickly. Adding medium-intensity work to improve yet keep something in reserve and occasionally increasing low-intensity work to fill the gaps can allow for more total work, but more realistically than haphazardly adding more volume to random exercises in the program or just trying to grind out more heavy stuff every session.

In our example, focusing on the total volume and breaking it down into three intensity zones creates a realistic plan like this:

Build week 1: 40 total sets of 12 low, 15 medium, 13 high

Build week 2: 44 total sets of 12 low, 17 medium, 15 high

Build week 3: 48 total sets of 15 low, 18 medium, 15 high

Build week 4: 52 total sets of 15 low, 20 medium, 17 high

Deload week: 28 total sets of 12 low, 10 medium, 6 high

Build week 1: 48 total sets of 15 low, 18 medium, 15 high

Build week 2: 52 total sets of 15 low, 20 medium, 17 high

Build week 3: 56 total sets of 20 low, 20 medium, 16 high

Build week 4: 60 total sets of 20 low, 20 medium, 20 high (big jump but likely low reps)

Deload week: 32 total sets of 12 low, 10 medium, 8 high

You can see how we add volume to the workout, but while the high-intensity volume doesn't increase too much compared to the starting point (outside of one week with a big spike), most of the big volume changes occur between the low- and moderate-intensity volumes. Those high-intensity sets are still fairly limited, even if we're constantly working on trying to add one or two more.

A simple rule of thumb is to drop volume on deload weeks to about 50 to 60 percent of your peak, while maintaining the loading intensity. Sometimes working to 100 percent isn't in the cards, so for very heavy efforts you might have to drop loading by 10 percent from the peak phase. Nevertheless, it should still be challenge, but with reduced volume.

Another wrinkle in adding volume to see gains is the dose–response relationship. Too low or too high volume produces less than the best results, but somewhere in the middle is the sweet spot. It's sort of like the Goldilocks story: this program is too easy, that program is too hard, but this one is just right. Finding that ideal volume is a challenge, and you'll probably go through some trial and error to find what works best. We can start with a basic workout template that seems like it'll hit the nail on the head, and in the following weeks add another set here and there as needed or add in another exercise if recovery goes well.

Let me pause here to point out that I know it may not be exciting to read about volume fluctuations and intensity markers and deloads, but I wouldn't be talking about this stuff if it wasn't important. You can choose to freestyle your workouts and train by feel and hope you're making progress, or you can write some things down, look back at the work you've done, and adjust accordingly to *know* you're making progress and know *where* you're making that progress. If you keep hurting yourself or find you're just not getting any stronger, this is the simplest and easiest way to figure out what's going on and see why you're not getting the results you're working so hard for. So pay attention to this last segment, start recording your workouts if you're not already doing so, and get ready to thank me for making you do the hard stuff that actually gets you stronger.

Light-Volume and Giant-Volume Days

Similar to how we track and change total volume over a given week, we can adjust volume on different days over a given week. There's some benefit to doing each workout with the same volume, like if your schedule is consistently the same and allows you the same amount of time each day for a workout, or if your frequency is low enough that you have ample recovery time between each workout so you don't have to worry about recovery days. If you're training four or more days per week, you might have some days that you can really push and some days that need to be a bit easier or shorter.

A light-volume day could be one where your goal is to do some activation, accessory, or medium-intensity work and get done relatively quickly. It could be a day after a bigger-volume day or a higher-intensity day or a day before a big-volume or high-intensity day. Either way, the benefit to not having a constant volume throughout the week is that you have short periods of recovery interspersed between heavier and harder days of training, without taking the day off entirely. There's nothing wrong with passive rest when needed, but on occasion, a better option is a lower-intensity or lighter-volume day. This is because an easier day allows you to move around and reduce possible soreness, shake off any grogginess, and maybe feel good when you leave the gym versus feeling like you need to prop yourself up against a wall or call your mom to come pick you up.

When going into a light or recovery workout, it's important to note that the point of the workout is to keep it short, move around, and not add more intensity or volume above what is outlined. Like the deload week, these workouts should leave you saying, "That was it?" at the end because of how short they feel compared to your other workouts. The shortness is a feature, not a bug, so keep them short, light, and happy, and fight the urge to add more and more to make them feel like a "real" workout. You'll have more opportunity for that when doing workouts with bigger volume, but a nice little break is a good thing once in a while. Training is about balancing stress and recovery, and these light workouts focus on recovery within a training week. They are primarily used during times of heavier volume and training intensity, so going slow and keeping it short is the point.

A giant-volume day is the exact opposite: the goal is to do a lot of work all at once. The added stress shifts your body's response, sort of like lifting a bigger weight than usual. Because there's more work, these workouts take longer, so pack a lunch, maybe bring some snacks, and work on getting through the time efficiently so you're not there all day, unless that's your thing.

Endurance athletes do this regularly—along with their other workouts they do long workouts weekly or every other week with significantly more volume than their average. You can get similar benefits from periodic lower-intensity, higher-volume gym sessions that train different components of the muscles' energy systems as well as the physiologic response to the workouts. Their main benefits are to build up endurance capacity while optimizing the body's use of workout fuel, such as carbs and creatine phosphate. If you can manage your fuels more efficiently, you can do more sustained work without hitting the wall, which means better gains over the long term.

Used throughout a regular training week, these giant and light workouts adjust the volume from workout to workout and allow you to hit the desired total volume, yet they also create microspikes in training and permit more recovery than if every workout were the same length. A challenge with having every workout of the same length and intensity is that fatigue will accumulate throughout the week, meaning your workouts toward the end of the week will suffer. You see the same effect during a Monday-to-Friday workweek. Monday you're starting fresh, ready to go, and only mildly panicked about what the rest of the week will bring. By Thursday, you're figuring out what you can push to the following week and what needs your barely present energy right now, and by Friday you're ready to call in sick or just sleep it off somewhere quietly at work.

We can switch things up through the workout week by adjusting the total volume in each workout to take advantage of a giant volume day and a light day. Using our original example of four workouts a week and 40 total sets, we could set up something like the following:

Workout 1: 10 sets

Workout 2: 14 sets (giant-volume day)

Off day

Workout 3: 7 sets (light-volume day)

Workout 4: 9 sets (can be heavier loading or max effort day)

Off day

The total volume is the same as it would be if we did four workouts with 10 sets each, but we can create more stress in workout 2 with big volume, and in workout 4 we can push the intensity a bit more. It can't be stated enough: There's more benefit to training this way than with unchanging volume and intensity in each workout.

This is a great way to incorporate more training variation through a week versus just adding more sets or lifting heavier weights each week. The higher-stress and lower-stress workouts allow short-term recovery from more challenging workouts, which better distributes training intensity over the course of the week. Plus, the bigger workouts will make you feel like you're working hard but not slowly dying as a result of cumulative fatigue throughout the week.

Age Considerations in Weight Training

Young lifters are awesome responders to weight training, as they can do pretty much anything in the gym and see results. They get to take advantage of all the pubertal hormones, tissues that are more elastic and resilient to stress, and not as many competing interests to take their time away from logging those crazy gains. The older folks (and for the purpose of this I'm defining "older" as anyone beyond their early 30s) have lower production and volume of circulating sex hormones, making it more difficult to gain muscle; less-elastic and less-hydrated tissues, making it a challenge to stretch without tearing; slightly slower recovery times that affect their weekly training volume and intensity; and other responsibilities such as work, family, hobbies, mortgages, and so forth that take time and energy that could otherwise be devoted to turning into an absolute unit.

Young Lifters

I make the joke that teenagers and people in their early 20s could get some strength and muscle gains simply by walking past the gym. Young people don't need the best program, just consistent applications of the fundamentals. For the rest of us, though, it's better to avoid the temptation to max out and see how much you can lift in favor of focusing on quality training.

A big reason why you shouldn't be maxing out every day is that very heavy workouts tire you out, and that fatigue can last for a few days, affecting your ability to put out big numbers in your subsequent workouts for up to two days.[13] Some very high-intensity training workouts—perhaps involving sprinting, max height or distance jumps, or max effort strength training—could mean you need up to 72 hours to fully recover from before you can produce similar force outputs.[14] These time frames get longer the older you are. Training heavy all the time might sound good in theory, but in practice, it's a good way to just get tired. If you do this, you risk sacrificing the strength improvements you're after.

In most training programs, you might have a few phases each year where your goal is to work up to max or near-max loading. The rest of the year typically involves training at a submax level where recovery is a bit easier, allowing you to make it to your next training session and put out sufficient numbers after adequate recovery. If you achieve peak loading only once or twice a year, there's no real point in testing your max weekly because your training program isn't geared toward getting you the biggest weights until those peak phases. It's like flexing in every mirror you pass: it might be fun but it won't produce new muscle mass or strength gains. (Worse, it might make you look weird to everyone else around you.) Most people don't even really need to peak their loading, because it won't help with their goals and will just increase their risk of injury more than using submax loading. If someone isn't training to be a strength athlete or isn't looking to go through any combine testing for their sport that would require max or near-max lifts, using this tool won't be all that useful for them compared to other lifting volumes and intensities.

Additionally, if you're a strength athlete always battling fatigue from lifting too much too frequently, your training will suffer. You might find you start missing lifts you'd otherwise get easily because you haven't allowed enough time to recover; you might wind up with more muscle aches and creaks than usual; and you might not see the kind of progress you want to see.

In your younger years, your ability to bounce back from hard training is pretty remarkable. Most young lifters can do multiple heavy workouts back to back and only really start feeling the effects when they're too tired to stay up late playing video games. They don't see the benefit or even the need for mobility work because they're still bendy and elastic, so most warm-up drills are better thought of as activation or ways to ramp up force generation in preparation for hitting the weights hard. Accessory work for younger lifters can focus on hypertrophy.

Older Lifters

Lifters with a few more years of training might need a different approach. Their bones and joints tend to change shape over time[15, 16]; connective tissues tend to become more stiff, less elastic, and carry less water content[17, 18]; and tissue changes in relation to increased stress or workloads tend to take longer to get to the same endpoints, such as vascular diameter or blood effusion to working muscles.[19, 20] It takes longer to recover from true max efforts or even just heavier training volumes and loads. Older folks' warm-ups might take a bit longer as the sticky joint capsules and fascia reluctantly slide and glide, blood crawls into working muscles, and ligaments and tendons agree to stretch and manage loading more effectively. Warm-ups focused on mobility with activation work can produce enough movement to prepare the older lifter for the heavier lifts to come. Accessory work can be about conditioning, working through or around previous injuries, producing higher-volume work, and leaving the gym feeling awesome.

In addition to the physiologic differences, older lifters may have a different psychological approach to the gym. They may have accumulated more injuries over time and know how much injuries suck, so they're more hesitant to overexert for the sake of overexertion, especially if there's a higher risk than they'd like. Their goal isn't to prove they're the best but to generally get more out of their life. Understandably, this can change the calculus of how much heavy or intense work they do. While training heavy and hard is still important for lifters who are more seasoned, it's less about "all at once" and more about "as much as needed," avoiding the need for a long recovery between sessions.

Adjusting for Age

While lifters of all ages can significantly benefit from strength training, sometimes you have to adjust a few variables to make it work best for each individual. When in doubt, try to address the biggest beneficial areas to see progress first, add loading to what you can tolerate, and make sure you can differentiate between productive soreness and work that needs to be fixed or skipped entirely to avoid soreness. Use lots of variety, have some fun, and leave enough in the tank to get back to the gym for your next session.

A realistic approach for younger lifters is to make more of the work done in the moderate range with some high-intensity work and a sprinkling of lower-intensity work used for pattern development or activation drills to prepare for the more intense work. Older lifters should use more low- and moderate-intensity work, with a smattering of higher-intensity lifting for seasoning and to give them something more exciting to look forward to without smashing them in the process.

Adjusting Intensity

It's pretty easy to get sucked into the trap of loading too much weight on the bar too often. It's really hard for people to admit they need to drop a few plates from their lifts, either because their technique isn't quite what it should be or because they're just not recovering effectively. It's pretty easy to avoid this trap by employing volume and load fluctuations, paying attention to detail on exercise technique, and chasing better-quality reps rather than lifting more weight with poor form.

That being said, it's always a possibility that as you add more stress in your workouts, you'll get to a point of over-reaching or overtraining, where your ability to recover from the previous workout isn't sufficient to prepare you for the next workout, and you wind up feeling more beat up than usual, see performance decreases, and generally have lower energy or a poorer quality of life outside of the gym.

Overreaching

Overreaching is a short-term push on loading or volume; the goal is to work really hard, then go through a recovery phase so your body can adapt to the challenge and emerge with considerably higher performance outcomes. It's a common stage of training for most competitive athletes in the lead-up to competitions. Some of the signs you're in this overreaching phase might include:

- You're going through or have just completed a notable increase in training volume, frequency, intensity, or all three.
- You feel tired after a full night's sleep—not exhausted, but just like it wasn't enough.
- You need an extra cup of coffee, tea, preworkout smoothie, or energy drink to get through the day or your training for the day.
- You experience an elevated resting heart rate, menstrual irregularities, or more acne than usual.
- You require a longer warm-up to get ready for training or feel more stiffness or soreness in muscles and joints that doesn't fully dissipate during the workouts and might accumulate over the course of the week's training.

- You experience lowered cognitive function or impaired focus. You wind up forgetting simple things or have some difficulty doing routine complex tasks, although they're still manageable.
- You spend less time with friends and family or have mild mood disturbances such as irritability, anger, or depressive episodes.

Some people will have some or all these symptoms fairly regularly and some might not have any. The big indicator is that exercise workload has increased significantly, and you might be feeling less than optimal for the short period in which it's elevated. This stress is meant to shift performance upward and should be used only for short training cycles, like a week or two before testing or competition or just before a break from training such as a vacation.

Overtraining

Overtraining can occur when someone has been overreaching for longer than a few weeks and starts to see a decline in performance and health. Symptoms might include:

- Sleep disturbances, such as the inability to get to bed at a regular time and wake up at a regular time, or feeling exhausted even after a full night's sleep
- A reliance on caffeine, energy drinks, or preworkout consumption to get through a day
- Menstrual dysfunction or amenorrhea (loss of menstrual cycle), hormonal dysregulation, or skin disturbances
- Pronounced effects on mental health such as more notable and severe depressive or anxious symptoms
- Development of overuse injuries or irritation of chronic injuries affect the ability to do workouts or use desired loading or volume
- More pronounced mood disturbances. Might become more socially isolative, cranky, overfocused on exercise to the exclusion or near exclusion of other pursuits
- Comments from friends, family, or coworkers that you seem run down or "different."

This obviously can be serious. However, it can be prevented with good tracking of volume and load, making sure any increases are followed with times of lower stress and tracking how you respond to the workouts over time. If you notice any of these signs or symptoms, it's time for a deload week, a short vacation, or a look back at your programming to figure out where you might need to make some adjustments.

Cutting down on how much heavy strength work or explosive training you do in a week, or reducing high- and moderate-intensity volume would be the first place to start. You don't have to go to extremes, but maybe start with a 25 percent reduction in either high- or moderate-intensity work, see how you feel after that, and if you're still not feeling recovered or ready to train or like you're still really beat up, cut another 25 percent the following week. This would be a 50 percent reduction over 2 weeks, which should have you feeling better by the end of that time frame.

If you're feeling really tired and beat up, maybe taking a week's vacation from training would be the best option. Find something different to do: go for some walks, get out of the house and into nature, do anything that will help you recharge and you'll be able to get back into the groove after that. Severe cases might take longer than a week, and you might need some additional treatments such as massage therapy, physiotherapy, or in some cases, changes in medication. Pay attention to how you're feeling, and if you notice any of these symptoms, try to cut it off early and program in a deload, even if the program you're following wants you to push for more. Everyone is different, and what one person can handle might not be close to what another person can, so be willing to adjust as needed to keep healthy. Focus on performance and don't just push for the sake of pushing.

Conclusion

There was a ton of info in this chapter. Here's a teller (although I hope you read the whole thing!):

- Training heavy builds strength faster than using lighter weights for more reps, but in terms of strength improvements, hypertrophy benefits, and relatively less risk, you could do lighter weights for more reps and still see solid progress.

- Maxing out isn't necessary, and testing too often might leave you more frustrated and possibly broken than looking for improvements in weight for reps, reps at a given weight, or total sets each week.

- Measures such as RPE and RIR are qualitative ways to track intensity and don't require pushing to failure. Leaving a few reps in the tank while still being able to maintain technique is the best course to staying healthy and seeing solid progress.

- Use build sets for your heavier compound lifts, as both a warm-up and self-audit of how you're feeling that day, to determine whether you push hard or dial it back.

- Adding volume in terms of sets per week can help you progress your programming, but there's a volume limit to what creates progress before it turns into overtraining. Finding that sweet spot can take time and require some playing with volume adjustments, so keep a log to see what's going on.

- Deloads need to happen after big increases in volume, load, or both. They allow your connective tissue to catch up to the strain and let your nervous system recover so you can see bigger performance gains when you get back to regular volume and intensity. Don't skip these, shorten them, or throw in additional work during them, since that would defeat their entire point.

- Higher-volume days and lower-volume days throughout the week can help you use smaller bursts in intensity and volume versus getting progressively beat up through a week of consistently hard training. This helps you see better overall results than you'd get by making all workouts the same length and intensity.

- True max effort training shouldn't be your focus unless you're a strength athlete gearing up for a competition or unless you have a job that requires fitness testing with max efforts. Otherwise, the benefits of testing don't exceed the risks of max efforts. Instead, think of doing maybe one or two max effort cycles per training calendar, but only if you want that data. Otherwise, it's not really necessary.

- Younger lifters can train with a higher intensity and recover faster with suboptimal conditions compared to older lifters. As you age, you should spend more time on warm-ups and build sets and budget for more time between intense training sessions to allow better recovery and regrowth of connective tissue. Spend more time on moderate-intensity work, and work on feeling awesome when you leave the gym versus beating yourself up and needing help to get off the toilet or get out of bed.

- Signs that you're training too hard need to be picked up relatively early to give you the best chance of bouncing back quickly and effectively. When you notice you're getting too sore and not recovering effectively, start by decreasing volume by 25 percent for 1 to 2 weeks, or take a full deload week and reassess how you feel after this time away from your regular training. Be willing to reduce either volume or intensity to find your sweet spot—don't try to force yourself to do more for the sake of doing more. The name of the game is progress, not simply staying busy.

Next up, we're going to look at filling in the gaps in your program by including side quests and more specific approaches to working through some of the challenges addressed in your assessment. We'll still have the big rocks in place, but if you also need to work on shoulder mobility or figuring out your cranky knees, the side quests will help you get those suckers worked up without taking away from the main program action.

7

Level-Up and Side Quest Accessory Approaches

Growing up I played a lot of video games. All the classic Nintendo and Super Nintendo games like *Super Mario Bros.*, *Contra*, *Legend of Zelda*, *Mega Man*, *River City Ransom,* and so many more ate up way too many hours of my childhood, as they did with a lot of kids my age as well as kids today. A big aspect of many of these games was the ability to upgrade your character with things like mushrooms or stars to improve their abilities or powers, or to use as keys to finish the level you were stuck on. These upgrades let you level up your character, making the new hero miles better than when you started.

Sometimes you had to go on a side quest to learn some new information, find a cool new weapon, or upgrade your character sufficiently so that they could take on the big boss at the end of the level. Often these side quests provided some exciting new options that helped you get more enjoyment out of the game than just progressing the story or moving through the regular levels. The Grand Theft Auto series was so packed with side quests that you could easily spend a year trying them after finishing the game. The side quests were half the fun of the games, so doing cool stuff outside the normal storyline made for a way better user experience.

Along those same lines, sometimes we need to level up our "main character" in the gym, upgrade some skills or abilities before challenging the big boss (the workout), or do some side quests to acquire new information or skills that might help us down the road. Classically, isolated mobility or strength work has been called *corrective exercise*, which is a poor choice of words for these valuable opportunities. You're building strength, improving range of motion, and expanding function in parts of the body that otherwise weren't doing what they needed to do to keep up with the workouts you were hoping to put them through. It sounds like they need a mushroom or star of their own, but instead of stealing those terms from video games, I prefer to call type of work *level-up exercises.* It sounds cooler, doesn't it?

Improving a certain element in our workout, say squat strength, can be achieved by including exercises that aren't squats but have a big carryover to squat performance, like lunges or other squat variations. Returning to video games, it's easy to consider them as side quests because they're improving the ability to do the main storyline work. But we're doing it outside the main story, as an accessory exercise that helps build up a character to keep pushing the progress. A solid warm-up before the training session gets more bang for your training buck, plus it makes the rest of the workout feel easier and better. It's a win-win, so let's begin our warm-up.

What Makes a Good Warm-Up?

"I don't think I'll be able to do too much today. Everything hurts." My client who has osteoarthritis in his knees, ankles, shoulders, and back would say this before every session. He'd get on the bike and start churning his legs slowly, making his knees and ankles grind through the range of motion to gradually pump some blood through the muscles and synovial fluid through the joint spaces. Every revolution was painful, but he soldiered through.

Then we'd start with an active warm-up to convince his joints to move as much as possible, using minimal load like body weight or even no load, with just his limbs up in the air. Gradually he would attain a larger range of motion as the pain reduced, as the temperature of his tissues increased, and as fluid started moving through his muscles and bones. His joints gradually became more lubricated and movement easier to tolerate, and by the end of the warm-up he was feeling pretty good.

Once we got into some strength work, we would gradually increase the loading from one set to the next, working within a tolerable range of motion. He began to feel better and better. By the time we were on his second strength series, about 30 minutes after he walked in the door, he felt unstoppable and ready to all but destroy everything I put in front of him.

It never ceased to amaze him that the warm-up could be so productive and help him feel so much better, just by gradually increasing movement and loading within his pain tolerances and being mindful of what felt productive for him and what he could do. Some days he felt at 100 percent after the warm-up, some days he felt just "better than when we started," but each day saw a notable increase in what he could do and how much discomfort he felt from the start of the session to the end of the warm-up.

A good warm-up should do a few key things:

- Prepare the muscles, joints, and movement patterns for what you're planning to do during the workout. If you're going to smash out some big squats, your warm-up should include some ramping intensities for training the squat movement (hip, knee, and ankle flexion and extension) and the muscles involved (quads, glutes, hamstrings, and core) and gradually increase pressure or load toward what you'll be using with your workout.

- Reduce tissue level restrictions to joint movement and fluid movement through the body. This can be blood flow into and out of muscles (via some form of cardio activity to increase the blood vessel diameter and heart rate); synovial fluid movement within a joint space (loading the joints and stretching the joint capsules to promote more fluid release and get the joints gliding); and easier oxygen transport (increasing bronchial dilation and driving more blood to lung tissues to pick up oxygen and drop off carbon dioxide).

- Act as a psychological bridge between the time before training and the time devoted to more intense training. Traversing this "bridge" can help you get into the mindset needed to train effectively, and it can also shake off any apprehension to training, as it did for my client who said everything hurt before the session. It can also be a time to check in with yourself to see how things are feeling and whether any element of training might need to be adjusted.

These physiological and psychological preparations can help to reduce the likelihood of an injury during the workout as well. Preparing the body to manage load and endurance requirements can go a long way to maintaining a more beneficial level of stress on the working tissues, without a sudden sharp rise in how much stress they're under or being unprepared to handle that stress. Both situations are strong predictors of possible tissue damage outside of what would be considered normal for a workout.

It may be tempting to skip the warm-up and go right into the meat and potatoes of the strength work, but the great thing about the warm-up is to the way it boosts your performance. Put another way, this means that warm-ups help you benefit more from your actual strength or performance workouts than if you skipped them. Wouldn't you want to be able to have a better workout if you could? And maybe see some better gains along the way because of it? I thought so.

I have a simple rule when my clients come in for a session and they're late: we cut back from the end of the workout, not from the beginning. Even if pressed for time, we're still going to go through a warm-up, even if it's slightly shortened or adjusted, but we don't skip it. If anything, we just reduce a series or two from the end of the workout or cut back a set or two on the main strength work, but the warm-up is vital to getting into the rest of the workout, so it's nonnegotiable. If you're concerned about improving your mobility, motor control, and overall ability to do the more complex compound exercises you may aspire to, why wouldn't you want to dedicate a portion of your workout to helping you get into a better position for exactly that?

Some key features of effective warm-up exercises are that they get the whole body moving, generally have low force applications, and take the joints being used through big ranges of motion with gradually increasing range and force based on what the individual feels is productive as they progress from one rep to the next. If a bodyweight squat is uncomfortable at a 90-degree knee bend on the first few reps, you can stop at roughly that range of motion, and if it starts to feel better as the warm-up goes on, you can expand the range as your comfort level gradually increases. If 90 degrees is all you have, use that as much as possible.

Warm-ups themselves benefit from a brief aerobic component at their beginning—something that permits the heart rate to rise gradually, over the span of 3 to 10 minutes, with any repetitive cardio tool. After that, you could run through the active mobility and warm-up drills. Let's look at a couple of compound movements that are effective warm-ups to start your workouts.

DOWNWARD DOG, LUNGE, AND ROTATION

This exercise has two distinct phases: the downward dog position and the lunge and rotation position. Start in a hands-and-toes position with your hands under your shoulders. Push your hips up and shoulders back, trying to keep the knees straight and the heels on or as close to the ground as possible, while pushing your shoulders into an overhead position (figure 7.1a). Bend from the hips, not from the lower back, and bend only as far as your hamstring flexibility allows. Hold for a half second to a full second, then bring the hips and shoulders forward and stride forward with one foot, trying to get the foot flat to the ground outside of the hand. If your left foot is coming forward, it's going to line up just outside of your left hand. With elbows still straight, push the hips forward and down until you can feel a stretch through the opposing leg hip flexor and quad, then rotate the arm on the same side as the forward leg up in the air, turning the torso and pointing your shoulder up to the ceiling (figure 7.1b). Hold for a half to a full second, and then return the hand to the ground and the forward leg back to the starting position, and return to the downward dog position before striding forward on the opposing leg. Make sure you breathe deeply and exhale fully as you get to each paused position in the movement.

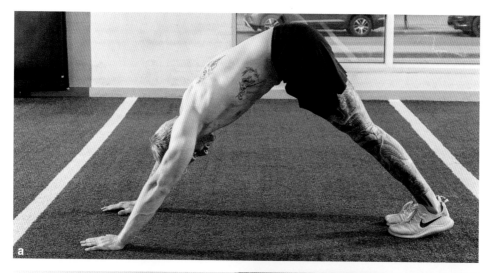

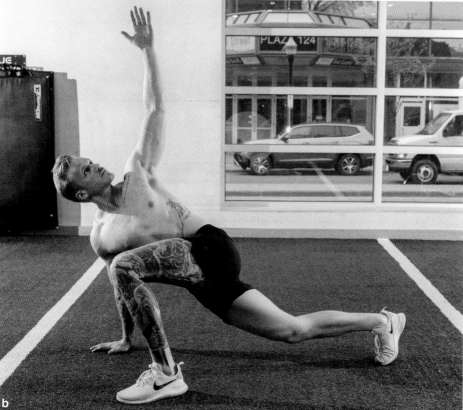

Figure 7.1 Downward dog lunge and rotation: *(a)* downward dog, *(b)* lunge and rotation.

SHIN BOX WITH PRESS-UP

From a seated position with feet approximately shoulder-width apart and knees bent, turn to one side so that both knees come down to the floor (figure 7.2*a*). If this is too difficult or you don't have the hip mobility to do this easily, place a hand on the ground behind your hips for support or sit on a block or step to reduce the hip flexion angle. Once both knees are on the ground and pointing in the same direction, push your hips forward and elevate off the ground, so the points of contact with the ground are the knees and feet (figure 7.2*b*). Press into hip extension with both hips, then lower back to the ground and rotate to the opposite side and repeat.

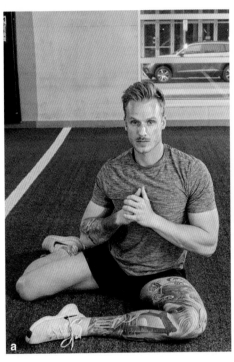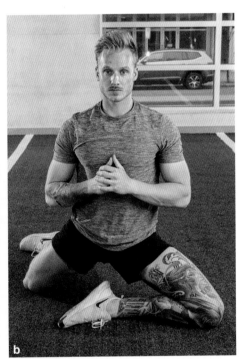

Figure 7.2 Shin box with press-up: *(a)* rotation and *(b)* press up.

LATERAL LUNGE WITH OVERHEAD DRIVER

From a standing position, take a big step out to the side, keeping the knee of the stationary leg as straight as possible. With the moving leg, bend the knee and lower into a lateral lunge as far as possible without rounding the spine or lifting the heel off the floor (figure 7.3a). At the bottom of the lunge position, drive both hands overhead as high as possible while maintaining straight elbows (figure 7.3b). Lower the hands, then return to the standing position, repeating on the opposite side.

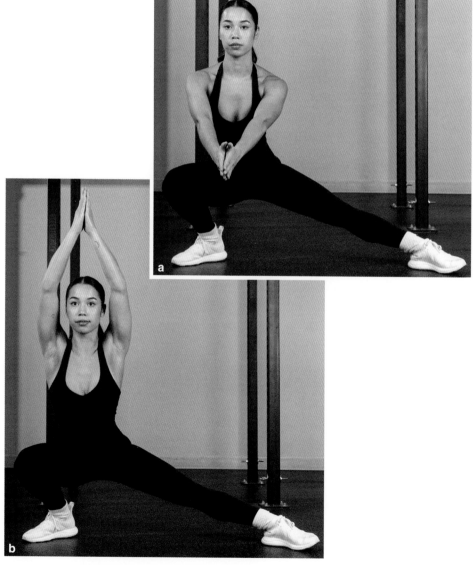

Figure 7.3 Lateral lunge with overhead driver: *(a)* step out and lunge, *(b)* finish.

PRONE HIP AND SPINE ROTATION

Lie on your belly with arms out to the sides. Lift one foot, rotating the hips and bringing the foot across the body (figure 7.4). Bring it as close as possible to the opposite hand. Let the hips and torso rotate as far as comfortable (you should feel a stretch in the pec of the nonrotating side), and bend the knee and extend the hip to bring the foot as close to the opposite hand as possible. Exhale slowly, and then return to the starting position, repeating on the opposite side. Don't push into any range of motion that is uncomfortable or painful. Go slowly enough to feel like you're getting the moving joints to easily stretch.

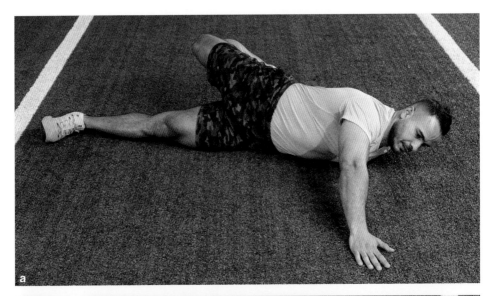

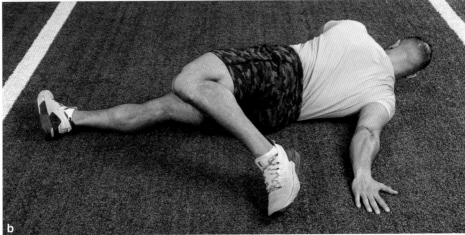

Figure 7.4 Prone hip and spine rotation: *(a)* right leg lifted and *(b)* left leg lifted.

OVERHEAD SQUAT

Standing in your preferred squat stance, hold a stick or dowel overhead with hands shoulder width apart, or wider based on your shoulder mobility and comfort (figure 7.5a). Use small wedges or plates under your heels if needed to assist in squat mobility. Squat as low as is comfortable (figure 7.5b), trying to keep the stick vertical over your feet and avoiding letting the stick move forward of your body position. Brace the abs and exhale as you rise to the starting position.

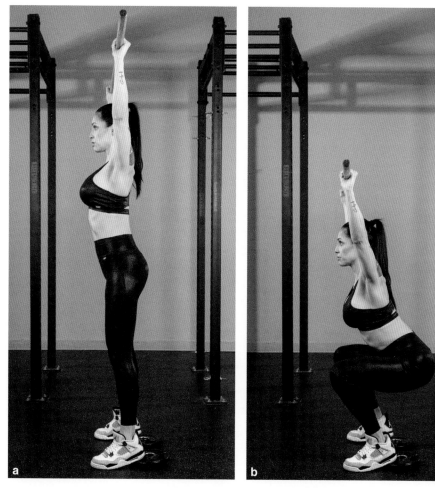

Figure 7.5 Overhead squat: *(a)* start position and *(b)* finish position.

This is a nonexhaustive list of possible movements, but doing even a brief series like this for a few sets before getting into your main workout will pay dividends in letting you move more easily and lift heavier for more reps than if you tried to go in cold.

Accessory Lifts

Similar to warm-ups, accessory work supports the main lifts but can be performed later in the workout. The benefit of accessory work is primarily that you spend some time on elements of the main efforts that might need a little more attention or that could benefit from a different angle or different equipment, ranges of motion, planes of action, or any combination of these. These are the side quests for your workout video game player 1 (you) and completing them can help to upgrade your skills for the levels to come, plus give you some sweet rewards, such as stronger and more aesthetic muscles, better work endurance, and improved joint stability in different ranges of motion.

For example, let's consider someone who wants to support their bench press. They could include some incline dumbbell presses to train the clavicular head of the pec muscle as well as tax the triceps and anterior delts a bit differently, then work on triceps press-downs to isolate triceps strength better than they could by just doing bench presses. These exercises directly benefit the main exercise in discussion and can fill in some of the gaps that the main exercise can't quite reach.

Accessory exercises are also the best way to increase moderate and higher-intensity volume in a program because they can be done for more reps and more sets without degradation to form. A back squat tends to wear an individual out faster than a split squat in terms of total loading and number of reps they can complete before fatigue affects the quality of the reps. Another set of a single-leg deadlift tends to be easier to complete than another set of barbell deadlifts as well, so pushing volume increases during build phases can be accomplished more easily with more accessory work. They're definitely a valuable tool to seeing the progressive overload you want.

Level-Up Exercises

Any level-up exercise should focus on gaining new skills or abilities that can be useful for getting after all the other fun stuff you want to do in the gym. Often this means improving joint-specific and direction-specific mobility, active control in specific ranges of motion, and localized strength in certain muscles or in muscles held at certain positions. An example would be someone who is weak through their lower back when pulling a deadlift off the floor. The level-up requirements are to strengthen the lower back to prevent it from rounding as soon as the bar begins to leave the floor and make it strong enough to hold that position from the start to the finish of the rep. Thus, the requirements of those level-up exercises would be anything that makes the muscles of the spine maintain position as either gravity or another external force (resistance of free weight, cable, band, etc.) tries to pull the spine into flexion or anything that helps build strength of the spine as it moves into extension.

Once those skills have leveled up, you're ready to go after the main quest again with new tools to help you be successful. You might have to revisit these level-up drills on occasion to maintain your abilities and keep your power meter on full, but their purpose is to give you the ability to do the harder stuff. Once you're there, you should be able to rock out with just occasional time spent working on those components.

A cool part of level-up and side quest drills is that they can be done daily, as skill development, and might require only minimal equipment, bodyweight positions, or stretches to get the job done. They make it easy to gain some low- and moderate-intensity volume through the week and keep your skills sharp.

Progressions and Regressions

Level-up and side quest drills come in two primary flavors: progressions and regressions. A progression is a way to make an exercise more challenging so it's appropriately difficult and beneficial. A regression is a way of reducing the challenge of the exercise to make it a better fit for an individual just learning the exercise or just beginning a program. Examples of progressions include increasing the amount of loading, changing the lever arm length, or changing the base of support to introduce a balance challenge. Examples of regressions are reducing the motor skill requirement of the exercise, reducing the number of moving parts, shortening the range of motion, or increasing the base of support to reduce the balance challenge.

The purpose of progressions and regressions is to find the right balance of challenge and competency so that the individual doing them can get the best benefits. This means not doing a drill that's too easy or too challenging. To get the full reward from the drill, an exercise should be challenging enough to make you use your mind and your muscles to complete the given number of reps but reasonable enough for you to do all the reps properly throughout the set. Progressions and regressions allow you to tailor the drill to your ability.

Breaking Down Complex Skills

One way to get a level-up benefit is to break down more complex movements into more manageable chunks, such as working on hip mobility to accomplish a better squat position or improving ankle stability for jumping and running. (We'll be addressing this later in the chapter. Working on segments or individual components of more complex skills makes them easier to learn while also focusing on areas that otherwise might compensate for a lack of motor control, strength, or mobility to do the desired exercise effectively. Putting all the pieces of a squat or deadlift together is a sophisticated act of coordination of the moving parts, muscles, and timing, so stepping back and working on less complicated or individual aspects can go a long way.

With upper-body movements, because of the complexity of thoracic extension, scapular upward rotation, humeral external rotation, and timing involved through each movement in conjunction with the other moving parts, using some regressed level-up drills can help improve an individual's ability to get into an overhead position more effectively compared to just hammering at overhead work and expecting those elements to improve as a part of the work being done. If the thoracic spine doesn't extend enough, the shoulder blades will be tilted forward and have difficulty going through proper upward rotation. The end result of this is a shoulder joint that doesn't move into an overhead position effectively and can pinch the supraspinatus tendon between the acromion on the shoulder and the humerus, the result being a sore shoulder and even a rotator cuff tear with enough use or pressure. You might be able to work through it for a while, but the risk is higher if the thoracic spine isn't moving the way it should to get into a better position for that overhead movement. We'll cover thoracic and shoulder movements in this chapter as well.

In some people the limited thoracic spine extension doesn't beat up the rotator cuff, but instead they wind up with a reduced range of motion, so the overhead press looks more like an "in front of the head" press. Maybe you find that overhead position by just extending your lower back, but you develop a sore lower back after a few reps. Each scenario means you're not getting the most benefit from the exercise, so improving thoracic spine mobility helps in that regard and poses fewer risks along the way.

Spending time on thoracic spine extension, using that extension to gain better control of scapular movement, and then using that to push into a more effective overhead position pays off big time. Building strength through the muscles that control these movements can help you to maintain those ranges of motion and positions when it comes to loading up an overhead press or other challenging movement. By working on motor control through those segments, you make them more resilient to challenging loads and volumes, since over time as they've had that training and now "know" what they should be doing. Those individual building blocks moving better, lining up better, and holding their positions more effectively are at the crux of what successful compound strength needs, so doing them is kind of an important thing that can't be skipped if you want to see progress and stay healthy in the gym.

Leveling Up Like Super Mario

In chapter 2, we identified a few key elements that affect how you go through your workouts. Things like joint mobility challenges, gross pattern aptitude, and localized strength issues might make bigger lifts less effective or downright detrimental. To find success with those exercises and within the program overall, we need to tailor the level-up approach you'll be using to your specific situation. Just as Mario needs the mushroom to challenge bigger opponents or jump higher, or needs the star to run roughshod through a series of goombahs, you need to upgrade your skills to find success and complete your own challenge.

Let's say you have limited ankle mobility. Logically, we would want to improve ankle mobility with ankle-focused level-up drills. We could still get some benefits from improving other regions, but in terms of biggest return for the time spent, the ankles would be the best place to work on until they're improved enough to retest successfully.

Similarly, if you find your performance limited during some of the gross pattern work, we might have to regress key movements to find success. For instance, in the example of tight ankles, if your squat was more of a hip hinge because of the limited movement, you might need to squat with a heel wedge to find that missing range of motion and make the squat fit your abilities. This is technically a regression, albeit one where you can find an easier position in which to work without secondary movements or compensatory patterns. Some people just don't have the joints or range of motion to complete certain movements, or maybe injury or age-related changes have made it next to impossible to do them without pain or problems, so using a regression on the gross pattern is their new way of getting the job done. Use regressions as needed for as long as needed.

Now if you went through the assessments and found no issues, you can still benefit from using some of the level-up drills as maintenance to keep that range of motion and motor control through the long term. A sprinkling of them here and there will go a long way to keep up those abilities as you age, so don't forget to use them on a semiregular basis. They won't be a big requirement to accessing the bigger lifts if you're already able to get into them, but will still be beneficial over time.

One thing I've encountered a lot in my career of working with people looking to improve their fitness or recover from some sort of injury is the belief that a program has to be super hard to be effective. Often people will say that a program isn't intense enough for them or isn't advanced enough, lacking new, exciting, challenging exercises. To be clear, these are usually people who haven't seen much progress in their fitness because they do a hard workout and get injured, burn out, or give up after a workout or two specifically because it's too difficult or too advanced for them to get the benefits they're after. Many of the most advanced lifters tend to pare their workouts back over time, focusing on ruthless efficiency and laser-like focus to perfect the basics rather than mixing things up all the time and throwing every variable at the wall to see what sticks. Their workouts become as basic as basic can be, yet they see progress over time. Weird how that works.

The goal of any program is to give *enough* stress to see positive adaptations. To get this stress, it's important to do the prescribed exercises properly. If you have trouble performing the movement well, use a regression to get into the right zone to see the benefits you're after. A big challenge with this is similar to workout complexity: people seem to think they're more advanced than they are and that they should be able to do every exercise perfectly right out of the gate. Never mind that some of these skills have to be honed effectively for a few decades for really experienced lifters to feel like they're doing them well. I've been lifting weights for close to 30 years and feel like I'm just starting to get the hang of it. I still have elements to improve and I still find limitations I have to keep working on.

Stepping outside your ego and making an unemotional decision about what will give you the best results lets you view regressions and progressions more realistically versus letting your emotions decide whether or not you'll force yourself to do an exercise that doesn't fit your abilities. Often this can be done with a simple (and totally unemotional) algorithm that can help make these decisions for you. Anything that helps to point you in the right direction can be massively useful and can be repeated, scaled, and easily deployed when needed.

We could even go through a simplified checklist for determining whether to proceed with the more complex compound strength work, whether to work in a regression (and if so, which one), and also whether to spend more time on level-up exercises to help unlock the ability to do the more complex work down the road.

Consider a regression as a different way of doing things. It's no better or worse, just different. It can let you focus on one or two key elements of a movement without all the movement complexity or dynamic demands, and help you improve your abilities with those elements before returning to the initial task. It's meant to simplify the application. It doesn't make the exercise less beneficial, just easier to get the benefits you're after.

The checklists shown in figures 7.6 and 7.7 take the mobility assessments from chapter 2 and build some of the functions you'll include in your own workouts. The goal is to tell you exactly what you'll need to work on to get the best results, set you up for success with a broad range of exercises, and outline whether certain exercises or movements will need a regression so that you can see the best benefits given your own unique abilities.

CHECKLIST

Bracing Strength Assessment: Leg Lowering Test (p. 31)

Your score _____

    Low core strength: 70 to 90 degrees from the floor

    Moderate core strength: 40 to 70 degrees from the floor

    High core strength: <40 degrees from the floor

Bracing Strength Assessment: Hollow-Body Hold Test (p. 33)

Your score _____

    Poor core endurance: Hold position for <30 seconds

    Moderate core endurance: Hold position for 30 to 59 seconds

    Excellent core endurance: Hold position for >60 seconds

Hip Flexion Assessment: Lying Knee to Chest (p. 36)

Your score _____

    Poor hip flexion ROM: Can't get knee to abdomen, regardless of rotation

    Moderate hip flexion ROM: Can get knee to abdomen with some hip rotation

    Excellent hip flexion ROM: Can easily get knee to abdomen

Ankle Dorsiflexion Assessment: Half-Kneeling Ankle Dorsiflexion Wall Test (p. 38)

Your score _____

    Poor ankle mobility: Can't get knee to wall without heel lifting or arch collapsing

    Moderate ankle mobility: Can get knee to wall with toes <4 inches from wall

    Excellent ankle mobility: Can get knee to wall with toes >4 inches from wall

Thoracic Extension Assessment: Prone Press-Up (p. 40)

Your score _____

    Poor thoracic spine ROM: Can't extend elbows without hips coming off the floor

    Moderate thoracic spine ROM: Can extend elbows and keep hips on the floor, but hands need to be moved forward and low back arches excessively

    Excellent thoracic spine ROM: Can fully extend elbows and keep hips on the ground without alterations

Shoulder Mobility Assessment: Overhead Test Against a Wall (p. 42)

Your score _____

    Poor shoulder ROM: Can't keep low back on floor or touch hands to the floor

    Moderate shoulder ROM: Can touch hands to floor, but elbows have to bend, thumbs have to separate, or lower back lifts off the floor

    Excellent shoulder ROM: Can touch hands to floor without elbows bending, thumbs separating, or lower back lifting off the floor

Figure 7.6 Mobility assessments and scoring.

CHECKLIST

Bracing Strength Assessment: Leg Lowering Test (p. 31)

If low core strength (70 to 90 degrees from the floor):

- Do any drills from chapter 5. Practice breathing with bracing.
- Avoid heavy strength work. Compound movements can be done with loads within technical fatigue limits.

If moderate core strength (40 to 70 degrees from the floor):

- Do any drills from chapter 5.
- Avoid loading outside of technical fatigue limits.

If high core strength (<40 degrees from the floor):

- Do any drills from chapter 5.
- Avoid nothing.

Bracing Strength Assessment: Hollow-Body Hold Test (p. 33)

If poor core endurance (hold position for <30 seconds):

- Do static hold exercises (planks) from chapter 5. Work on increasing duration of hold.
- Avoid loaded drills outside of technical fatigue or endurance exercises under loading.

If moderate core endurance (hold position for 30 to 59 seconds):

- Do static hold exercises (planks) from chapter 5. Work on increasing duration of hold.
- Avoid loaded drills outside of technical fatigue.

If excellent core endurance (hold position for >60 seconds):

- Do any drills from chapter 5.
- Avoid nothing.

Hip Flexion Assessment: Lying Knee to Chest (p. 36)

If poor hip flexion ROM (can't get knee to abdomen, regardless of rotation):

- Do quadruped posterior hip stretch, goblet pry stretch, and hip level-up drills.
- Avoid squats, cleans, snatches, pistol squats, and single-leg squats.

If moderate hip flexion ROM (can get knee to abdomen with some hip rotation):

- Do hip level-up drills.
- Avoid squats, cleans, snatches, pistol squats, and single-leg squats into end range positions.

If excellent hip flexion ROM (can easily get knee to abdomen):

- Do any or all hip drills as needed.
- Avoid nothing.

Figure 7.7 Actions based on mobility assessments and scoring.

Ankle Dorsiflexion Assessment: Half-Kneeling Ankle Dorsiflexion Wall Test (p. 38)

If poor ankle mobility (can't get knee to wall without heel lifting or arch collapsing):
- Do toe-to-wall soleus stretch and ankle level-up drills.
- Avoid squats, cleans, snatches, lunges, step-ups, pistol squats, and single-leg squats.

If moderate ankle mobility (can get knee to wall with toes <4 inches from wall):
- Do ankle level-up drills.
- Avoid squats, cleans, snatches, lunges, step-ups, pistol squats, and single-leg squats into end range positions.

If excellent ankle mobility (can get knee to wall with toes >4 inches from wall):
- Do ankle level-up drills as needed.
- Avoid nothing.

Thoracic Extension Assessment: Prone Press-Up (p. 40)

If poor thoracic spine ROM (can't extend elbows without hips coming off the floor):
- Do weighted thoracic extension on roller, thoracic spine level-up drills.
- Avoid military press, push press, jerks, handstands, front squats, cleans, snatches.

If moderate thoracic spine ROM (can extend elbows and keep hips on the floor but hands need to be moved forward and lower back arches excessively):
- Do thoracic spine level-up drills.
- Avoid military press, push press, jerks, handstands, front squats, cleans, and snatches into end ranges.

If excellent thoracic spine ROM (can fully extend elbows and keep hips on the ground without alterations):
- Do thoracic spine level-up drills as needed.
- Avoid nothing.

Shoulder Mobility Assessment: Overhead Test Against a Wall (p. 42)

If poor shoulder ROM (can't keep lower back on floor or touch hands to floor):
- Do close grip chin-up stretch, feet on wall dumbbell pull-over on roller, shoulder flexion level-up drills.
- Avoid miliary press, push press, jerks, handstands, front squats, cleans, snatches.

If moderate shoulder ROM (can touch hands to floor but elbows have to bend, thumbs have to separate, or lower back lifts off the floor):
- Do shoulder flexion level-up drills.
- Avoid military press, push press, jerks, handstands, front squats, cleans, and snatches into end ranges.

If excellent shoulder ROM (can touch hands to floor without elbows bending, thumbs separating, or lower back lifting off the floor):
- Do shoulder flexion level-up drills as needed.
- Avoid nothing.

Figure 7.7 *(continued)*

Keep in mind that getting to a specific exercise or graduating past the level-up or accessory work shouldn't be the goal. The goal is to get the best training stimulus you can, which means you might need to stick with certain variations of exercises for the long term and might have to skip certain other variations because they just don't work for you or aren't ones you can successfully do to a minimum technical proficiency. We all have limits, and as much as I might want to do something cool like contortionist training, even their most basic requirements would likely cripple me because I'm just not built to do that specific thing. In fact if you ever see me doing anything that resembles a back bridge or pancake splits, please do me a favor and call for an ambulance because something has gone horribly wrong in my life.

Doing a squat with a heel wedge or pulling a deadlift from some small blocks versus off the floor is a small switch to allow for the training volume and intensity within your technical and physical abilities that creates the progress you want to see. It's not a lower-quality exercise, it just adjusts a variable to make it more effective for you. The result is going to be the same: you'll get the training stress you want without putting yourself into a disadvantageous position that might cause more problems than it would fix.

Once you figure out what needs work, whether you need mobility, stabilization, regressions, or some combination of those, you can add the exercises for those characteristics into your workouts, do a few months of training, and then retake the assessment to see if you've had any changes in your potential limitations. If you haven't, that's fine; just stay the course and keep working. Sometimes physiological changes are slow, especially if the limit is something like a joint shape or capsule tightness, or if change is fighting a competing demand from some occupational requirement or other lifestyle consideration. Not seeing fast progress in certain things doesn't mean you're not working toward something good, it just means it might take more time than you thought it would, so be patient.

If there have been positive changes, that's awesome, and you can adjust accordingly by adjusting which level-up exercises, regressions, or progressions you keep in your training program. Occasionally you can see some fast progress in a few movements with some good cueing, waking up some different muscles, and building some practice in certain movements. These rapid changes are more about improving the motor program driving those movements or joint capacities, which can sometimes be seen within a single training block and even possibly within a single training session for some.

Once you've run through the checklist, figured out what level-up exercises and regressions or progressions to plug into your workouts, trained your butt off for a training cycle, retake the assessment and adjust the drills for the following cycle. This new cycle might be different from the previous one based on the changes resulting from the previous cycle, which is the entire point of training. As you progress, the workouts should adjust to allow you to continue seeing progress versus being the same all the time or changing so frequently that you can't track progress over time. Progress might normally be measured in how much weight you lift or how far you run, but another good metric is whether you're seeing any improvements in how well you can move your different joints and whether you're crushing your ability to perform complex motor skills with better precision and efficiency.

With each of these assessments, the first result (low) shows a region that needs more mobility to successfully perform exercises associated with it; the second result (moderate) shows a region that could benefit from some regular mobility training to maintain or slightly improve range of motion to keep those exercises available; and the third result (high) shows regions with no restrictions on the exercises available. For any regions in which you check the first result, you can include the daily stretches outlined in chapter 2 along with the assessments, as well as the mobility drills within the workouts themselves. For regions in which you check the second result, doing the mobility within the workouts would be a good choice and sufficient for most. For any regions in which you checked the third result, there's no specific requirement to doing mobility work, but it would be good to train for long-term maintenance, and there's no limit to the exercises you're able to go through.

If you complete the test and find a region-specific limit, include the mobility drill and daily stretch for that region into your workouts and scale back the exercises that require the full mobility from that region. If you have no limit to that region, you fist pump and party on with the unscaled exercises as you see fit, working on mobility drills as more maintenance versus a need to see bigger ranges of motion. After training for a few months, reassess that region, and if you've seen progress you can adjust your workouts accordingly. If movement into certain ranges of motion is uncomfortable or painful, refer to chapters 1 and 8 to figure out what's going on and how to adjust training to keep you in the game or to know whether to consult a medical professional for a deeper evaluation.

The level-up drills will be outlined later in this chapter, and the good thing is you don't need to do all of them all the time but can pick and choose which ones you want to play with as you go through the programming. It would be a good idea to switch between different ones to allow some variety and keep things interesting instead of doing the same drill every time you work out.

If you're scoring in the poor categories, try to do the level-up drills in each workout. If you're in the moderate categories, rotating the joint-specific work at least once a week is recommended, and more if possible, but make sure you get all the spots at some point each week.

Mobility Level-Up Drills

The following section outlines how we prefer to address specific mobility limitations you might have found with the assessment. The big key to consider here is we're not doing a lot of static stretching, which has a strong place in a lot of programs. Rather we're opting for more active range-of-motion drills that not only improve site-specific mobility but allow you to train the structure as well as the motor pattern that might be limiting your ability to access those ranges. What's more, you can sprinkle them throughout the workout without compromising strength or power. Static stretching still plays a role, but it's not the entire program.

All right, let's talk about level-up drills. When you went through the assessment you identified key regions of the body (ankles, hips, thoracic spine, or shoulders) that might have limited mobility and that might affect your ability to get the best results from your workouts, so now we're going to show you some of the best methods to boost your mobility for those tasks.

When performing any of these level-up drills, a key concept to think about is trying to maximize tension and muscle activity into the end ranges of each rep. A static stretch is fine if you enjoy just hanging out on the end of a muscle, but you can see some significantly larger mobility increases by getting into that stretch end range position, and then contracting a muscle to either pull deeper into the range of motion or move out of that range of motion.

A good example is a simple standing quad stretch (figure 7.8). Standing tall, grab the top of one foot and bring the heel to your butt, trying to keep the knee pointing toward the floor. You should feel a stretch through the front of your thigh. Once you're in this position, contract the hamstring as if you're trying to get the heel closer to your butt and then hold that contraction for 5 to 10 seconds. Once you release the hamstring contraction, contract the quad as if you're trying to straighten your knee. Hold this contraction for another 5 to

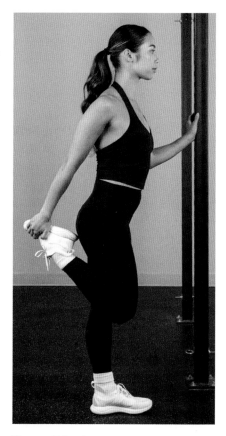

Figure 7.8 Standing quad stretch.

10 seconds, and then release the leg and try to walk out any cramps that may have occurred along the way.

This contractile element during a static hold can be an easy way to upgrade any mobility drill, even ones that aren't held in one position for any length of time. When you get into an end range position, contract associated muscles to squeeze a little extra range of motion out of the movement. The muscle contraction into that range of motion has a few important benefits. First, it puts a bit more tension into the position and can help to stretch out some of the tissues that are involved in the movement, rather than just settling into it. Second, the contractile element can help to train the neural input into the muscle, thus improving active range of motion more than static stretches would. Training the nerve to more effectively contract the muscle while in that range of motion will make it easier to use that range later. Third, using the contraction makes the movement feel more intense, meaning you're less likely to get bored and skip it, plus it might give you some fun delayed-onset soreness the following day, so it will feel more productive than just easy stretching.

The more frequently you can train mobility, the faster it's going to improve for you. Making it a part of your day—or, at the very least, a component of every workout—ensures it gets done. Think of it like brushing your teeth: you don't want to wait until a medical professional tells you it's something you should have been doing all this time because now here you are with tight muscles and joints and really bad breath. Ignoring or underutilizing mobility training is the best way to stay exactly where you are and see no progress, so making sure you're diligent and consistent at getting into those end ranges can be a great way to see improvements.

Let's jump into some of the region-specific level-up drills.

Ankle Level-Up Drills

Why do you need ankle mobility when the movement for most of the exercises you're looking to do will predominantly come from the hips and knees? A major reason is that there should be some forward movement from the shin (tibia) during movements like a lunge, squat, or jump, and not having that movement come from the ankle limits the overall mobility of the movement. If the knee can't move forward on a movement like the squat, it's harder to keep your center of mass over your base of support, and you might wind up shifting your weight back and feel like you're losing your balance. This will artificially limit the depth you can get to on a squat, which limits your performance on the exercise. At the end of the day, it's a pretty important part of the process, so we don't want to overlook it. In reality, we want to get as much from it as possible, so let's jump into the specific drills.

KNEELING ACTIVE ANKLE ROCKBACK

From a half-kneeling position, lean on your forward thigh to add loading to the position. Keeping some tension through the arch of the foot, slowly lean forward to flex the ankle, making sure you aren't letting the arch collapse to gain more range of motion, and making sure the kneecap tracks in line with the middle toe (figure 7.9a). Move into ankle flexion as far as possible without letting the arch fall or the heel lift off the floor, then actively lift the toes and ball of the foot off the ground in the end range position. Maintain this tension and slowly rock back (figure 7.9b), trying to maintain the ankle flexion angle as you pull the knee back from over the toes. The goal is to maintain the angle that you can get into passively by leaning your weight on your leg with the angle you can maintain while rocking back and actively trying to pull the ball of the foot up as high as possible.

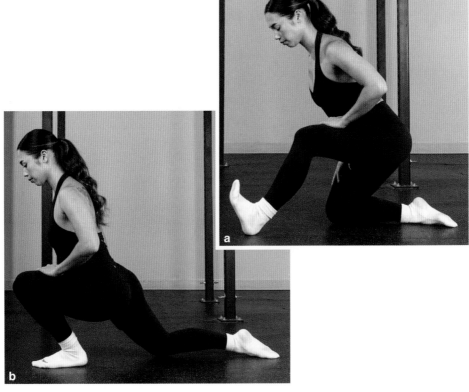

Figure 7.9 Kneeling active ankle rockback: *(a)* lean forward, *(b)* lift toes and rock back.

ECCENTRIC HEEL DROP

Stand with the ball of your foot on a slightly elevated surface such as a weight plate, 2 × 4, or low step. Rise on the ball of the foot as high as possible to squeeze the calf muscle, then slowly lower, trying to get the heel as low as possible below the ball of the foot (figure 7.10). Hold in the bottom stretched position for a full second. Ideally, do this on one foot, not both, but if you don't feel you have the calf strength to do it with one foot, two is fine. Start close to something you can hold on to for balance assistance throughout the exercise.

GOBLET SQUAT WITH LATERAL ROCK

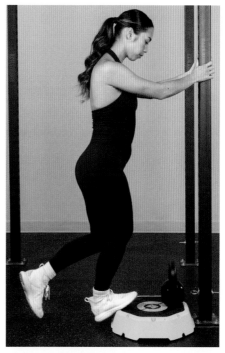

Figure 7.10   Eccentric heel drop.

Hold a light-to-moderate weight dumbbell at your chest in a goblet position. Squat as low as possible without letting your low back round or letting your heels lift off the ground. At the bottom of your squat, shift your hips over one ankle and let the knee move ahead of the foot as much as possible (figure 7.11a), then shift your weight over the other foot (figure 7.11b) and return to standing. Throughout the set, try to maintain the foot arch.

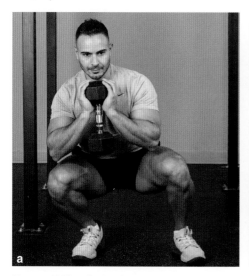
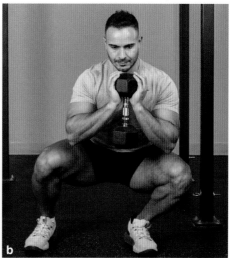

Figure 7.11   Goblet squat lateral rock: (a) squat and (b) lateral rock.

Hip Flexion Level-Up Drills

All the power for most athletic movements comes from hip extension. However, it's getting into hip flexion that allows hip extension. Without enough hip flexion range of motion, it's difficult to get into a bottom squat position, control the core and pelvis to generate tension to drive up, and to do something simple like sit on the floor without feeling like your back might explode. Training hip flexion directly is often overlooked but should still get some regular love within your program, even if you can squat without feeling any restrictions. Those muscles play a role in your strength development, so let's get them fired up.

WALL-SUPPORTED KNEE TO CHEST

Stand with your back against the wall and feet slightly forward from the wall. Ensure you have little to no flexion through the lower back. Bend one knee and bring the knee toward your chest as far as possible without letting your lower back round or letting your back leave the wall (figure 7.12). Ideally you should be getting the knee above the height of your belly button. If you can't do this active movement with a straight spine and your back against the wall, practice by sitting on a riser or yoga block to reduce the hip flexion requirements and over time you can progress to sitting on the floor.

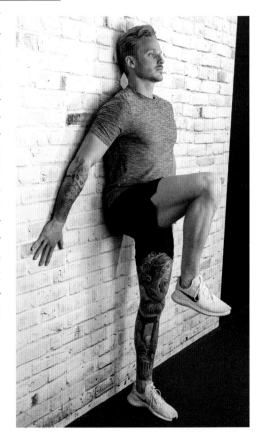

Figure 7.12 Wall-supported knee to chest.

HALF-KNEELING HIP FLEXION

Begin in a half-kneeling position with something you can hang onto for balance. Brace the core, keeping your torso tall, and try to raise the forward foot as high as possible off the ground (figure 7.13), making sure you aren't shifting your hips or rounding your lower back to get the knee higher. Squeeze the hip flexor hard in the top position for a full second and return to the ground. Complete desired number of reps and then repeat on the other side.

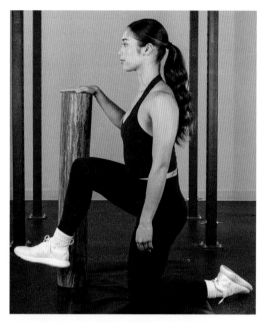

Figure 7.13   Half-kneeling hip flexion.

SUPPORTED SQUAT HIP PRY

Using the squat rack as a hand support, sink into the bottom of your squat, making sure you aren't letting your lower back round and trying not to hang back off your hands. Your weight should be in the middle of your feet with your hands holding on to assist your balance as you move into the bottom position. Try to press your knees out as wide as possible in the bottom of the squat position (figure 7.14), using your elbows to press out on the inside of your knees if needed. Complete all reps before returning to the standing position.

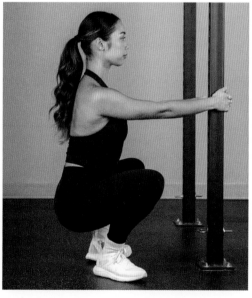

Figure 7.14   Supported squat hip pry.

Thoracic Spine Level-Up Drills

The thoracic spine is the foundation for the shoulder blade and shoulder joint, so if you can move it freely, your shoulder blade will also be able to move freely, much more so than if the thoracic spine was stiff and rigid. Finding sufficient thoracic extension and rotation is a challenging process for many, given how much time we spend sitting, staring at a computer screen, or looking down at our phones. We lock into flexion and lose extension over time, so we should try to improve shoulder blade rotation and overhead shoulder positioning in order to gain a new range of motion that will be useful for any overhead movements. Besides, more extension tends to make your posture look better and make you look more jacked, so of all the mobility work you could do, this one has the most aesthetic payoff in daily life. Time to get those ribs moving!

KNEELING BENCH THORACIC SPINE STRETCH

Kneel in front of a bench. Place your elbows on the bench and sit back into your hips so that you can lower your head between your shoulders, ideally below the height of the bench (figure 7.15). With your elbows on the bench, either clasp your hands together or hold a stick with palms facing toward you at roughly shoulder-width apart. Sit back and lower your shoulders as far as possible to get the biggest stretch possible from the lats, shoulders, and thoracic spine. When in the bottom position, try to inhale and exhale by expanding your ribs laterally as much as possible, and lightly press your elbows down into the bench through the stretch. Return to starting position after the number of breath reps have been completed.

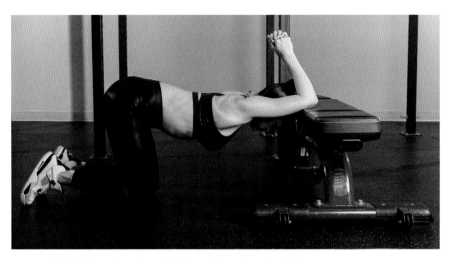

Figure 7.15 Kneeling bench thoracic spine stretch.

HALF-KNEELING WALL THORACIC SPINE ROTATION

Assume a half-kneeling position beside a wall, hands together and pointing out from your chest. Keeping your hip against the wall, turn the head and shoulders away from the wall, opening your arms (figure 7.16). Try to keep your hip against the wall. Keep your elbows pulled back and turn the ribs as far as possible on the pelvis, exhaling at the end range position. Return to the starting position. Complete the set and then switch sides.

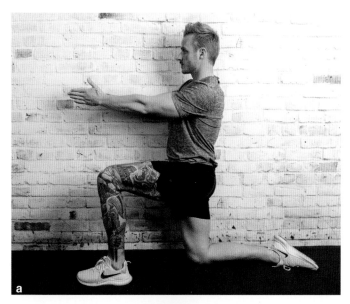

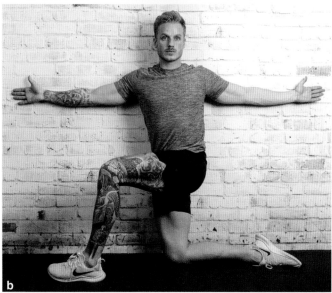

Figure 7.16 Half-kneeling wall thoracic spine rotation: *(a)* start and *(b)* finish.

SPHINX ARM SLIDE

Lying on your belly with your arms under your shoulders and hands pointing forward over your head, press up to your elbows so your back is extended (figure 7.17a). In this position, you'll look like the Sphinx, so try to be majestic. Try to press the shoulders down away from your ears, and maintain an active tension between and below the shoulder blades to hold you in this position. Slowly reach an arm out, away from your starting position, along the floor (figure 7.17b). Don't sink into the supporting shoulder or rotate the torso to find more range of motion. Now slide the arm back to the starting position and reset from any positional change that may have happened. Keep your neck long and stay pressed up through the shoulders. Alternate arms on each rep.

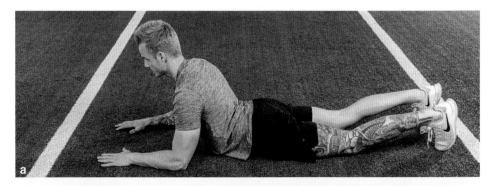

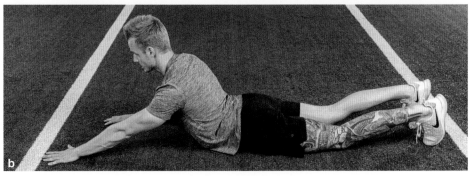

Figure 7.17 Sphinx arm slide: *(a)* start position and *(b)* slide arm.

Shoulder Level-Up Drills

After we've built the foundation of thoracic mobility, we have to build all of the downstream movements for the shoulder blades and shoulder joint itself to help you get more from the workouts and regain that overhead movement. The shoulder blade itself is a pretty complex device that moves in a bunch of different directions, so getting more movement variability out of it can help direct where the shoulder goes more effectively, and help reduce the stress on the shoulder joint to complete the exercises you're looking to smash out. Once the shoulder can move effectively, the shoulder joint can direct force more effectively and not demolish your rotator cuffs in the process. Hands up if you're ready for some shoulder shenanigans.

WALL SHOULDER SLIDE AND LIFT-OFF

Face a wall. Start with your forearms on the wall and feet staggered so you can brace the abs and not let the lower back arch as you do the movement (figure 7.18a). Slowly slide the hands up the wall (figure 7.18b), letting the forearms come off the wall as you go higher, making sure you aren't arching through the lower back to get higher up the wall. Once your elbows are straight, try to maintain your torso positioning and pull the hands off the wall into an overhead position (figure 7.18c). If this movement seems very difficult, slide your hands up the wall in a wider angle versus straight up overhead. Once the hands are off the wall, return them to the wall and slide down, repeat-

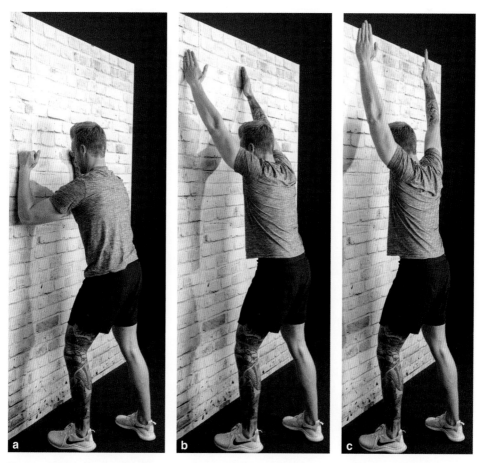

Figure 7.18 Wall shoulder slide and lift-off: *(a)* start position, *(b)* slide forearms, and *(c)* overhead position.

ing for the given number of reps. When doing this drill, think not only of sliding the hands up but also of pressing the hands into the wall and trying to get the shoulder blades to scoop forward and push the hands up from underneath. This focus on shoulder blade rotation can make getting into overhead positions much easier.

DUMBBELL PULL-OVER

Set one dumbbell on a bench for easier loading and unloading. Begin with your feet on the ground and shoulders on the bench with your torso at a 90-degree angle to the bench so that your hips are unsupported and maintaining a bridge position. Grab the dumbbell with both hands and bring it over your chest, keeping your elbows as straight as possible (figure 7.19*a*). Brace the core and start to reach your arms overhead, stretching the shoulders into flexion as far as

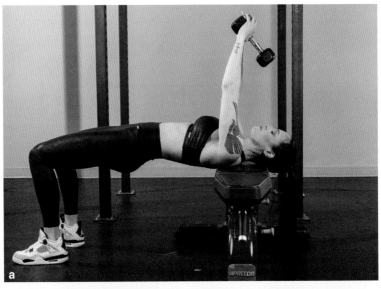

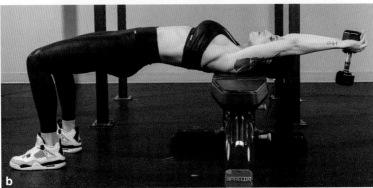

Figure 7.19 Dumbbell pull-over: *(a)* start position and *(b)* arms overhead.

comfortable (figure 7.19*b*). Come back to the starting position and repeat. Use a weight that allows you to get the biggest stretch possible without feeling like it's pulling you into an uncomfortable position. This might be fairly light to start, but remember, this is a mobility drill and not a max-effort loading exercise.

INCLINE BENCH Y RAISE

Lie face down on a bench on a mild incline (30 to 45 degrees, depending on how your bench adjusts). Lift your head and chest slightly off the bench, but don't arch high. Focusing on the shoulder blades, tilt the shoulders back and down, letting the arms raise up in a Y position in front of you, until they're at least parallel to the floor (figure 7.20). If you can raise the arms high enough to be in line with

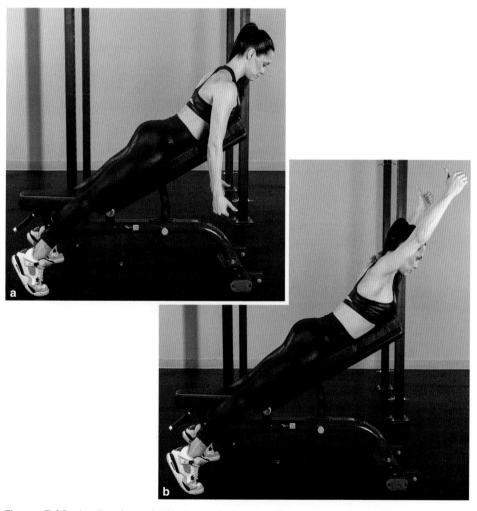

Figure 7.20 Incline bench Y raise: *(a)* start position and *(b)* Y position.

your torso, that's awesome, but don't do it if it means you're using your neck or feeling like your upper traps are doing all the work. Try to maintain a relatively soft neck through the rep. If these feel way too easy for you, and you can tell you're doing them perfectly, you could grab a couple small dumbbells to use during the movement, but for most people using just arm weight is enough to get what they need from the movement.

These level-up drills are definitely not exhaustive of all the possibilities that could help you get into better positions to dominate your main lifts and keep healthy as long as possible, but they do cover a lot of ground toward that outcome. These drills can accomplish a lot in a very short time but are still fairly general, meaning if you need something more specific it would still be worthwhile to connect with a good physical therapist who can instruct you in more exercises or mobility drills or a fantastic trainer who knows how to get you to move more effectively and easily. Always listen to what your body is telling you. If any exercise doesn't feel like it gives you what you need or creates some new discomfort or pain, there's no need to keep doing it, and it would be worthwhile to either swap it out for a different exercise or to get coaching, treatment, or a diagnosis on what might be happening to prevent something from going awry.

Cardio Training

Yes, you need to do some form or multiple forms of cardio on a semiregular basis. Some people seem to believe that doing anything outside of strength training will sap your energy and reduce your potential for strength or muscle gains. While this may be the case for top-level powerlifters or bodybuilders entering their peak phases prior to competition, if you're not in their situation, trying to copy their programming likely won't give you any real benefits. Maximizing anything typically requires cutting out everything else, but there's always a cost of doing business when it comes to anything related to fitness. Sure, you might cut back on any non-exercise activity, but then you'll wheeze when you have to climb a flight of stairs. A hard set might be really heavy, but you won't be able to do your next set for about 10 or 15 minutes because it takes that long for your muscles to get new oxygen and for your heart rate to come back to normal.

Cardio is one of the easiest ways to get better results from your strength training. (Well, easiest outside of any pharmaceutical interventions, that is.) The main benefits of cardio come down to a few key features:

- Improved blood flow to working muscles. This helps increase oxygen delivery to and waste removal from those regions, so you can do more work and recover more quickly compared to if you didn't have that blood flow.

- Increased work capacity. You can do things throughout your day with greater ease, which makes your stress tolerance higher, and therefore allows you to get after it in the gym with more effort and intensity to see some progress. You can also bounce back from small aches and pains more easily.

- Improved recovery from harder training sessions. As with improved blood flow, having muscle tissue that can more easily reoxygenate and get more of the nutrients it needs to repair and recover, as well as being able to more easily remove waste products and restore normal pH values, can significantly hasten recovery, which means you can hit it hard again, sooner than if you weren't doing any cardio training.

So better recovery in the workout, between workouts, and easier ability to do work plus living your life with less stress all sound like pretty awesome benefits. Then there's the whole improved cardiopulmonary function bit of making healthier heart, lungs, and blood vessels, which can all make you less likely to need to go to a cardiologist (or a mortician). All this is a pretty good argument for including some amount of cardio in your weekly rotation.

So why do so many people rail against cardio training? They believe it saps your strength, it's boring, and it makes you fatter. Yes, there are actually people out there who'll try to tell you that doing more exercise makes you gain weight. What a time to be alive.

Let's break down these three big myths one at a time.

First, it's a myth that cardio will sap your strength or reduce your energy. A big reason this myth got started was that people were comparing the outcomes of individuals training for marathons and their body types against sprinters and other jacked individuals who didn't do long-duration aerobic work. The (very shoddy) reasoning was that the marathoner isn't jacked and is likely weak, so doing cardio will make you weak and not jacked too!

There are a few reasons this is ridiculous. First, the marathoner is likely logging 12 to 15 hours or more of cardio each week for their sport. Comparing the outcomes of that to someone trying to add in two or three 30-minute cardio sessions each week is wildly different in terms of stress, outcomes, and physiological requirements. Should we also discourage people from starting to lift weights two or three times a week who don't want to get too big because they might wind up looking like the Olympia competitors who spend 8 to 12 hours a week in the gym?

In terms of energy, I'd wager if you did an hour or two of very intense interval training you'd likely not have much energy to do weights right afterward. However, those intervals can do some really cool things to your ability to turn carbs or fats into usable energy. They let you become more efficient at producing energy in the form of ATP, meaning you can actually wind up with *more* energy. If you doubt me, do a search on the Krebs cycle for me, and see how biochemistry can give you the win you're looking for. Also, you don't have to do two hours of intervals, and doing cardio before your weights might actually get you into the zone if the time frame is relatively short (10 to 20 minutes) and the intensity isn't max. Also, if you're really worried about maxing out your weight training intensity, you could just do cardio after your weights. Simple solution—problem solved.

The second main argument against doing cardio: It's boring. Sure, riding a stationary bike and staring at a wall might suck. Same with walking on a treadmill or pedaling an elliptical without going anywhere. The equipment can be big, bulky, expensive, and limited in utility, but the good thing is that these aren't the only ways to do cardio. There's a big wide world out there that you can actually do lots of stuff in, and being outside might actually be as good for you as doing the cardio itself. Go for a bike ride, a walk, a run, climb a mountain, skate, or even find a group of people to play a sport with and make cardio something that isn't boring.

Admittedly, there are times when outdoors might not be the best option. I live in a climate where six months of the year you could die from freezing cold, and for the other six months of the year there's a 50 percent chance that it's either too hot or too smoky to work hard outside for long. Getting outside might not be the easiest, but there are still lots of options for getting active and getting the heart rate up. The key is to find something, anything, that lets you work for an extended period of time and not die, and that elevates your heart rate and breathing rate enough to feel like you're getting a good training effect.

Last, and definitely least, it's a myth that cardio will make you fatter. This is a weird one where people made some absolutely massive leaps in correlation to infer causation, which all somehow violate the laws of thermodynamics and common sense. A big reason given was that cardio tended to spike stress hormones and impair your ability to burn fat and use carbs for energy. To be fair, all exercise tends to spike your stress hormones. That's the point. You get some physical stress, and your body has to adapt to it and make some changes. This thought process implied that this stress would cause your body to not "want" to break down body fat and to actually store more, which, let's be fair, doesn't happen unless you have excess calories to store.

Further, there was the belief that doing cardio would cause you to want to take in more calories, especially carbs, which we've been taught are the devil. To be fair, if you did some cardio and wound up feeling hungry and overate as a result, you'd likely gain some weight. However, the same could be said for overeating after strength training. Or overeating after sitting, or watching a movie, or literally doing anything. Properly refueling after a workout will make sure you're managing your weight effectively. Along this same line, people would claim that cardio was being done for weight loss but note that the most effective way to lose weight is through dietary restriction. But, and this is a big but, if you actually want to lose weight, dietary restriction combined with some additional calorie burn, like from cardio, can help you lose weight too, and the combined effort can be more beneficial than just calorie restriction, plus it gives you all the good stuff we've discussed previously.

I can honestly say that in all the years of training others, I've never had a client gain weight with the simple addition of cardio to their week. Even clients who train for endurance sports can usually train 12 to 20 hours a week in their given endurance activity and still see some decent strength gains. The biggest limiter for them is recovery from their endurance activities and warming up so that they feel like they can put out some effort on a barbell instead of only on the track or bike pedals. Non-endurance athletes can safely and easily add 2 to 5 hours of cardio work to their week and still recover well enough to get the benefits from their strength training. Additionally, this cardio work typically helps them see better results from strength training, so the arguments against it are typically not all that great and easy to counter.

Now how should you add cardio training to your workouts? There are three different ways you could make this happen. First, you could do cardio on your workout days. When you get to the gym, do a few minutes of cardio to warm up, ideally 5 to 10 minutes, to get a sweat going and feel like your body is ramped up and ready. If you really want to, you could go for a bit longer at an easy intensity. From there, you complete your strength work and then follow it with some cardio. This post-strength cardio won't negatively affect the intensity of your workouts, and it also will help to move blood through the working muscles to aid recovery. Just 20 to 30 minutes of steady-state or interval training can go a long way.

Second, you could do cardio on days when you're not doing strength training. There are obvious benefits to having days off from the iron, and those days can include some aerobic work or intervals, or even sports or more competitive conditioning work. This can be a great way to establish the habit of daily activity.

Third, you could work out twice a day: strength training in one workout and cardio training in another. Some people prefer to start their day with steady-state aerobic work and finish with heavier strength work; some people prefer the reverse. Either way, it can break up your day and allow you to get in the work you're looking for.

How much cardio should you add in? If you're just getting started, two workouts a week of 20 minutes each is a good start. From there you can add 5 more minutes each week as you get used to it. When you're doing two workouts of 30 minutes each, you could add in another workout to split up the time frame, gradually building to 2 to 4 hours a week, depending on your schedule. If you do four workouts of 30 minutes each week, you're rocking. Any more and you're an absolute rock star.

Again, find ways to do cardio that you actually enjoy, do it for the benefits to your other strength workouts and life in general, and make sure you're not crushing the left side of the IHOP menu after each workout, and you should see some pretty awesome results.

Conclusion

With all the info we've gone through and how we approach training, level-up applications, and exercise accommodations, you might be thinking this sounds all too reasonable and not too insane or intense. You're right. We're not pushing a quick-hit program that'll smash you to bits and maybe leave just enough left over for you to exist outside of the gym. We want you to work out, see steady, realistic progress, not push into problems, and know how to fix simple stuff on your own. And we want you to be able to do that for decades without needing to take time off for recovery or surgery because the program didn't fit you properly.

Some of the best programs will show you measurable results over the span of years, not simply days. If you can look back 10 years from now and say you showed up consistently, put out good effort, and still feel like all your joints, muscles, and tendons are working as they should, you're very likely to have made some serious improvements in strength, range of motion, and body composition. You should also feel like you can do things like put on socks, climb a flight of stairs, and turn your neck without much effort. These outside-the-gym benefits are part of why you spend your time in the gym. Adding in some cardio will help you recover between sets, recover between workouts, and enjoy different activities you might want to do outside the gym, plus keep your heart, lungs, and blood vessels healthier than they would be without it.

In the next chapters, we'll outline how to know when to train hard, when to back off, and how to adjust your program to make it fit what you need at a given moment, plus we'll show you simple work-arounds for common issues that might make certain exercises uncomfortable, and how to get the most bang for your buck.

Training With Common Injuries

Understanding pain and how to navigate it is of paramount importance to the weightlifter. If you have been weight training for long enough, you've no doubt sustained some sort of injury or pain problem. Statistically speaking, participation in a weight training sport is going to average one injury every one to two years if you train five days per week for an hour or so.[1]

What we also know is that training through pain is just plain risky. If we choose to train through minor pain or smaller injury, we increase the chance of that injury worsening or a whole new injury occurring that's worse than the initial problem.[2]

It's also important to understand the difference between pain that's related to an injury and pain associated from muscular soreness. Muscular soreness, or more specifically delayed onset muscle soreness (DOMS), is a natural phenomenon that occurs after strenuous (and also unaccustomed) exercise.[3] It generally peaks 24 to 72 hours after training and feels like pain and stiffness in the muscles that were worked in the prior training session.[3] I think everyone experiences DOMS the first time they go down the stairs the day after a really tough squat session. I know I stayed upstairs for a full day after my first squat session because I couldn't face the pain.

Kidding aside, some soreness after training is OK and often expected if the prior day's session was more intense than usual or when beginning a new training program. However, extreme soreness is also a sign you may have pushed yourself a bit too hard and attempting to train hard again when excessively sore may also lead to problems (or, at the very least, reduced performance).[4] This extreme soreness may be a sign the muscles need a bit more recovery before we hit the weights hard again.

In addition, exercise is just plain uncomfortable, especially if you're pushing hard. Go run a mile as fast as you can or perform a heavy set of 20 rep breathing squats. How did it feel? Probably horrendous.

We've known for a long time that exercise produces changes in acids, ions, proteins, and hormones within our bodies that may be responsible for the discomfort felt during exercise.[5] This is all normal, natural, and often embraced by masochistic meatheads around the globe.

So what about other types of pain and injury in the weight room? Generally speaking, any sort of pain *not* associated with DOMS or the discomfort that comes with being a savage on the leg press is a more serious concern. It could be a sharp pain in a muscle or dull ache in a joint. Once you get a feel for what is normal pain associated with training, anything that falls outside of DOMS and training discomfort I'd classify as an injury—or at least some pain we should attend to and make changes for in our training.

I know as lifters we identify as tough and able to push through pain in our training. The old saying "no pain, no gain" comes to mind. *However*, blowing through pain regularly is a great way to eventually derail your training and end up with longer-term issues. Trust me, as a physical therapist I see this happen all the time with my patients. Pain starts as an annoyance that pops up only during maximal sets of bench press. Over time it can start limiting the weight we use on our top sets. Eventually you have to scrap bench press altogether because it's too painful. Lifting through pain is just risky business. The best way to handle pain like this in the gym is to listen to your body and make smarter decisions when pain problems pop up. The rest of this chapter will focus on strategies to do this.

Understanding Pain

Before we go over specific strategies, it's vital to have a chat about what pain is because that will set the stage for understanding why we should make better training decisions when injuries happen.

Pain is a defense mechanism in the body. Generally, your brain produces pain whenever it feels like your body is at risk of injury or has been injured. Nearly everywhere in the body you have receptors known as nociceptors. Their job is to send information about potentially damaging input back to the brain. If enough nociception information finds its way to the brain, your brain may eventually say, "OK, something is wrong and we have to do something about this." So it creates pain as a protective response to prevent any further harm to your body.

Think about sitting on a hard rock to take a break while hiking. If you sit there long enough, your butt gets sore as your brain tries to get you to move. You get to a point where the brain doesn't want you to sit any longer because it's afraid you're going to get a pressure ulcer if you sit for too long on the hard rock.

Pain is also protective after an injury. Let's say you strain your pec while bench pressing. In this case the load exceeded your pec's ability to handle the stress and you've got a tear in the muscle. The brain responds by creating a bunch of pain in that area. It sensitizes the area by activating more nociceptors in the region and making the already active ones much more sensitive.[6] In this case, after the injury just a light stretch really aggravates the pec. This doesn't mean that light stretch is necessarily damaging the area further (although it's certainly possible if you're a bonehead and go too far), but your body is attempting to keep you from doing anything stupid in the future by making the area especially tender and sore. The idea is that this will keep you from benching heavy for a while and give the body some time to recover.

So if you have some pain while training, it's your brain's attempt to tell you, "Hey, stupid, don't do anything dumb. We've got an issue going on over here." Now, this doesn't mean that you have to stop training. Being sedentary is bad for your health and an individual's poor health has enormous implications for the society we live in. On top of this we know that exercise can be very beneficial from a rehabilitation standpoint for most orthopedic injuries. In my opinion, you should never stop exercising in some capacity (barring some extreme circumstances), but you do have to train smarter and listen to your body when pain rears its ugly head.

So what do you do when pain or injury happens? The safest thing is to get it checked out by a licensed health care professional. Small tweaks of pain in the gym are usually nothing to be concerned about, but there are sometimes red flags that need medical attention. It's also useful to have someone guide you through the rehab process, prescribing beneficial exercises and giving you an idea of what movements are helpful and which ones to avoid temporarily.

Back when I was a CrossFit coach (and also a physical therapist) I would get swarmed at the end of every class with questions about injuries. My generic answer was to temporarily back off exercises that hurt, and as the area improves, slowly start ramping back into those movements. If the pain doesn't go away in a few weeks, get it checked out. This would help most folks.

Of course, major injuries, such as a pec tear or a pop in the knee with swelling, require immediate attention. If you're ever in doubt about a given injury, it's never a bad idea to get it checked out. Mild tweaks or more chronic aches and pains can be dealt with through an understanding of exercise modifications.

Identifying Your Trainable Menu

When dealing with pain in the gym, the last thing you want to do is stop training. You don't want your biceps to turn into mashed potatoes just because you have some shoulder pain, right? Instead, it's smart to focus on what you can still train. A good friend, the super-smart strength coach Tony Gentilcore, calls this the *trainable menu*. Basically, this means you stick to the movements in your program that you can still perform comfortably.

An easy example is shoulder pain while bench pressing. Let's say your shoulder is currently not enjoying heavy barbell bench pressing. However, dumbbells actually tend to feel really good. Also, all rowing exercises in the gym seem to feel absolutely fine. Arm work feels decent as well. As much as you wish it didn't, leg day is also absolutely fine from a pain perspective. You can also hit the core, log some cardio, and do those weird neck exercises. Turns out your trainable menu is quite large, maybe even as robust as Taco Bell's impressive selection. You also may need only a few weeks away from bench press to let the shoulder get over itself and then you can slowly ramp back into barbell work.

Modifying Load

Another useful strategy for continuing training while respecting a healing injury is to modify the load or intensity. Intensity is how close a given weight is toward your 1 rep max. If your 1 rep max bench press is 1,000 pounds (454 kg)—reasonable, right?—and your working sets are 800 pounds (363 kg), you're using 80 percent of your 1 rep max. For most folks, an injury is load intolerant. Basically, this means they can lift lighter weights comfortably but once the weights get too heavy, the exercise becomes intolerable. Simply speaking, too much intensity is *no bueno*. What's important to keep in mind is that we can tweak the exercise intensity (lower it) to keep working toward training goals while simultaneously respecting the injured area. There are a bunch of ways to do this.

Reduce the RPE or Increase the RIR

Rating of perceived exertion, or RPE, is a subjective measure of perceived intensity after completing a set. You rank the set on a scale of 0 to 10, where 0 is super easy and 10 is the hardest set of all time. For example, if you got close to failure on a given set, you would rank the set 9 out of 10 on an RPE scale.

Reps in reserve, or RIR, refers to how many reps you feel like you have left in the tank after completing a given set. Let's say you did a set of 10 bench presses but felt you could have completed 2 more reps; that's a 2 RIR set.

What's important to keep in mind is that you don't have to go to absolute failure when training to maximize both strength and hypertrophy. What this also means is that if you drop a little weight off the bar and keep a few reps in the tank, it makes almost no difference in your progress over time. This is nice for anyone in pain who is load intolerant. If we simply lower the RPE or increase the RIR, we can often train quite comfortably and make zero change in our long-term progress from a strength and hypertrophy perspective. We may even end up with better long-term outcomes because we're being *smart* and not blowing through pain and getting injured further. (I've always said that one of the best ways to get weaker and smaller is by getting hurt.)

Increase the Repetitions

Where can you use more weight: doing reps of 3 or doing reps of 15? Obviously your 3-rep max will be much higher than your 15-rep max. Increasing the reps used for a given training session will also force you to reduce the load, just as changing RPE and RIR does.

Increasing reps does reduce the strength training effect slightly. Reps in the 1 to 5 range are generally more effective than reps over 10 for increasing strength. However, if heavier loads are not an option due to pain, then increasing reps is still a great way to keep working toward your training goals. You'll still increase strength and hypertrophy (hypertrophy at the same rate as heavier loads) as long as you're getting close to failure, but note that absolute failure is not needed.

So if the day calls for sets of 5 and the shoulder simply is not feeling it (or is feeling it too much), you can still get in some great work with sets of 10 to 15 reps.

Slow-Down Repetitions

Have you ever tried lifting with a tempo? It's godawful. If you've never tried it, lifting with a tempo consists of slowing down the movement to a tempo (1 to 5 seconds, for example) during the lockout, lowering, bottom, or ascent of the lift. Imagine loading up a barbell and descending into a squat with a 3-second lower, 1-second pause in the hole, and then another 3-seconds on the way up. Godawful, right? What happens? Besides hating the speed of movement, you have to lower the load. Tempo lifting simply makes each rep harder and the weights have to decrease as a result.

This provides another option for those who can't handle heavier loads. What's good about tempo lifts is that they're hard. You get a solid training effect with them and they're great for really solidifying exercise technique to boot. It's another good training option I love to hate for lifters in (mild) pain.

Modifying Training Due to Injury

What happens if you can't perform a given movement even at a lower intensity? Well, you can always try a new exercise variation that mimics the movement that's aggravating. For example, you could use a barbell floor press instead of a barbell bench press. The reduction in range of motion can be just what the doctor ordered for a painful shoulder.

We can modify all the major movements in the gym that can be troublesome. In the following sections, we'll go over shoulder, lower-back, and knee pain and find ways to deal with pain during the most common gym movements. We'll cover what to know for each movement and then give you some modifications to try. The goal is to use the exercise variation that is most similar to your regular exercise but is well tolerated from a pain perspective.

Bench Press and Shoulder Pain

Before listing the principles to remember when bench pressing is painful, I want to explain my use of the word *stress* in this section. It's important to understand that stressing a structure is not a bad thing; quite the opposite. You have to stress your biceps with curls to stretch out those medium-sized T-shirts, right? With an injury, we're attempting to modify the stress to produce a positive adaptation to the area while respecting the injury.

When bench pressing is painful, remember these principles:

- **Greater loads increase stress to the shoulder.** More weight on the bar generally equates to more stress on the shoulder. Faster lifting speeds also increase stress on the shoulder.

- **The shoulder is very prone to overuse issues.** Unlike the hip and knee, the shoulder was not designed to bear weight. For this reason, the shoulder may be more prone to overuse issues if bench-press frequency is too high.

- **Specific bar paths, ranges, and positions can become overused**. Overusing specific grips, angles of press, and specific ranges of motion can create overuse problems within the shoulder.

- **Wider grips and deeper pressing increases stress to the shoulder (AC joint).**[10] The farther away the elbow gets from the body and the farther it travels toward the floor, the more stress on the shoulder.

Here are some tips for reducing shoulder pain during bench press.

First, decrease the total load or slow down the speed of movement. Lowering total load decreases the stress on the shoulder. To achieve this, you can increase the number of reps (decreasing the total load you can use for the set), slow down the speed of the lift, or add pauses at the bottom of the bench press.

Second, press less frequently and for fewer reps throughout the course of the week. Often, decreasing total pressing volume will be enough to end shoulder pain. Reduce the total sets of bench press in a given session or substitute one or two rowing exercises for pressing exercises in your program.

Third, vary the pressing exercise. Changing the angle, grip, or implement is often enough to remove or reduce pain while pressing. You can try changing to an incline or decline press, changing your grip width or switching to a neutral-grip bar, or using dumbbells.

Fourth, narrow the grip and limit the range of motion. A narrower grip and less depth will decrease stress on the AC joint. Switch to a closer grip or try a floor press, board press, or Spoto press.

Finally, if all else fails, try substituting a rowing variation for a pressing variation. Consider the seal row, chest-supported row, or single-arm dumbbell row.

If you are unable to eliminate pain by slowing down reps or attempting a higher rep range, use the bench press modification ladder for shoulder pain (figure 8.1) to find a pain-free bench press variation.

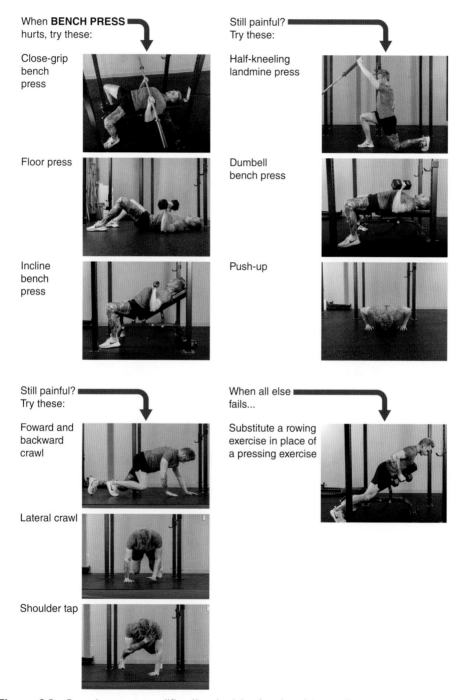

When **BENCH PRESS** hurts, try these:

Close-grip bench press

Floor press

Incline bench press

Still painful? Try these:

Half-kneeling landmine press

Dumbell bench press

Push-up

Still painful? Try these:

Foward and backward crawl

Lateral crawl

Shoulder tap

When all else fails...

Substitute a rowing exercise in place of a pressing exercise

Figure 8.1 Bench press modification ladder for shoulder pain.

Overhead Press and Shoulder Pain

The overhead press is generally one of the toughest things to perform when the shoulder is painful. It often has to be taken out of the program temporarily to allow the shoulder to heal before being included again. Here are five things to keep in mind when overhead press is painful:

- **Greater loads increase stress to the shoulder.** More weight on the bar generally equates to more stress on the shoulder. Faster lifting speeds also increase stress on the shoulder.

- **The shoulder is very prone to overuse issues.** Unlike the hip and knee, the shoulder was not designed to bear weight. For this reason, the shoulder is more prone to overuse issues if too much overhead pressing is done.

- **Different grip widths and pressing implements can help with pain.** Often, switching grip widths or pressing implements (barbell versus dumbbell versus kettlebell) is enough to eliminate pain during overhead press.

- **When overhead pressing is painful, sometimes horizontal pressing is well tolerated.** For this reason, different angles of pressing can substitute for overhead pressing to get your training in for the day.

- **Substituting a row variation for pressing is often helpful.** When you can't find a pressing variation that can be accomplished without pain, often substituting a rowing variation is well tolerated.

Here are some tips for reducing shoulder pain during overhead press.

First, decrease the total load or slow down the speed of movement. Less total load decreases stress on the shoulder. Achieve this by increasing the number of reps (decreasing the total load you can use for the set) or slow down the speed of the lift.

Second, press less frequently throughout the course of the week for fewer reps. Often decreasing total pressing volume will be enough to lessen shoulder pain. You can reduce the total sets of overhead press in a given session or substitute one or two rowing exercises for pressing exercises in your program.

Third, vary the grip. A narrower grip may help with shoulder pain.

Fourth, vary the pressing implement. Switching from a barbell to dumbbells, kettlebells, or a landmine is often enough to eliminate pain.

Fifth, vary the plane of pressing. Switching from an overhead press to a more horizontal press such as an incline press can be effective for reducing pain and continuing to train for the day.

Finally, if all else fails, substitute rowing for pressing. Try a seal row, chest-supported row, or single-arm dumbbell row.

If you are unable to eliminate pain by slowing down reps or attempting a higher rep range, use the overhead press modification ladder for shoulder pain (figure 8.2) to find a painless overhead press variation.

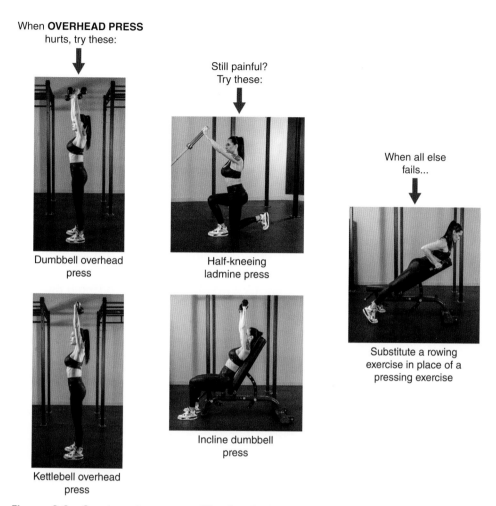

When **OVERHEAD PRESS** hurts, try these:

Dumbbell overhead press

Kettlebell overhead press

Still painful? Try these:

Half-kneeing landmine press

Incline dumbbell press

When all else fails...

Substitute a rowing exercise in place of a pressing exercise

Figure 8.2 Overhead press modification ladder for shoulder pain.

Pull-Up and Shoulder Pain

Fortunately for us, pull-ups are generally not as difficult for the injured shoulder than are other shoulder-dominant exercises, such as bench press and overhead press. However, when pull-ups are painful, we need to know how to work around it. Here are few things to keep in mind:

- **Greater loads increase stress to the shoulder.** More weight simply increases stress to the shoulder joint (think of performing a weighted pull-up). Faster lifting speeds also increase stress on the shoulder.
- **Different grips can help with pain.** Often, changing to an underhand or neutral grip is enough to make the movement painless.
- **When pull-ups are painful, sometimes more horizontal pulling is well tolerated.** Try a horizontal rowing motion.

Here are some tips for reducing shoulder pain during pull-ups.

First, decrease the total load or slow down the speed of movement. Less total load decreases stress on the shoulder. You can achieve this by increasing the number of reps (decreasing the total load you can use for the set via dropping any additional weight you were planning to use). Add band assistance or use the lat pull-down. You can also slow down the speed of the lift.

Second, vary the grip. A neutral or chin-up grip may help with shoulder pain.

Third, vary the plane of pulling. Switching from a pull-up to a more horizontal pull can be effective in reducing pain and continuing to train for the day. Try a half-kneeling overhead pull-down or other horizontal rowing variation.

If you are unable to eliminate pain by slowing down reps or attempting a higher rep range (dropping any additional weight added), use the pull-up modification ladder for shoulder pain (figure 8.3) to find a painless pull-up variation.

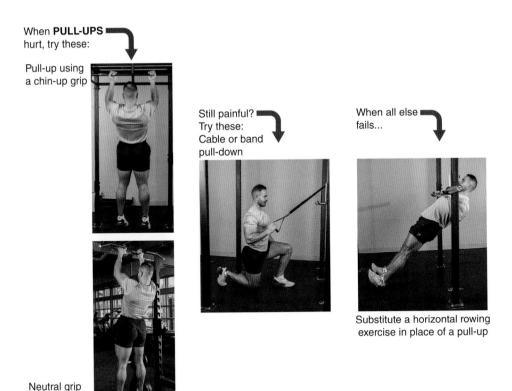

When **PULL-UPS** hurt, try these:

Pull-up using a chin-up grip

Still painful? Try these: Cable or band pull-down

When all else fails...

Substitute a horizontal rowing exercise in place of a pull-up

Neutral grip pull-up

Figure 8.3 Pull-up modification ladder for shoulder pain.

Deadlift and Lower-Back Pain

Generally, the elements that increase stress to the lower back when deadlifting are as follows:

- **Going too far outside of neutral spine.** The muscles around the spine fire best and the stresses on the spine are minimized when the spine is kept in a neutral position while deadlifting. Deeper deadlifts (rack pull versus deadlift from the floor) can be more stressful because they require more lower-back rounding than shallower deadlifts do. Mobility issues in the hamstrings can create more lower-back rounding. Stance affects this as well; for some, a neutral spine is much easier to maintain in a sumo stance.

- **Greater loads.** More weight on the bar generally equates to more stress on the spine. Faster lifting speeds also increase stress on the spine.

- **More forward torso inclination**. Inclining the torso forward and sending the hips farther back during a deadlift increases stress to the spine. Think of the difference between a Romanian deadlift and a trap bar deadlift.

Here are some tips for reducing lower-back pain during deadlifts.

First, learn to maintain a neutral spine and brace appropriately during deadlifts. Decrease the depth of the deadlift to reduce lower-back rounding at the bottom of the squat. Some exercises to try are rack pulls, partial-range dumbbell deadlifts, or elevated-handle trap bar deadlifts.

Second, decrease the load lifted or the speed of the lift. Taking weight off the bar or slowing down the lift will help to decrease stress on the spine. Try slowing the pace of your tempo lifts. Adding 2 or 3 repetitions to your working sets with less weight on the bar will still allow a training effect. Use a deadlift variation that forces you to use less load, like a dumbbell Romanian deadlift.

Third, use a deadlift variation that keeps you more upright to decrease stress on the spine. Pick sumo and trap bar deadlifts over conventional deadlifts.

Fourth, try hip thrusts. Hip thrusts work the lower back, hips, and hamstrings similarly to a deadlift but have less compressive force through the spine and are generally well tolerated by those with painful lower backs.

Finally, substitute single-leg strength work. If all else fails and all movements are painful, then try using single-leg exercises. These allow some leg strength training while decreasing stress on the spine. Try single-leg deadlifts, kickstand Romanian deadlifts, and good mornings.

When you are unable to eliminate pain by slowing down reps, attempting a higher rep range, or modifying technique, use the deadlift modification

Deadlift	Low handle trap bar deadlift	High handle trap bar deadlift	Elevated kettlebell deadlift	Hip thrust	Single-leg deadlift

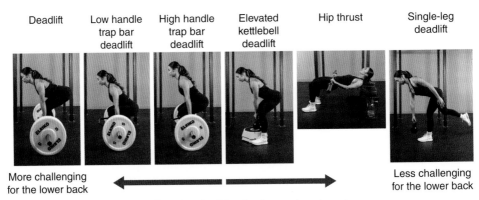

More challenging for the lower back ←——————————————→ Less challenging for the lower back

Figure 8.4 Deadlift modification ladder for lower-back pain.

ladder for lower-back pain (figure 8.4) to find a deadlifting variation that should hurt less.

Squat and Lower-Back Pain

Generally, elements that increase stress to the lower back when squatting are as follows:

- **Going too far outside of neutral spine.** The muscles around the spine fire best and the stresses on the spine are minimized when the spine is kept in a neutral position while squatting. Deeper squats are more stressful because they require more lower-back rounding than do shallower squats. Mobility issues at the hips and ankles can increase lower-back rounding. Squat stance affects this as well; for some, a neutral spine is much easier to maintain with a wider stance or toes pointed farther out.

- **Greater loads.** More weight on the bar generally equates to more stress on the spine. Faster lifting speeds also increase stress on the spine.

- **More forward torso inclination**. Inclining the torso forward and sending the hips back farther during a squat stresses the spine (think of the difference between a barbell box squat and an upright front squat).

Here are some tips for reducing lower-back pain during squats.

First, maintain a neutral spine and brace appropriately during squatting. Decrease the depth of the squat to reduce lower-back rounding at the bottom of the squat.

Second, decrease the load lifted or the speed of the lift. Taking weight off the bar or slowing down the lift will help to decrease stress on the spine. Try tempo lifts or add a pause to the bottom position of the squat. Adding 2 or 3 repetitions to your working sets with less weight will still allow a training effect. Use a squat variation, such as a front squat or goblet squat, that forces you to use less load.

Third, stay more upright during squats or use a squat variation that keeps you more upright. A more upright squat variation decreases stress on the spine. Pick front squats over back squats, high-bar back squats over low-bar back squats, or try goblet squats and double kettlebell front rack squats. These challenging variations keep you upright with minimal spinal stress.

Fourth, correct mobility limitations in the hips and ankles. Mobilize both hips and ankles prior to squatting. Use a heel lift or Olympic lifting shoes. Ensure you use your full mobility to stay neutral while squatting after mobilizing.

Fifth, try hip thrusts. Hip thrusts work the lower back, hips, and hamstrings similarly to a squat but have less compressive force through the spine and are generally well tolerated by those with painful lower backs.

Finally, substitute leg strength work. If all else fails and all movements are painful, try using single-leg exercises. These allow some leg strength training while decreasing stress on the spine. Choose split squat, lunge, step-up, and hip thrust variations.

When you are unable to eliminate pain by slowing down reps, attempting a higher rep range, or modifying technique, use the squat modification ladder for lower-back pain (figure 8.5) to find a squatting variation that should hurt less.

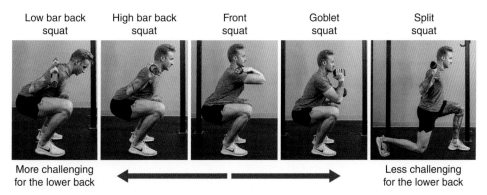

| Low bar back squat | High bar back squat | Front squat | Goblet squat | Split squat |

More challenging for the lower back ← → Less challenging for the lower back

Figure 8.5 Squat modification ladder for lower-back pain.

Olympic Weightlifting and Lower-Back Pain

Generally, elements that increase stress to the lower back when Olympic weightlifting are as follows:

- **Going too far outside of neutral spine.** The muscles around the spine fire best and the stresses on the spine are minimized when the spine is kept in a neutral position while lifting. For the pull phase of an Olympic lift, pulling from the floor is more stressful than pulling from a hang or elevated surface (blocks) because it requires more lower-back rounding. Mobility issues at the hamstrings can create more lower-back rounding. In the catch and squat, deeper squats are more stressful because they require more lower-back rounding than do shallower squats (think of the difference between catching a clean in a full squat versus a half squat). Mobility issues at the hips and ankles can create more lower-back rounding. Squat stance affects this as well; for some, a neutral spine is easier to maintain with a wider stance or toes pointed farther out.

- **Greater loads.** More weight on the bar generally equates to more stress on the spine.
- **More forward torso inclination**. Inclining the torso forward and sending the hips back while coming up out of the hole in a clean or snatch increases stress to the spine.

Here are some tips for reducing lower-back pain during Olympic lifts.

First, limit lumbar flexion (rounding) by improving technique and modifying squat and pull depth. Ensure you keep a braced, neutral spinal position throughout the lift. To adjust the starting depth for the pull, use hang variations and pull from blocks instead of pulling from the floor. For the catch and squat, limit the depth of the squat or use power variations over full squat variations.

Second, decrease the load. Taking weight off the bar helps decrease stress on the spine. Using hang variations and pauses (at knee or mid-thigh) within reps decreases load on the bar but still works technique and allows a training effect. Similarly, you can add 2 or 3 repetitions to your working sets with less weight on the bar and still get a training effect.

Third, stay more upright when coming out of the hole in a clean or snatch. A more upright squat variation decreases stress on the spine. This may require you to reduce the load on the bar.

Fourth, correct mobility limitations in the hips and ankles. Mobilize both hips and ankles prior to lifting. Use a heel lift or Olympic lifting shoes. Ensure you use your full mobility to stay neutral while squatting after mobilizing.

When you are unable to eliminate pain by cleaning up your exercise technique, use the Olympic weightlifting modification ladder for lower-back pain (figure 8.6) to find an Olympic weightlifting variation that should hurt less.

Squat and Knee Pain

Generally, elements that increase stress to the knee when squatting are as follows:

- **Increased depth of the squat.** Deeper squats are generally more stressful than shallower variations.
- **Forward knee translation**. The more the knee travels forward during squatting, the more stress is placed on the knee.

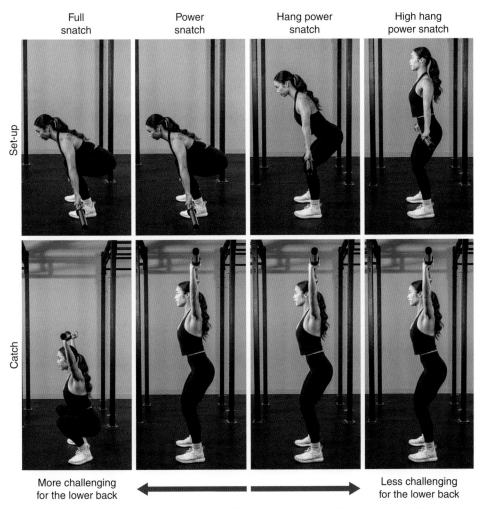

Full snatch | Power snatch | Hang power snatch | High hang power snatch

Set-up

Catch

More challenging for the lower back ⟵——————————⟶ Less challenging for the lower back

Figure 8.6 Olympic weightlifting modification ladder for lower-back pain.

- **Increased quadriceps contraction**. The more the quads contract during a squat, the more stress is placed on the knee. More upright squat variations and more forward knee translation both contribute to this. Faster lifting speeds and greater loads also increase this.

- **Dynamic valgus or knee in.** If the knee travels inward in relationship to the second toe during a squat, the knee joint takes additional stress.

Here are some tips for reducing knee pain during squats.

First, limit the depth of squats. Try box squats with limited depth or quarter squats.

Second, make squatting movements more hip dominant. Send your hips back farther when you squat. Choose squat variations that require a less upright position, such as back squats and box squats.

Third, decrease total load or slow down the speed of movement. Less total load decreases stress on the knee. You can increase the number of reps (decreasing the total load you use for the set), slow down the speed of the lift, or add pauses in the bottom of the squat.

Fourth, maintain proper alignment of knee over toe. This means ensuring the knee is aligned over the second toe at all points during the squat. Groin muscle, calf muscle, and ankle joint tightness can cause these issues and may require mobilization if tight to align properly during squats.

Finally, substitute squat variations for hip hinge variations. If all else fails, limiting knee bend and quad contraction by switching to hinge variations should allow you to train for the day with less pain or even pain free. Some exercise examples are deadlifts and good mornings.

When you are unable to eliminate pain by slowing down reps, attempting a higher rep range, or modifying technique, use the squat modification ladder for knee pain (figure 8.7) to find a squatting variation that should hurt less.

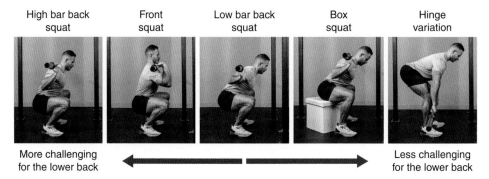

| High bar back squat | Front squat | Low bar back squat | Box squat | Hinge variation |

More challenging for the lower back ⟵⟶ Less challenging for the lower back

Figure 8.7 Squat modification ladder for knee pain.

Olympic Weightlifting and Knee Pain

Generally, the elements that increase stress to the knee when Olympic lifting are as follows:

- **Increased depth of squatting or pulls**. Deeper squats (and pulls from the floor versus hang) are generally more stressful than shallower variations.

- **Greater loads.** More weight on the bar generally equates to more stress on the knees.

- **Dynamic valgus or knee in**. If the knee travels inward in relationship to the second toe during a clean or snatch, additional stress is placed on the knee joint.

Here are some tips for reducing knee pain during Olympic lifts.

First, limit the depth of Olympic variations through power variations. Going from full to partial range of motion limits the amount of stress on the knee.

Second, decrease the total load or slow down the speed of movement. Less total load decreases stress on the knee. Achieve a decrease in total load by increasing the number of reps (decreasing the total load you can use for the set), slowing down the speed of the lift, or adding pauses at the bottom of the squat or during the pull phases of the lift.

Third, ensure proper alignment of the knee over the second toe at all points during the lift. Hip and ankle joint tightness can cause alignment issues and may require mobilization if tight to align properly during lifts (particularly the catch portion).

When you are unable to eliminate pain by slowing down reps, attempting a higher rep range, or modifying technique, use the Olympic weightlifting modification ladder for knee pain (figure 8.8) to find an Olympic lift variation that should hurt less.

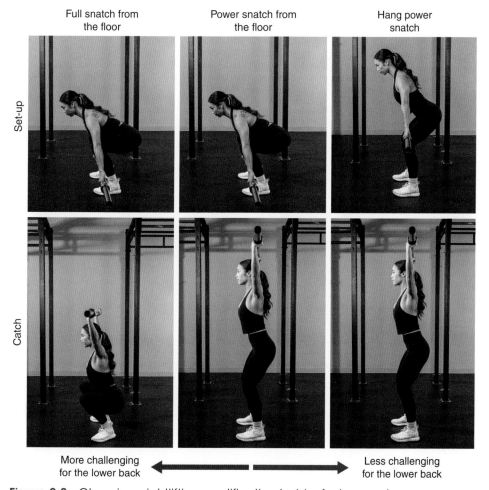

Figure 8.8 Olympic weightlifting modification ladder for knee pain.

Conclusion

Knowing exactly what to do when pain rears its ugly head during training is of paramount importance. A few smart modifications here and there in your training are key to maintaining steady progress toward your goals. Ignoring these issues and not respecting pain can eventually force you to take off extended periods of time if you sustain a serious injury.

In the next chapter we'll go over another one of my favorite strategies to keep you training in the gym—auto-regulation. Buckle up!

9

Autoregulation

Autoregulation is a vital aspect of lifelong progress in the weight room while minimizing your risk of injury. *Autoregulation* refers to the way your body automatically adjusts to maintain its normal state. In this instance, we're talking about the goal of continued progress over time without an injury. In this chapter we'll talk about how we can use autoregulation to accomplish this goal. Before we discuss how to do this, first some explanation.

One of the biggest issues we face as humans is that we generally have stressors in our lives other than training. Maybe some of you have completely cut out all competing stressors like family, friends, relationships, and work. Perhaps you get to train in a completely stress-free bubble, getting massages between training sessions while being fed grapes. However, most of us don't have this luxury. We still have a mortgage to pay, family to tend to, school exams, work deadlines, traffic, and annoying coworkers who don't understand boundaries.

We're constantly being bombarded with stressors that compete with our sweet, sweet gains in the gym. Unfortunately, these can also limit what our bodies can handle before an injury pops up. These life stressors are often referred to as *allostatic load*. Allostatic load refers to the cumulative burden of chronic stress and life events.[11] When environmental challenges exceed the individual's ability to cope, then allostatic overload ensues.[11] This overload may show up as an injury or unfortunately manifest as something of a muscle vampire, leading us down a shameful pathway of wearing kids' size medium T-shirts for the rest of our days.

As discussed in chapter 1, we know that mental health has a profound impact on injury.[1] Mental health disorders in athletes are not only associated with an increased injury risk but also predict poorer outcomes after injury (like prolonged recovery times), increased rates of injury recurrence, decreased rates of return to sport after injury, and reduced performance on return.[1] We also know that high perceived stress levels, high academic pressure (which peaks around exam times for students), and self-reported low energy levels also correlate with injury in athletes.[2] In fact, Hamlin et al. showed that every unit increase in perceived stress (on a 1 to 5 scale, where 1 is the highest level) came with a 10.8 percent increase in injury risk.[2]

We also discussed how total volume of training as well as spikes in training volume are risk factors of injury.[3,4] If we train more frequently, we simply are exposed to more opportunities to get injured in the gym. On top of that, when we expose our bodies to a harder challenge than we are accustomed to dealing with (i.e., a training spike), our risk of injury increases.

On the flip side of things, we know that recovery also plays a very important role in injury risk. Crucial factors in successful recovery are sleep and nutrition. In university athletes, reduced sleep duration correlates with the onset of a new injury.[2] In a study by Huang et al. (2021), sleeping less than 7 hours per night for at least 2 weeks increased risk of injury by 1.7 times.[14] Poor sleep is also a predictor of who goes on to develop chronic pain after the onset of a new injury.[5,6] Clearly, it stands to reason that if you're getting enough high-quality sleep, you're more likely to undertake more training with less risk of injury.

Nutrition is also an important factor in both injury prevention and rehabilitation from injury. A diet low in calories, calcium, and vitamin D increases the risk of bone stress injuries and low bone-mineral density in cross country runners.[7] Adequate dietary protein and carbohydrates is important to combat loss of muscle following injury.[8] Quite simply, if we aren't fueling appropriately for our training, we may also be increasing our risk of injury.

In short, we need to find the optimal training volume and couple it with optimal recovery for best results. How do we know if we're on the right track? On top of this, how do we know if we're about to veer off the path from muscle greatness? Lastly, how do we adapt our training when stress punches us in the face? What do we do on days when we slept for a total of 30 minutes because our newborn hasn't figured out the difference between day and night? Here's where autoregulation comes into play.

Tracking Variables

I recommend that all lifters keep a training journal to help with autoregulation. The goal is to track all the variables that influence injury. When stress levels are high and recovery is low, we probably need to pull back on our training (more on how to do this later). When stress is low and we feel great, business can proceed as per usual.

Here is what I recommend tracking regularly:

- Total calories
- Sleep (weekly average and last night)
- Perceived stress
- Energy level
- Pain
- Acute to chronic workload ratio (ACWR): daily, weekly

Total Calories

This one is pretty straightforward. If you're an athlete who's pushing the envelope in training, you're going to need the raw materials to fuel your training and recover afterward. If you're behind on your calorie goals for the past few days and you're planning on a barnburner workout, you might want to dial the workout back a bit. You simply haven't earned the right to have an enormous session. Or, to put it another way, you haven't recovered and fueled appropriately.

Now, this isn't a book on nutrition. Obviously, more goes into a solid nutrition plan than total calories. It's probably worse to consume 3,000 calories in chocolate bars than in salmon with fruits and vegetables, but writing down your calories each day is a great start and can lead you to make smarter training decisions regularly.

Although it can be a pain in the butt, I recommend learning to count calories. You can find plenty of tutorials and apps online to teach you. I recommend tracking how much you eat daily; that way, you can figure out how many calories you need to maintain your body weight and what amounts result in weight gain or loss. This number obviously varies from person to person and activity levels, so it will take some time to figure out.

This also means that if you're dieting for weight loss, you may want to err on the side of less training in the gym, or at least caution while training. If you're finding that you aren't recovering well from workouts, you're not progressing from a strength perspective, or you've been losing weight that you don't want to lose it may be time to bump up your calories.

Sleep

Sleep is also relatively straightforward. I recommend that you write down how much sleep you get each night. Our goal is 7 or more hours per night. If you're routinely getting less sleep than this, you aren't earning the right to crush those tough workouts. I'd also add that if you have one really bad night of sleep prior to a tough training session, it's probably wise to scale back that session as well.

Just as with my calorie recommendation, if you're finding that you aren't recovering well from workouts, try adding another 30 minutes to your nightly sleep routine or consider improving your sleep hygiene with some of these tips.[9]

1. Go to bed only when sleepy. Stay out of bed and do something boring until you feel sleepy.
2. Create regular bedtime routines like taking a warm bath or reading something relaxing like a book or magazine. If you read, go old school, with books or magazines made out of paper—no e-books or devices. Screen time at bedtime is widely believed to impair healthy sleep.

3. Set a regular wake-up time even on weekends and holidays.

4. Sleep 7 or more hours every night and don't take naps during the day, since these can interfere with the next night's sleep. If you find it necessary to nap, keep all naps to less than an hour and get them done before 3 p.m.

5. The bedroom is used only for sleeping or intimacy—nothing else. Watching TV and using other electronics interferes with sleep.

6. Don't drink caffeinated beverages. If you really can't live without them, stop consumption after noon.

7. Don't drink alcohol, particularly prior to bedtime, since it interferes with sleep.

8. Cigarettes are bad for a myriad of things, sleep included, so quit.

9. Avoid strenuous exercise prior to bedtime. This can raise your level of cortisol (a stress hormone), which disrupts quality sleep.

10. Make your bedroom a cave. Your sleep environment should be cool, dark, and quiet. Consider earplugs and an eye mask if needed.

I recommend tracking the amount of hours you sleep the night prior to a training session as well as keeping a weekly average of hours per night. Training should be modified (more on this later) if your weekly average or prior night's sleep is less than 7 hours.

Perceived Stress

Hamlin et al. found that high levels of both perceived stress and academic stress correlated with an increased rate of injury.[2] What was really great about this study was that they simply used a 1 to 5 scale to grade stress level. A score of 1 indicated you felt very stressed and under a lot of pressure. A score of 5 indicated very little stress and pressure.

We can use the same 1 to 5 scale and grade our current level of stress right before training. If you score a 3 or greater, you're likely ready to roll for your training session. If you're at 1, 2, or 3, then you may want to take it a little bit easier.

Typically, it takes some time to figure out your average score. Once you have an average, you can make informed decisions moving forward. Someone who scores a 2 but is routinely at a 5 should most likely back off because they're substantially below their average. Someone at a 2 who always ranks themselves as a 3 may not have to back off quite as much.

Lastly, if you're always rating yourself at 1, 2, or 3 (remember, 1 is the most stressed and 5 is the least), you may want to take a minute to figure out why you're so stressed. Keep in mind that mental health issues significantly affect your risk of injury just like myriad other health issues, so getting some professional help is never a bad idea.

Energy Levels

Hamlin et al. also found that low energy levels correlated with an increased rate of injury.[2] They used the 1 to 5 scale for determining stress to also determine energy level. A score of 1 constituted extremely low energy and a score of 5 constituted high or excellent energy level. I recommend grading your energy level just prior to training. As with stress, a score of 2 or below may indicate your body just isn't ready to train at your top level.

Also, if you're chronically at a low energy level even while minimizing and managing stress, eating well, and sleeping 7 or more hours per night, it may be a good idea to consult a health care professional to see what's going on.

WEARABLE DEVICES FOR SLEEP, HEART RATE, AND HEART RATE VARIABILITY

Several wearable devices are marketed to measure sleep, heart rate, and heart rate variability (HRV). They use this data to create scores indicating how ready individuals are to train.

Heart rate variability is a measure of how much variance an individual has from one heartbeat to the next. This variety is believed to be a positive. The theory is that the more varied the heart rate is, the better rested you are as an athlete and thus more ready to tackle challenging training sessions.

Some preliminary research shows that HRV may be a predictor of who is more susceptible to injury.[15] Some of these wearables use HRV among other variables (like sleep and heart rate) to provide a score that's meant to suggest how hard athletes can push in the gym on any particular day. Just keep in mind that these wearable devices are not perfect and the validity of the measurements changes from device to device.[13] On top of this, research is in its infancy as to whether HRV and these "readiness" scores are valid.

These devices may show promise in their ability to give feedback about recovery status.[12,13,15] However, there are simpler and cheaper alternatives that have been validated by research to help guide the intensity of training and indicate when we may be more at risk of getting injured.

Pain

Obviously, if you have an injury or any sort of pain problem, it's wise to consult a professional who can figure out a plan for rehabilitation and make sure nothing more serious is going on. However, some pain is common during training and it is something we should take notice of during each session.

For example, from time to time my shoulder will act up during heavier sets of bench press. This is my reminder to modify the movement, so I respect the injured area and track my progress from week to week to make sure the pain is moving in the right direction.

Remember that "training through" a current injury is a great predictor of either worsening said injury or creating another injury.[10] It's up to us to make smarter decisions when pain and injury pops up so that we can continue training and progressing for the long haul.

Now, I'm a big fan of simplicity and making this journaling task easy to perform. Asking people to warm up prior to training is hard enough, let alone asking them to spend precious time keeping a journal about sleep and stress. However, the more specific you can get about the pain, the better. It's a good idea to track where the pain is, which movements aggravate the area, the modifications used in the past to continue training and the severity of the pain (on a simple 0 to 10 scale in which 10 is the worst pain imaginable and 0 is no pain).

With this information we can continue to make smart modifications, easily tell if we're making progress from week to week, and in general listen to our bodies to continue making smarter training decisions over time.

Acute to Chronic Workload Ratio

Tim Gabbett's research on the acute to chronic workload ratio (ACWR) highlighted the importance of preparing your body well for whatever demands you throw at it.[3] Imagine trying to run a marathon but never going for a training run beforehand. That's the best example of a training spike. There's a good chance you'll get hurt during that marathon. We can minimize the spike by slowly and progressively building up our running volume over time so we're prepared for the marathon.

The way to calculate this is by taking the session length and multiplying it by the session's perceived difficulty. Let's say you train for 60 minutes and rate the workout as a 6 out of 10 difficulty. You'd multiply 60 × 6 for a total workload of 360. Our goal is to keep future training sessions around the 360 mark. If we start extending 1.5 times beyond this mark, we might be getting ourselves into hot water.

Let's say your buddy trains with you one day and you decide to do three extra exercises at the end of the session. The workout is now 90 minutes, and you rate the workout as an 8 out of 10. Your workload is now calculated at a 720 (acute workload), representing double the average (chronic workload). This is a training spike, something to be avoided if long-term health is our main goal.

Workloads are also measured across a given training week. Using the previous example, let's say we have four sessions per week, all calculated at 360 workload. That's a total of 1,440 units spread across the week. This would be your acute workload for the week. Our goal is to ensure that each week we have somewhere near 1,440 units of workload total in one week.

We calculate chronic workload by taking the weekly workload from the past 4 weeks and dividing it by 4. This gives us an average (chronic) workload to which our body is accustomed from the past month. Let's say the past four weeks of training have yielded acute weekly ratios of:

Week 1: 1,450 training load

Week 2: 1,620 training load

Week 3: 1,700 training load

Week 4: 1,370 training load

If we add all of these numbers together and divide by 4, we get a chronic workload of 1,535 units.

The way we calculate acute to chronic work ratios (ACWR) is by taking the acute weekly workload and dividing it by the chronic workload. Let's use the prior example and say our acute workload for the week is 1,440 and our chronic workload is 1,535:

$$1,440 / 1,535 = 0.94 \text{ ACWR}$$

Our goal is to keep the ACWR below 1.5. Our number here, 0.94, is far below 1.5, so we're doing a great job. Our goal is to keep our numbers from week to week consistent and try our best not to break 1.5.

ACWR becomes particularly important when we have time off from training or when we decide to ramp things up. Whenever we take some time off from the gym (let's say you drop down to two times per week or go on vacation for a week or two), we have to reduce our total training volume when we return because fitness (chronic workload) has decreased.

Another consideration is that a lot of folks will suddenly ramp up their training volume by adopting a more challenging program or starting something new (like beginning a running program). These are generally good things because we're adding more fitness to our lives but care should be taken to slowly ramp into each activity and respect the ACWR over time. A weightlifter who switches over to only running may have a similar ACWR based on time training and effort, but the areas stressed and the manner in which they're stressed is completely different.

Keep in mind that these ACWR principles apply to every novel movement you perform in the gym. Snatching when you haven't before (even if you're used to training) represents a spike in training for that new movement. Just because you're "trained" doesn't mean you're prepared for new activities that impose new stress on the body.

Also keep in mind that where the stress is applied becomes relevant as well. Let's say you train 4 days per week with a perceived intensity of 6 out of 10. The next week you do exactly the same thing. However, week 1 was lower-body dominant and week 2 was upper-body dominant. The

ACWR is exactly the same from week to week, but the area stressed is completely different. In this example, week 1 saw a spike in training volume of the lower body (and a decrease for the upper body) and week 2 saw a spike in upper body training volume (and a decrease for the lower body).

It may also make sense to track the volume of particular lifts in the gym, like squats, deadlifts, and Olympic lifts. This way we can track higher-stress movements and make sure we're being consistent over time. However, you can easily see how complex this can get. Calculating ACWR regularly is time intensive, and I know people are much more apt to give up if the process is too complex.

At the end of the day I think the goal is consistency. Try your best to make small changes from week to week and month to month. It may be fun to have wide variety in your training but unfortunately this may spike your training volume and increase injury risk as well. By all means try to use ACWR to its fullest extent, but I highly recommend just keeping things simple at the start and making it a healthy habit along with the rest of the variables discussed in this chapter.

There is no magic number where an injury is imminent when it comes to exceeding our typical workload. However, if we're staying close to our typical chronic workload and making changes slowly over time, then we're probably doing everything in our power to stay safe.

My recommendation is to calculate your workload at the end of each session and to keep track of your workload over the course of a week. If you notice your acute workload is starting to get much larger (using 1.5 times as a benchmark) than your chronic workload, it makes sense to back down. The goal is consistent workload over time. If you want to increase your fitness, make sure you do it very gradually, over time, to avoid spikes.

ACWR EXAMPLE 1

Tom currently trains 3 times per week for about 60 minutes at a 6 out of 10 RPE (60 x 6 x 3). His chronic weekly workload is generally around 1,080. He's been feeling good and decides to add in another day and push a little bit longer on some of his other training days. Here's his training log for this week.

Monday: 60 minutes x 7/10 = 420

Tuesday: 45 minutes x 8/10 = 360

Thursday: 90 minutes x 7/10 = 630

Friday: 60 minutes x 6/10 = 360

Tom's acute workload for this week is 1,770. His chronic workload is 1,080. His ACWR ratio is 1,770 / 1,080 = 1.64, which is above the recommended 1.5 number discussed previously. Tom should have dialed back somewhere within his training week.

ACWR EXAMPLE 2

Meghan trains consistently 5 times per week for 75 minutes at a 7 out of 10 perceived intensity. Her chronic workload is 2,625. She decides to go on a two-week vacation and she doesn't train at all during that time. When she returns, her goal is to resume her previous schedule exactly. Is she violating the ACWR guidelines? Let's re-calculate her chronic workload:

Week 1: 2,625 acute workload

Week 2: 2,625 acute workload

Week 3 (vacation): 0 acute workload

Week 4 (vacation): 0 acute workload

Meghan's chronic workload is now 5,250 / 4 = 1,313. Her two-week vacation means she has detrained. Attempting to continue her normal training as though the vacation never happened represents a 2,625 acute load. So, compared to her current chronic workload of 1,313, she'll have an ACWR of 2. Her ACWR is now over 1.5 and therefore she may be more at risk of injury upon return.

Meghan could consider starting back to training with 3 sessions per week, 4 the following week, and lastly 5 as a way to slowly reintroduce training stress and reduce the chance of injury.

Modifying Your Program

The next logical question is: How do you modify your training program if one of these variables is off? The easiest way is simply to back off somewhere. This can be achieved in a variety of ways:

- Reduce the weights used in your top sets (lower the RPE).
- Reduce the total number of sets for each exercise in a workout (for instance, 3 versus 4 total sets).
- Reduce the total number of exercises in a session (eliminate some of the less important accessory movements at the end of a session).
- Reduce the challenge of the exercises chosen (swap pull-ups for ring rows or squats for leg presses).

How much you back off will depend entirely on how bad your numbers are. If you went on a weekend bender consisting of hot dogs, beer, and cigarettes (not recommended!) or slept an average of 4 hours per night while getting a divorce (also not recommended!), you'll probably have to back off training by a *lot*. But if you just have a low energy level one day and are otherwise doing great, then maybe do one or two fewer deadlifts on your lower-body day.

What's also nice about tracking this information regularly is that you can use this data to more accurately improve your health and performance. Each parameter is obviously important for reducing your risk of injury, but it's also vitally important for both your health and performance in the gym. You can bet your bottom dollar that better sleep and nutrition are going to help build a bigger bench and those gigantic pythons you've been dreaming about.

With this data you can direct your efforts more accurately. Maybe your nutrition is on point but your sleep is terrible. You don't need to spend more time cooking, you need more time sleeping. Or maybe you never realized how stressed out you feel, and that may be the missing link in getting some of those chronic aches and pains to go away once the stress is resolved.

Intraworkout Monitoring by Data or Feel

It can be challenging to monitor how intense a training session is, and even harder to figure out if a specific set of an individual exercise was hard enough, too hard, or too easy, just by feel or qualitative measures alone. There have been some significant advancements made in tracking intensity during an exercise, and one of the most common and easily implemented technologies is velocity-based training (VBT). This involves measuring the speed of the bar, dumbbell, kettlebell, or whatever implement you might be using, and tracking changes in velocity from rep to rep.

As loading goes up, the velocity of the lift goes down in a near-perfect linear manner. At maximum load (expressed as 1RM), the velocity needed to move the weight and complete the rep is the lowest possible speed. At submaximal loads done for reps, the ability to maintain velocity across all reps tends to decrease as fatigue begins to set in. (To put it in simpler terms, you slow down as you get tired, even with a submax load.) Between sets, as fatigue begins to limit muscular force and neural input into the working muscles, velocity decreases. The decrease can be as much as 30 percent, and this figure can be used to determine how much volume the individual can successfully perform before fatigue-related changes set in, essentially giving an idea of how much work is needed to see an overreach that will produce the desired gains.

For example, let's say you're able to complete 5 reps of a back squat with 220 pounds (100 kg), and you do this for 5 sets. For the first 3 sets, the velocity is the same from the first rep to the last. For the sake of argument, we'll say you're cruising at around 2.2 feet per second (0.7 m/s). On the fourth set, the first rep is fast, but then, as you go through the set, bar speed slows down by about 0.3 feet per second (0.1m/s) by the end of the set. For the fifth set, you start at 2.2 feet per second (0.7 m/s), and then on the second rep you're already down to 2.0 feet per second (0.6 m/s), and by the last rep you're grinding at 1.6 feet per second (0.5 m/s). This represents a drop in velocity of almost 30 percent from the start of the work, which shows you're getting pretty tired. So how much volume can you manage effectively to get the benefits you're looking for? In this example we can see it would be 5 sets, because your velocity notably dropped on the last set. If you tried to do a sixth set, you'd likely hit failure by the third rep, or you would grind such an ugly rep that people would come over to ask if you're okay and your gym crush will never talk to you again.

In this same example, let's say your last workout with 220 pounds (100 kg) back squat for 5 sets of 5 had you moving at 2.2 feet per second (0.7 m/s). Today you come into the gym and want to use the same weight for the same number of reps and sets. That first set feels pretty light, and you find you were moving at 2.9 feet per second (0.9 m/s). What gives? Well, you moved the same weight faster, which is an indicator of greater muscle strength and power. That being said, you could take this info and assume you could manage a bit more weight on the bar to get you to that 2.2 feet per second (0.7 m/s) velocity, so using this info can help you adjust your training load, training volume, and rest between sets to maximize your training benefits.

The cool thing about VBT is you can use it to produce some flexibility in your programming and give you specific, real-time metrics to gauge how and where to switch things up and keep getting maximum benefits without having to guess what's going to work. You could set a goal of maintaining the same average velocity on all reps, stopping the set or number of sets when you see velocity drop by a certain number. You can perform as many sets as possible within a given velocity. You can start with a given load and add load until velocity meets a specific target. You can reduce weight over sets to maintain a specific velocity. You can change rest time between sets to try to maintain velocity at a given load over multiple sets. The sky is the limit, and all options figure in to what you're looking to do.

Compared to 5 or 10 years ago, the number and quality of VBT training tools has expanded significantly. For only a few hundred dollars you can now get devices that measure precisely and sync to your phone or tablet for real-time readouts and data tracking over time. If you want to get really detailed with your training and have the disposable cash, they're a great individual investment, and they're also great for coaches who want to provide more data for their clients or athletes.

If you don't want to spend any money, there are "soft signs" that the bar is moving well. For speedier sets, try to make the plates clink on the bar, where the bar moves so fast the plates push up and click on the bottom of the bar. As your speed drops, this clink sound will be harder and harder to create. When you start to notice that the bar pauses in your range of motion and you have to dig deep to start it moving in the right direction again, you might be at your lowest velocity. Finding the sweet spot between the clink of the plates on the bar and the pause at the sticking point of the lift can help give some info on where your fatigue point of volume is and whether or not you're lifting more weight for the same plate clink to determine increases in power output.

All of this is assuming that you're able to perform the exercises well under load and that fatigue isn't causing a breakdown in technique as you go through the reps. If you find that your positioning or movement starts to break down even if you're moving with a good velocity, you should stop there and reassess how you're performing the exercise before trying to push deeper into fatigue and seeing further breakdown in technique. Always, always, always stop at mechanical fatigue, even if you feel good, the bar is moving fast, and you want to show off for your social media channels. Trust me, no one will want to see those poor quality reps, and your results won't be what you'd want from performing them, so focus on good-quality, technique-oriented reps before you start pushing speed under load for specific volumes.

The use of VBT in your training is just another way to track progress or gauge whether you can change things up or not. The big question to consider is always, "How did that feel?" If it felt harder than you thought it would or you're not happy with the performance, the data validates that, saving you the risk of pushing through just for the sake of pushing. Keep in mind, though, that data isn't everything. The data can facilitate decisions about changing things or it could become a crutch if you rely on it and don't take into account how you feel. If you're feeling good and want to add more, give it a shot and see what happens. You can always change back if needed. If you're feeling under the weather or sense that the workout won't be your best today, take some weight off the bar or strip a set off each exercise. You're in charge—just use the data to help you decide what might be available for you to do in your workouts and track progress over time.

Conclusion

How do you know when you're on the right track with your training? Here are some general principles to determine when your training is moving in the right direction:

- The weight you use on the major lifts are going up in the gym.
- Your mood and energy level for training is consistent and moderate or high.
- You don't have injuries popping up or persisting.

How do you know if you're starting to overdo it or are at risk for injury? Here are some general principles to determine when your training is moving in the wrong direction:

- Your loads are stagnating or decreasing.
- You feel highly stressed or have low energy levels.
- You're dreading upcoming workouts.
- You start acquiring new injuries, or old injuries persist and become chronic.

If you're moving in the right direction, that's great! Keep going. If you aren't moving in the right direction, you can use some of the information you've gleaned from your training journal to help get you back on the right path.

If you feel you've maxed out on improving all the parameters I suggested earlier and you still feel run down, it may also mean your body is ready for a deload, a change of exercises, or potentially a reduction in training volume.

I have found myself in training slumps from time to time. These are periods when I just don't feel that motivated to train. They typically occur during periods of higher life stress but can also happen for what seems like no reason at all. I recommend continuing to modify based on how you feel (as outlined in this chapter) and start ramping back up once you start feeling better again.

Lastly if you ever feel like you need extra help from a medical provider due to excessive fatigue or mental health issues then definitely reach out and get some help, so we can keep pumping those biceps for life.

10

Sample Programs

Now we can get into the nitty gritty of what the workouts actually involve. But first, the standard disclaimers and legal stuff. The workouts shown in tables 10.1 to 10.21 at the end of this chapter are just examples. You can choose to do them or not, but they're not matched to *your* strengths, weaknesses, injuries, or medical concerns. There's no way for a book to match all of those criteria to someone we've never met or assessed, or if we haven't seen their medical history, and any exercise has a potential risk of injury. This program is no different. We can't assume any liability to any possible injuries that might result from attempting this program, so contact your doctor, physical therapist, qualified trainer, or strength coach and see if any of the following programs might be a good fit for you, or if you might need further adjustments or specializations to make sure you have the best risk-to-reward potential you could ask for.

With that out of the way, let's discuss how we've put this all together. As we've discussed throughout the book, many of the adjustments derive from the assessments in chapter 2, and take into account movement limitations that might come from the ankle, hip, thoracic spine, or shoulder. These aren't meant to diagnose any injuries; rather, they're just to say these areas might need special attention or adjustments if you weren't able to show full movement or control over them, and definitely do if that was the case and you want to add loading.

The workouts are designed to be doable with equipment you find at any commercial gym. In some situations, you might need to adjust based on available equipment, or if you work out in a home gym and don't want to buy something like a giant cable machine. You can easily use an elastic tube or a band anchored to a door or other sturdy structure to replicate any of the band exercises. If you don't have a kettlebell, dumbbells work well. If you don't have a barbell and plates, dumbbells will work in a pinch. If you have only a yoga mat and a dusty old treadmill, well, we can do only so much with that, especially if your goal is to get stronger, so you'll probably need to shell out for a gym membership.

We've built three different workout tracks—Low Everything, Medium Everything, and Unrestricted Everything—based on the results of the assessment. There's a good chance you'll have some variation of these, with your own assessment showing some combination of the three options. Don't feel like you have to fit into any of these, just use them as guidelines for your own workouts. If you have Medium Everything but one or two assessments show low mobility, add in a few more of the Level Up exercises for those regions, as discussed in chapter 7.

As a refresher, here are some of the Level Up exercises we went through in chapter 7:

Ankle Dorsiflexion

- Kneeling Active Ankle Rockback
- Eccentric Heel Drop
- Goblet Squat with Lateral Rockback

Hip Flexion

- Wall-Supported Knee to Chest
- Half-Kneeling Hip Flexion
- Supported Squat Hip Pry

Thoracic Spine

- Kneeling Bench Thoracic Spine Stretch
- Half-Kneeling Wall Thoracic Spine Rotation
- Sphynx Arm Slide

Shoulders

- Wall Shoulder Slide and Lift Off
- Dumbbell Pull-Over
- Incline Bench Y Raise

If any of these come up as part of your programming, give them a try, but feel free to switch and substitute based on what feels best and gives you the biggest benefits. There are also a ton of other exercises that can get you some serious mobility and motor control benefits, so if you feel others are better suited to your needs, or you'd rather use ones recommended to you by a coach or physical therapist you've worked with before, you can use those instead.

The metrics for the workout are minimal but provide enough detail to give you the information you need to get a quality workout in the volume and intensities desired, while letting you easily refer to the data to monitor your progress. In the workouts, you'll track the following variables:

• **Exercises**: This section outlines the different exercises to be performed. We've discussed them all in this book, so there shouldn't be any surprises.

• **Sets**: This is the number of times you'll perform the exercise within the workout. For whatever number is listed in the program, consider it as a suggested range. If it says to perform 4 sets, you might find the best option for you is to complete 3, 4, or even 5 sets, depending on your fitness level, energy level, endurance, and the load being used.

• **Reps**: Short for *repetitions*, this is the number of times you perform the exercise in a single set. This value will be presented as either a single number or as a range (i.e., 6-10). In either case, the goal is to get the number of reps within the set to be roughly this many, while also following the other metrics of the workout, like RPE and RIR.

• **Weight**: This will be the amount of weight used in specific exercises. It might be body weight, a specific elastic tension, or a certain dumbbell or barbell weight. We purposely left this metric blank because everyone is unique and so the weight will vary. Your job is to pick the weight that will allow you to complete the outlined number of reps within the range of the RPE and RIR given.

• **RPE**: Short for *rating of perceived exertion*, this is a qualitative (subjective) measure. It measures your perception, after finishing a set, of how hard the set was, using with a number from 1 to 10, 1 being super easy and barely challenging and 10 being the hardest thing you've ever done in your life. Some exercises might require you to think a lot but aren't as physically taxing; for those the RPE may feel really high due to the mental challenge, but RPE is a physical rating, not a mental one.

• **RIR**: Short for *reps in reserve*, this is a qualitative measure of how many reps you feel like you could still complete at the end of the set. If you finished a set with a 10 RPE, you probably couldn't have completed any more reps, whereas with an RPE around 4 or 6, you would likely have a higher number of reps in reserve. If you were supposed to complete only 3 reps and your RPE was 8 or 9, you likely would be able to do only one more rep with good technique, so your RIR would be 1.

- **Rest**: This is the amount of time to take as passive recovery between each set. It's important to rest, so don't be in a hurry to start the next set. Insufficient rest time could negatively affect your ability to perform the next set with enough work output. You might even need *more* rest to see enough output, so adjust this as needed, but make sure you still have some rest between sets.

We've outlined the exercises based on intensity as well. In addition to the qualitative metrics, there are three different intensity levels that can give you an idea of how hard you should be working. They can also help you to see how much volume of each is included in the workouts. The low-intensity work, shown highlighted in light green, can be done pretty much all the time, whereas the high-intensity work, shown highlighted in light red, will be limited to only a few exercises in each workout, as they make it harder to recover if you attempt too many of them at once. The moderate-intensity exercises (shown highlighted in light yellow) require more volume and endurance.

The workouts are outlined as supersets, with an A and B pairing. This means you would complete a full set of the A exercise, immediately go into a full set of the B exercise, and then rest before repeating A and B. This can help you fit more work into a workout versus just doing a single exercise at a time, plus it lets you get in some more of the Level Up exercises as an active recovery from some of the strength work.

Each month has a progression of volume or loading from the first to last week. The third month of each program includes one giant-volume day and one lower-volume day, as well as a deload week in week 5. The progressive build in volume and intensity also means a change in the weight used within each workout, so make sure you adjust loading based on the number of reps to be performed, as well as the RPE and RIR outlined for each exercise.

Besides the listed exercises for the workouts, it's important to do an effective warm-up before each workout, as well as to do some form of aerobic exercise outside of these workouts. In chapter 7, we outlined some sample warm-up exercises, which include the following:

Downward Dog, Lunge, and Rotation

Shin Box With Press-Up

Lateral Lunge With Overhead Driver

Prone Hip and Spine Rotation

Overhead Squat

You could run through each of these exercises, or any other exercises you feel help you to move easier and get a general sense of preparation for the coming workouts, plus get your heart rate up without creating any serious discomfort. Ideally the warm-up should include at least one set for each major body part, and more for high-output individuals who plan to lift heavy, or for people who have more miles on their training due to either lots of time in the gym or lots of time on Earth in general. For those people, 2 to 4 sets per body part might be needed, but an effective warm-up should take 5 to 15 minutes, regardless of how awesome or creaky you might feel.

Aerobic work can be done 1 to 3 times each week and won't take anything away from your strength work as long as it's not performed to maximal exertion or to serious fatigue. Workouts of 20 to 40 minutes will be enough for many to see some physiologic benefits, but if you're used to clocking a lot more time with your aerobic work, you can add in a bit more. Be sure, though, that you're still focusing on strength training. The aerobic work is to support the strength work, not the other way around, so make sure it's benefiting your ability to lift more weight, move more easily, or recover better between sets and between workouts.

If some exercises just don't jibe with you, maybe because of previous injury, discomfort during the movement, or lack of available equipment, you might benefit from using a regression or a different exercise. Review the information on the trainable menu in chapter 8 to see what we mean by finding what you can do in lieu of that movement, and pinpoint ways to get the training response you're looking for, even if it's not with the outlined exercise. There's always a way to get in the work you're trying to do, so find what will work and use that option. Don't force something that might not be as easy or consistent with your own situation.

Here's an example of how you could switch things up. Let's say the workout calls for doing a bench press, but bench press makes your shoulders scream bloody murder after each set. Instead of forcing yourself to push through and then hating life for the next three days, you could work on a few different things. First, you could spend more time getting your shoulders set up into the bench with a tighter position so there's less anterior shoulder strain, and if that doesn't work, maybe opt for some dumbbell movements with a rotated hand position instead. You could also do a floor press, where you lie on the floor and press the dumbbells, using the ground to prevent you from lowering the weights too far, or try different pressing options such as a standing cable press, push-up, or decline press that will give you most if not all of the benefits you're after but with a different approach.

For a movement like a deadlift, you could switch from a straight bar to a trap bar, or to a kettlebell, or work with a single-leg deadlift or a hip thrust to get some of the hip extension benefits. For a barbell squat, you could switch to a front squat or goblet squat, put some wedges under your heels, use a belt squat machine, or even jump on a leg press or hack squat machine, whatever will give you the stimulus and effort you're looking for without making you feel awful in the process.

When you start on the workouts, you can adjust things as you go, but try to keep them as close to the original outline as possible. Think of them like a recipe for a certain dish. If you start making a ton of substitutions left, right, and center, it's going to change the outcome pretty substantially, but adjusting one or two ingredients or a bit of cooking time won't alter the end result too much.

I'm sure after looking through the workouts you'll think to yourself, "Wait, these don't seem all that complicated, and there aren't any funky exercises or advanced options. These actually look kinda basic!" And you'd be right. The purpose of this book isn't to give you 50 novel exercises that have never been done before and that are so complex learning how to dance would have fewer steps. The purpose is to give a solid foundation with proven fundamentals that give great results, while also providing options that you can use to work through common issues that might hold you back. And of course, we've outlined some programming elements to help you adjust the program to fit your needs. In spite of what many Instagram posts might have you believe, some of the fittest people on the planet have built their bodies with basic exercises. The big reason why these workouts include these fundamental exercises without a lot of fluff is pretty simple: they work.

Exercises don't need to be complex or complicated to be beneficial. Mastery of the basics can take decades or longer, so while it might be fun to try new stuff all the time and it might make you feel like you're crushing yourself in the process (which in theory would produce some results), it's hard to look back and see where you've come from and what progress you've made if you're constantly switching things around. Seeing your squat or deadlift go up by 200 or 300 pounds (91-136 kg) in 5 years is real, tangible, and trackable progress that comes only from steady application of that exercise and unwavering focus on technique over years of repeated efforts. So yes, the exercises and workouts aren't complicated, because they don't need to be.

Once you've had a chance to run through the three months of programming, give the assessment another shot and see if you've made any changes. Also, look back on the progress you've made since week 1 and make some notes on whether you're moving more weight, completing more reps, or simply just feeling any better or worse throughout your day. While good training should be something that shows up as results in the weight room, it should also show some results outside of the weight room too, and with long-term programming you want to feel better and better as you progress, not feel like you're getting repeatedly run over and barely able to function in the real world. Once you reassess, you can jump back into week 1 on another training run that correlates with the outcome of the assessments and keep those gains coming.

Table 10.1 Low Everything Month 1, Weeks 1 and 2

Exercises	WEEK 1						WEEK 2					
	Sets	Reps or time	Weight	RPE	RIR	Rest	Sets	Reps or time	Weight	RPE	RIR	Rest
Day 1												
1A Medicine Ball Seated Rotation (p. 133)	2	8		3	NA		3	8		3	NA	
1B Wall-Supported Knee to Chest (p. 202)	2	6		4	NA	1 min	3	6		4	NA	1 min
2A Dumbbell Goblet Squat (p. 62)	3	8		5-7	5-7		4	8		5-7	5-7	
2B Dead Bug Squeeze (p. 127)	3	8		4	NA	1 min	4	8		4	NA	1 min
3A Bird Dog (p. 126)	3	10		4	NA		3	10		4	NA	
3B Dumbbell Row (p. 108)	3	12		5-7	5-7	1 min	3	12		5-7	5-7	1 min
Day 2												
1A Kneeling Active Ankle Rockback (p. 200)	2	6		2-3	NA		3	6		2-3	NA	
1B Cable Split Stance Chop (p. 137)	2	8		4-5	NA	1 min	3	8		4-5	NA	1 min
2A Trap Bar Deadlift (p. 74)	3	8		6-7	5-7		4	8		6-7	5-7	
2B Dumbbell Bench Press (p. 94)	3	6-10		6-7	5-7	1 min	4	6-10		6-7	5-7	1 min
3A Half-Kneeling Wall T-Spine Rotation (p. 205)	3	8		2-3	NA		3	8		2-3	NA	
3B Medicine Ball Seated Rotation (p. 133)	3	10		5-6	NA	1 min	3	10		5-6	NA	1 min

Exercises	WEEK 1						WEEK 2					
	Sets	Reps or time	Weight	RPE	RIR	Rest	Sets	Reps or time	Weight	RPE	RIR	Rest
Day 3												
1A Hardstyle Plank (p. 146)	2	30 sec		4-5	NA		3	30 sec		4-5	NA	
1B Dumbbell Pull-Over (p. 208)	2	10		4-5	NA	1 min	3	10		3-4	NA	1 min
2A Dumbbell Goblet Squat (p. 62)	3	12		6-8	4-5		4	5		6-8	45	
2B Medicine Ball Standing Rotational Throw (p. 139)	3	8		3-4	NA	1 min	4	8		3-4	NA	1 min
3A Seated Row (p. 106)	3	8		6-7	5-7		3	8		6-8	4-5	
3B Barbell Overhead Press (p. 99)	3	8		6-7	5-7	1 min	3	8		6-8	4-5	1 min
Day 4												
1A Cable Split Stance Chop (p. 137)	2	8		2-3	NA		3	6		2-3	NA	
1B Half-Kneeling Wall T-Spine Rotation (p. 205)	2	8		4-5	NA	1 min	3	8		4-5	NA	1 min
2A Standing Horizontal Press (p. 93)	3	12		6-7	5-7		4	8		6-7	5-7	
2B Bench Leg Lift (p. 144)	3	6-10		6-7	5-7	1 min	4	6-10		6-7	5-7	1 min
3A Trap Bar Deadlift (p. 74)	3	8		2-3	NA		3	8		2-3	NA	
3B Kneeling Active Ankle Rockback (p. 200)	3	10		5-6	NA	1 min	3	10		5-6	NA	1 min

Table 10.2 Low Everything Month 1, Weeks 3 and 4

Exercises	WEEK 3						WEEK 4					
	Sets	Reps or time	Weight	RPE	RIR	Rest	Sets	Reps or time	Weight	RPE	RIR	Rest
Day 1												
1A Medicine Ball Seated Rotation (p. 133)	3	8		3	NA		3	8		3	NA	
1B Wall-Supported Knee to Chest (p. 202)	3	6		4	NA	1 min	3	6		4	NA	1 min
2A Dumbbell Goblet Squat (p. 62)	4	8		5-7	5-7		4	6		6-8	4-5	
2B Dead Bug Squeeze (p. 127)	4	8		4	NA	1 min	4	8		4	NA	1 min
3A Bird Dog (p. 126)	3	10		4	NA		3	10		4	NA	
3B Dumbbell Row (p. 108)	3	12		5-7	5-7	1 min	3	12		5-7	5-7	1 min
Day 2												
1A Kneeling Active Ankle Rockback (p. 200)	3	6		2-3	NA		3	6		2-3	NA	
1B Cable Split Stance Chop (p. 137)	3	8		4-5	NA	1 min	3	8		4-5	NA	1 min
2A Trap Bar Deadlift (p. 74)	4	8		6-7	5-7		4	6		6-8	4-5	
2B Dumbbell Bench Press (p. 94)	4	6-10		6-7	5-7	1 min	4	6-10		6-7	5-7	1 min
3A Half-Kneeling Wall T-Spine Rotation (p. 205)	3	8		2-3	NA		3	8		2-3	NA	
3B Medicine Ball Seated Rotation (p. 133)	3	10		5-6	NA	1 min	3	10		5-6	NA	1 min

Exercises	WEEK 3						WEEK 4					
	Sets	Reps or time	Weight	RPE	RIR	Rest	Sets	Reps or time	Weight	RPE	RIR	Rest
Day 3												
1A Hardstyle Plank (p. 146)	3	30 sec		4-5	NA		3	30 sec		4-5	NA	
1B Dumbbell Pull-Over (p. 208)	3	10		3-4	NA	1 min	3	10		3-4	NA	1 min
2A Dumbbell Goblet Squat (p. 62)	4	5		6-8	4-5		5	3		6-8	4-5	
2B Medicine Ball Standing Rotational Throw (p. 139)	4	8		3-4	NA	1 min	5	8		3-4	NA	1 min
3A Seated Row (p. 106)	3	8		6-8	4-5		3	8		6-8	4-5	
3B Barbell Overhead Press (p. 99)	3	8		6-8	4-5	1 min	3	8		6-8	4-5	1 min
Day 4												
1A Cable Split Stance Crop (p. 137)	3	6		2-3	NA		3	6		2-3	NA	
1B Half-Kneeling Wall T-Spine Rotation (p. 205)	3	8		4-5	NA	1 min	3	8		4-5	NA	1 min
2A Standing Horizontal Press (p. 93)	4	8		6-7	5-7		4	5		7-8	4-5	
2B Bench Leg Lift (p. 144)	4	6-10		6-7	5-7	1 min	4	6-10		6-7	5-7	1 min
3A Trap Bar Deadlift (p. 74)	4	5		2-3	NA		4	5		2-3	NA	
3B Kneeling Active Ankle Rockback (p. 200)	3	10		5-6	NA	1 min	3	10		5-6	NA	1 min

Table 10.3 Low Everything Month 2, Weeks 1 and 2

Exercises	WEEK 1						WEEK 2					
	Sets	Reps or time	Weight	RPE	RIR	Rest	Sets	Reps or time	Weight	RPE	RIR	Rest
Day 1												
1A Bird Dog (p. 126)	2	8		3	NA		3	8		3	NA	
1B Supported Squat Hip Pry (p. 203)	2	6		4	NA	1 min	3	6		4	NA	1 min
2A Barbell Back Squat (p. 63)	4	5		6-8	2-4		4	5		7-8	2-3	
2B Dead Bug Squeeze (p. 127)	4	6		5	NA	1 min	4	8		4	NA	1 min
3A Medicine Ball Standing Rotational Throw (p. 139)	3	10		4	NA		3	10		4	NA	
3B Seated Row (p. 106)	3	12		5-7	5-7	1 min	3	12		5-7	5-7	1 min
4A Suitcase Carry (p. 122)	3	30 sec		7-8	NA		3	10 sec		5-7	NA	
4B Eccentric Heel Drop (p. 201)	3	8		4-5	NA	1 min	3	8		4-5	NA	1 min
Day 2												
1A Kneeling Active Ankle Rockback (p. 200)	2	6		2-3	NA		3	6		2-3	NA	
1B Plank Rotation (p. 128)	2	8		4-5	NA	1 min	3	8		4-5	NA	1 min
2A Kettlebell Deadlift (p. 73)	3	8		6-7	5-7		4	8		6-7	5-7	
2B Push-Up (p. 91)	3	6-10		6-7	5-7	2 min	4	6-10		6-7	5-7	2 min
3A Kneeling Bench T-Spine Stretch (p. 204)	3	8		2-3	NA		3	8		2-3	NA	
3B Cable Split Stance Chop (p. 137)	3	10		5-6	NA	1 min	3	10		5-6	NA	1 min
4A Farmer's Carry (p. 121)	3	30 sec		7-8	NA		3	30 sec		7-8	NA	
4B Half-Kneeling Hip Flexion (p. 203)	3	8		3-4	NA	1 min	3	8		3-4	NA	1 min

Exercises	WEEK 1						WEEK 2					
	Sets	Reps or time	Weight	RPE	RIR	Rest	Sets	Reps or time	Weight	RPE	RIR	Rest
Day 3												
1A Hardstyle Plank (p. 146)	2	30 sec		4-5	NA		3	30 sec		4-5	NA	
1B Dumbbell Pull-Over (p. 208)	2	10		3-4	NA	1 min	3	10		3-4	NA	1 min
2A Dumbbell Goblet Squat (p. 62)	3	5		6-8	4-5		4	5		6-8	4-5	
2B Cable Split Stance Chop (p. 137)	3	8		3-4	NA	1 min	4	8		3-4	NA	1 min
3A Seated Row (p. 106)	3	8		6-8	4-5		3	8		6-8	4-5	
3B Barbell Bench Press (p. 96)	3	8		6-8	4-5	1 min	3	8		6-8	4-5	1 min
4A Incline Bench Y Raise (p. 209)	3	8		4-5	NA		3	8		4-5	NA	
4B Kneeling Active Ankle Rockback (p. 200)	3	8		3-4	NA	1 min	3	8		3-4	NA	1 min
Day 4												
1A Medicine Ball Seated Rotation (p. 133)	2	6		2-3	NA		3	6		2-3	NA	
1B Kneeling Bench T-Spine Stretch (p. 204)	2	8		4-5	NA	1 min	3	8		4-5	NA	1 min
2A Dumbbell Bench Press (p. 94)	3	8		6-7	5-7		4	8		6-7	5-7	
2B Cable Lunge and Press (p. 136)	3	8-12		6-7	5-7	1 min	4	6-10		6-7	5-7	1 min
3A Suitcase Carry (p. 122)	3	8		2-3	NA		3	8		2-3	NA	
3B Goblet Squat With Lateral Rock (p. 201)	3	6		5-6	NA	1 min	3	10		5-6	NA	1 min
4A Bench Leg Lift (p. 144)	3	6		6-8	NA		3	6		6-8	NA	
4B Dumbbell Goblet Squat (p. 62)	3	10		6-8	4-5	1 min	3	12		6-8	4-5	1 min

Table 10.4 Low Everything Month 2, Weeks 3 and 4

	Exercises	WEEK 3						WEEK 4					
		Sets	Reps or time	Weight	RPE	RIR	Rest	Sets	Reps or time	Weight	RPE	RIR	Rest
Day 1													
1A	Bird Dog (p. 126)	3	8		3	NA		3	8		3	NA	
1B	Supported Squat Hip Pry (p. 203)	3	6		4	NA	1 min	3	6		4	NA	1 min
2A	Barbell Back Squat (p. 63)	4	5		7-8	2-3		4	5		8-9	1-3	
2B	Dead Bug Squeeze (p. 127)	4	8		4	NA	1 min	4	8		4	NA	1 min
3A	Medicine Ball Standing Rotational Throw (p. 139)	3	10		4	NA		3	10		4	NA	
3B	Seated Row (p. 106)	3	12		5-7	5-7	1 min	3	12		5-7	5-7	1 min
4A	Suitcase Carry (p. 122)	3	10		5-7	NA		3	10		5-7	NA	
4B	Eccentric Heel Drop (p. 201)	3	8		4-5	NA	1 min	3	8		4-5	NA	1 min
Day 2													
1A	Kneeling Active Ankle Rockback (p. 200)	3	6		2-3	NA		3	6		2-3	NA	
1B	Plank Rotation (p. 128)	3	8		4-5	NA	1 min	3	8		4-5	NA	1 min
2A	Kettlebell Deadlift (p. 73)	4	8		6-7	5-7		4	6		6-8	4-5	
2B	Push-Up (p. 91)	4	6-10		6-7	5-7	2 min	4	6-10		6-7	5-7	2 min
3A	Kneeling Bench T-Spine Stretch (p. 204)	3	8		2-3	NA		3	8		2-3	NA	
3B	Cable Split Stance Chop (p. 137)	3	10		5-6	NA	1 min	3	10		5-6	NA	1 min
4A	Farmer's Carry (p. 121)	3	30 sec		7-8	NA		3	30 sec		7-8	NA	
4B	Half-Kneeling Hip Flexion (p. 203)	3	8		3-4	NA	1 min	3	8		3-4	NA	1 min

		WEEK 3						WEEK 4					
	Exercises	Sets	Reps or time	Weight	RPE	RIR	Rest	Sets	Reps or time	Weight	RPE	RIR	Rest
Day 3													
1A	Hardstyle Plank (p. 146)	3	30 sec		4-5	NA		3	30 sec		4-5	NA	
1B	Dumbbell Pull-Over (p. 208)	3	10		3-4	NA	1 min	3	10		3-4	NA	1 min
2A	Dumbbell Goblet Squat (p. 62)	4	5		6-8	4-5		5	3		6-8	4-5	
2B	Cable Split Stance Chop (p. 137)	4	8		3-4	NA	1 min	5	8		3-4	NA	1 min
3A	Seated Row (p. 106)	3	8		6-8	4-5		3	8		6-8	4-5	
3B	Barbell Bench Press (p. 96)	3	8		6-8	4-5	1 min	3	8		6-8	4-5	1 min
4A	Incline Bench Y Raise (p. 209)	3	8		4-5	NA		3	8		4-5	NA	
4B	Kneeling Active Ankle Rockback (p. 200)	3	8		3-4	NA	1 min	3	8		3-4	NA	1 min
Day 4													
1A	Medicine Ball Seated Rotation (p. 133)	3	6		2-3	NA		3	6		2-3	NA	
1B	Kneeling Bench T-Spine Stretch (p. 204)	3	8		4-5	NA	1 min	3	8		4-5	NA	1 min
2A	Dumbbell Bench Press (p. 94)	4	8		6-7	5-7		4	5		7-8	4-5	
2B	Cable Lunge and Press (p. 136)	4	6-10		6-7	5-7	1 min	4	6-10		6-7	5-7	1 min
3A	Suitcase Carry (p. 122)	4	5		2-3	NA		4	5		2-3	NA	
3B	Goblet Squat With Lateral Rock (p. 201)	3	10		5-6	NA	1 min	3	10		5-6	NA	1 min
4A	Bench Leg Lift (p. 144)	3	6		6-8	NA		3	6		6-8	NA	
4B	Dumbbell Goblet Squat (p. 62)	3	12		6-8	4-5	1 min	3	12		6-8	4-5	1 min

Table 10.5 Low Everything Month 3, Weeks 1 and 2

Exercises	WEEK 1						WEEK 2					
	Sets	Reps or time	Weight	RPE	RIR	Rest	Sets	Reps or time	Weight	RPE	RIR	Rest
Day 1												
1A Medicine Ball Standing Rotational Throw (p. 139)	2	8		3	NA		3	8		3	NA	
1B Wall-Supported Knee to Chest (p. 202)	2	6		4	NA	1 min	3	6		4	NA	1 min
2A Dumbbell Goblet Squat (p. 62)	4	5		6-8	2-4		4	5		7-8	2-4	
2B Hardstyle Plank (p. 146)	4	20 sec		5	NA	1 min	4	20 sec		4	NA	1 min
3A Bird Dog (p. 126)	3	10		4	NA		3	10		4	NA	
3B Seated Row (p. 106)	3	12		5-7	5-7	1 min	3	12		8-9	1-2	1 min
4A Rack Carry (p. 123)	3	30 sec		5-7	NA		3	30 sec		5-7	NA	
4B Eccentric Heel Drop (p. 201)	3	8		4-5	NA	1 min	3	8		4-5	NA	1 min
Day 2												
1A Kneeling Active Ankle Rockback (p. 200)	2	6		2-3	NA		3	6		2-3	NA	
1B Cable Split Stance Chop (p. 137)	2	8		4-5	NA	1 min	3	8		4-5	NA	1 min
2A Trap Bar Deadlift (p. 74)	3	8		6-7	5-7		4	8		6-7	5-7	
2B Dumbbell Bench Press (p. 94)	3	6-12		6-7	5-7	2 min	4	6-10		6-7	5-7	2 min
3A Sphinx Arm Slide (p. 206)	3	8		2-3	NA		3	8		2-3	NA	
3B Plank Rotation (p. 128)	3	10		5-6	NA	1 min	3	10		5-6	NA	1 min

Exercises	WEEK 1						WEEK 2					
	Sets	Reps or time	Weight	RPE	RIR	Rest	Sets	Reps or time	Weight	RPE	RIR	Rest
Day 3												
1A Dead Bug Squeeze (p. 127)	2	8		4-5	NA		3	8		4-5	NA	
1B Incline Bench Y Raise (p. 209)	2	10		3-4	NA	1 min	3	10		3-4	NA	1 min
2A Barbell Back Squat (p. 63)	3	5		6-8	4-5		4	5		6-8	4-5	
2B Bench Leg Lift (p. 144)	3	8		3-4	NA	1 min	4	8		3-4	NA	1 min
3A Dumbbell Row (p. 108)	3	8		6-8	4-5		3	8		6-8	4-5	
3B Barbell Bench Press (p. 96)	3	8		6-8	4-5	1 min	3	8		6-8	4-5	1 min
4A Wall Shoulder Slide and Lift-Off (p. 207)	3	8		4-5	NA		3	8		4-5	NA	
4B Goblet Squat With Lateral Rock (p. 201)	3	8		3-4	NA	1 min	3	8		3-4	NA	1 min
5A Lat Pulldown (p. 111)	2	15		7-8	3-4		2	15		7-8	3-4	
5B Ab Wheel Rollout (p. 145)	2	8		7-8	3-4	1 min	2	8		7-8	3-4	1 min
Day 4												
1A Medicine Ball Slam (p. 140)	3	6		7-8	NA		3	6		7-8	NA	
1B Kneeling Bench T-Spine Stretch (p. 204)	3	8		4-5	NA	1 min	3	8		4-5	NA	1 min
2A Standing Horizontal Press (p. 93)	3	8		6-7	5-7		4	8		8-9	1-2	
2B Angled Barbell Straight-Arm Rotation (p. 134)	3	6-10		6-7	5-7	1 min	4	6-10		6-7	5-7	1 min
3A Suitcase Carry (p. 122)	3	8		2-3	NA		3	8		2-3	NA	
3B Kneeling Active Ankle Rockback (p. 200)	3	10		5-6	NA	1 min	3	10		5-6	NA	1 min
4A Medicine Ball Seated Rotation (p. 133)	3	12		6-8	NA		3	12		6-8	NA	
4B Dumbbell Goblet Squat (p. 62)	3	12		6-8	4-5	1 min	3	12		8-9	1-2	1 min

Table 10.6 Low Everything Month 3, Weeks 3 and 4

	Exercises	WEEK 3						WEEK 4					
		Sets	Reps or time	Weight	RPE	RIR	Rest	Sets	Reps or time	Weight	RPE	RIR	Rest
Day 1													
1A	Medicine Ball Standing Rotational Throw (p. 139)	3	8		3	NA		3	8		3	NA	
1B	Wall-Supported Knee to Chest (p. 202)	3	6		4	NA	1 min	3	6		4	NA	1 min
2A	Dumbbell Goblet Squat (p. 62)	4	5		7-8	2-3		4	5		8-9	1-3	
2B	Hardstyle Plank (p. 146)	4	20 sec		4	NA	1 min	4	20 sec		4	NA	1 min
3A	Bird Dog (p. 126)	3	10		4	NA		3	10		4	NA	
3B	Seated Row (p. 106)	3	12		8-9	1-2	1 min	3	12		8-9	1-2	1 min
4A	Rack Carry (p. 123)	3	30 sec		5-7	NA		3	30 sec		5-7	NA	
4B	Eccentric Heel Drops (p. 201)	3	8		4-5	NA	1 min	3	8		4-5	NA	1 min
Day 2													
1A	Kneeling Active Ankle Rockback (p. 200)	3	6		2-3	NA		3	6		2-3	NA	
1B	Cable Split Stance Chop (p. 137)	3	8		4-5	NA	1 min	3	8		4-5	NA	1 min
2A	Trap Bar Deadlift (p. 74)	4	8		6-7	5-7		4	6		7-8	4-5	
2B	Dumbbell Bench Press (p. 94)	4	6-10		6-7	5-7	2 min	4	6-10		8-9	1-2	2 min
3A	Sphinx Arm Slide (p. 206)	3	8		2-3	NA		3	8		2-3	NA	
3B	Plank Rotation (p. 128)	3	10		5-6	NA	1 min	3	10		5-6	NA	1 min

Exercises	Week 3 Sets	Reps or time	Weight	RPE	RIR	Rest	Week 4 Sets	Reps or time	Weight	RPE	RIR	Rest
Day 3												
1A Dead Bug Squeeze (p. 127)	3	8		4-5	NA		3	8		4-5	NA	
1B Incline Bench Y Raise (p. 209)	3	10		3-4	NA	1 min	3	10		3-4	NA	1 min
2A Barbell Back Squat (p. 63)	4	5		6-8	4-5		5	3		6-8	4-5	
2B Bench Leg Lift (p. 144)	4	8		3-4	NA	1 min	5	8		3-4	NA	1 min
3A Dumbbell Row (p. 108)	3	8		6-8	4-5		3	8		6-8	4-5	
3B Barbell Bench Press (p. 96)	3	6		7-8	2-3	1 min	3	6		7-8	2-3	1 min
4A Wall Shoulder Slide and Lift-Off (p. 207)	3	8		4-5	NA		3	8		4-5	NA	
4B Goblet Squat With Lateral Rock (p. 201)	3	8		3-4	NA	1 min	3	8		3-4	NA	1 min
5A Lat Pulldown (p. 111)	2	15		7-8	3-4		2	15		7-8	3-4	
5B Ab Wheel Rollout (p. 145)	2	8		7-8	3-4	1 min	2	8		7-8	3-4	1 min
Day 4												
1A Medicine Ball Slam (p. 140)	3	6		7-8	NA		3	6		7-8	NA	
1B Kneeling Bench T-Spine Stretch (p. 204)	3	8		4-5	NA	1 min	3	8		4-5	NA	1 min
2A Standing Horizontal Press (p. 93)	4	8		8-9	1-2		5	3		8-9	1-2	
2B Angled Barbell Straight-Arm Rotation (p. 134)	4	6-10		6-7	5-7	2 min	5	6-10		6-7	5-7	2 min
3A Suitcase Carry (p. 122)	4	5		2-3	NA		4	5		2-3	NA	
3B Kneeling Active Ankle Rockback (p. 200)	4	10		5-6	NA	1 min	4	10		5-6	NA	1 min
4A Medicine Ball Seated Rotation (p. 133)	3	12		6-8	NA		3	12		6-8	NA	
4B Dumbbell Goblet Squat (p. 62)	3	12		8-9	1-2	1 min	3	12		8-9	1-2	1 min

Table 10.7 Low Everything Month 3, Week 5, Deload Week

	Exercises	WEEK 5 DELOAD						
		Sets	Reps or time	Weight	RPE	RIR	Rest
Day 1							
1A	Medicine Ball Standing Rotational Throw (p. 139)	2	8		3	NA	
1B	Wall-Supported Knee to Chest (p. 202)	2	6		4	NA	1 min
2A	Dumbbell Goblet Squat (p. 62)	2	5		6-7	3-5	
2B	Hardstyle Plank (p. 146)	2	20 sec		4	NA	1 min
3A	Bird Dog (p. 126)	2	10		4	NA	
3B	Seated Row (p. 106)	2	12		6-7	3-5	1 min
4A	Rack Carry (p. 123)	3	30 sec		5-7	NA	
4B	Eccentric Heel Drop (p. 201)	3	8		4-5	NA	1 min
Day 2							
1A	Kneeling Active Ankle Rockback (p. 200)	2	6		2-3	NA	
1B	Cable Split Stance Chop (p. 137)	2	8		4-5	NA	1 min
2A	Trap Bar Deadlift (p. 74)	2	6		7-8	4-5	
2B	Dumbbell Bench Press (p. 94)	2	6-10		6-7	3-5	2 min
3A	Sphinx Arm Slide (p. 206)	3	8		2-3	NA	
3B	Plank Rotation (p. 128)	3	10		5-6	NA	1 min

WEEK 5 DELOAD

	Exercises	Sets	Reps or time	Weight	RPE	RIR	Rest
Day 3							
1A	Dead Bug Squeeze (p. 127)	2	8		4-5	NA	
1B	Incline Bench Y Raise (p. 209)	2	10		3-4	NA	1 min
2A	Barbell Back Squat (p. 63)	3	3		6-7	3-5	
2B	Bench Leg Lift (p. 144)	3	8		3-4	NA	1 min
3A	Dumbbell Row (p. 108)	2	8		6-7	3-5	
3B	Barbell Bench Press (p. 96)	2	6		7-8	2-3	1 min
4A	Wall Shoulder Slide and Lift-Off (p. 207)	3	8		4-5	NA	
4B	Goblet Squat With Lateral Rock (p. 201)	3	8		3-4	NA	1 min
Day 4							
1A	Medicine Ball Slam (p. 140)	2	6		7-8	NA	
1B	Kneeling Bench T-Spine Stretch (p. 204)	2	8		4-5	NA	1 min
2A	Standing Horizontal Press (p. 93)	3	3		8-9	1-2	
2B	Angled Barbell Straight-Arm Rotation (p. 134)	3	6-10		6-7	5-7	2 min
3A	Suitcase Carry (p. 122)	2	5		2-3	NA	
3B	Kneeling Active Ankle Rockback (p. 200)	2	10		5-6	NA	1 min
4A	Medicine Ball Seated Rotation (p. 133)	3	12		6-8	NA	
4B	Dumbbell Goblet Squat (p. 62)	3	12		8-9	1-2	1 min

Table 10.8 Medium Everything Month 1, Weeks 1 and 2

	Exercises	WEEK 1						WEEK 2					
		Sets	Reps or time	Weight	RPE	RIR	Rest	Sets	Reps or time	Weight	RPE	RIR	Rest
Day 1													
1A	Plank Rotation (p. 128)	2	8		3	NA		3	8		3	NA	
1B	Wall-Supported Knee to Chest (p. 202)	2	6		4	NA	1 min	3	6		4	NA	1 min
2A	Dumbbell Goblet Squat (p. 62)	3	8		5-7	5-7		4	8		5-7	5-7	
2B	Suitcase Carry (p. 122)	3	30 sec		6	NA	1 min	4	30 sec		6	NA	1 min
3A	Medicine Ball Seated Rotation (p. 133)	3	10		4	NA		3	10		4	NA	
3B	Half-Kneeling Wall T-spine Rotation (p. 205)	3	12		5-7	5-7	1 min	3	12		5-7	5-7	1 min
Day 2													
1A	Dumbbell Row (p. 108)	2	12		6-8	4-5		3	12		6-8	4-5	
1B	Medicine Ball Standing Rotational Throw (p. 139)	2	8		4-5	NA	1 min	3	8		4-5	NA	1 min
2A	Trap Bar Deadlift (p. 74)	3	8		6-7	5-7		4	8		6-7	5-7	
2B	Push-Up (p. 91)	3	6-10		6-7	5-7	1 min	4	6-10		6-7	5-7	1 min
3A	Kneeling Bench T-Spine Stretch (p. 204)	3	8		2-3	NA		3	8		2-3	NA	
3B	Bench Leg Lift (p. 144)	3	10		5-6	NA	1 min	3	10		5-6	NA	1 min

Exercises	WEEK 1						WEEK 2					
	Sets	Reps or time	Weight	RPE	RIR	Rest	Sets	Reps or time	Weight	RPE	RIR	Rest
Day 3												
1A Dead Bug Squeeze (p. 127)	2	10		4-5	NA		3	10		4-5	NA	
1B Incline Bench Y Raise (p. 209)	2	10		3-4	NA	1 min	3	10		3-4	NA	1 min
2A Barbell Back Squat (p. 63)	3	5		6-8	4-5		4	5		6-8	4-5	
2B Near Overhead Presses (p. 100)	3	8		6-8	3-4	1 min	4	8		6-8	3-4	1 min
3A Standing Horizontal Press (p. 93)	3	8		6-8	4-5		3	8		6-8	4-5	
3B Rack Carry (p. 123)	3	30 sec		6-8	NA	1 min	3	30 sec		6-8	NA	1 min
Day 4												
1A Cable Split Stance Chop (p. 137)	2	8		5-6	NA		3	8		5-6	NA	
1B Sphinx Arm Slide (p. 206)	2	8		4-5	NA	1 min	3	8		4-5	NA	1 min
2A Barbell Overhead Press (p. 99)	3	8		6-7	5-7		4	8		6-7	5-7	
2B Dumbbell Pull-Over (p. 208)	3	10		6-7	NA	1 min	4	10		6-7	5-7	1 min
3A Barbell Deadlift (p. 75)	3	6		6-8	3-4		3	6		2-3	NA	
3B Dumbbell Goblet Squat (p. 62)	3	10		5-6	4-5	1 min	3	10		5-6	NA	1 min

Table 10.9 Medium Everything Month 1, Weeks 3 and 4

Exercises	WEEK 3						WEEK 4					
	Sets	Reps or time	Weight	RPE	RIR	Rest	Sets	Reps or time	Weight	RPE	RIR	Rest
Day 1												
1A Plank Rotation (p. 128)	3	8		3	NA		3	8		3	NA	
1B Wall-Supported Knee to Chest (p. 202)	3	6		4	NA	1 min	3	6		4	NA	1 min
2A Dumbbell Goblet Squat (p. 62)	4	8		5-7	5-7		4	6		6-8	4-5	
2B Suitcase Carry (p. 122)	4	30 sec		6	NA	1 min	4	30 sec		6	NA	1 min
3A Medicine Ball Seated Rotation (p. 133)	3	10		4	NA		3	10		4	NA	
3B Half-Kneeling Wall T-spine Rotation (p. 205)	3	12		5-7	5-7	1 min	3	12		5-7	5-7	1 min
Day 2												
1A Dumbbell Row (p. 108)	3	12		6-8	4-5		3	12		6-8	4-5	
1B Medicine Ball Standing Rotational Throw (p. 139)	3	8		4-5	NA	1 min	3	8		4-5	NA	1 min
2A Trap Bar Deadlift (p. 74)	4	8		6-7	5-7		4	6		6-8	4-5	
2B Push-Up (p. 91)	4	6-10		6-7	5-7	1 min	4	6-10		6-7	5-7	1 min
3A Kneeling Bench T-Spine Stretch (p. 204)	3	8		2-3	NA		3	8		2-3	NA	
3B Bench Leg Lift (p. 144)	3	10		5-6	NA	1 min	3	10		5-6	NA	1 min

Exercises	WEEK 3						WEEK 4					
	Sets	Reps or time	Weight	RPE	RIR	Rest	Sets	Reps or time	Weight	RPE	RIR	Rest
Day 3												
1A Dead Bug Squeeze (p. 127)	3	10		4-5	NA		3	10		4-5	NA	
1B Incline Bench Y Raise (p. 209)	3	10		3-4	NA	1 min	3	10		3-4	NA	1 min
2A Barbell Back Squat (p. 63)	4	5		6-8	4-5		5	3		6-8	4-5	
2B Near Overhead Presses (p. 100)	4	8		6-8	3-4	1 min	5	8		6-8	3-4	1 min
3A Standing Horizontal Press (p. 93)	3	8		6-8	4-5		3	8		6-8	4-5	
3B Rack Carry (p. 123)	3	30 sec		6-8	NA	1 min	3	30 sec		6-8	NA	1 min
Day 4												
1A Cable Split Stance Chop (p. 137)	3	8		5-6	NA		3	8		5-6	NA	
1B Sphinx Arm Slide (p. 206)	3	8		4-5	NA	1 min	3	8		4-5	NA	1 min
2A Barbell Overhead Press (p. 99)	4	8		6-7	5-7		4	5		6-8	2-3	
2B Dumbbell Pull-Over (p. 208)	4	10		6-7	5-7	1 min	4	10		6-7	5-7	1 min
3A Barbell Deadlift (p. 75)	4	5		2-3	NA		4	5		2-3	NA	
3B Dumbbell Goblet Squat (p. 62)	3	10		5-6	NA	1 min	3	10		5-6	NA	1 min

Table 10.10 Medium Everything Month 2, Weeks 1 and 2

Exercises	WEEK 1						WEEK 2					
	Sets	Reps or time	Weight	RPE	RIR	Rest	Sets	Reps or time	Weight	RPE	RIR	Rest
Day 1												
1A Medicine Ball Seated Rotation (p. 133)	2	8		6	NA		3	8		6	NA	
1B Half-Kneeling Hip Flexion (p. 203)	2	6		4	NA	1 min	3	6		4	NA	1 min
2A Dumbbell Goblet Squat (p. 62)	4	5		6-8	2-4		4	5		7-8	2-4	
2B Suitcase Carry (p. 122)	4	6		7	NA	1 min	4	8		7	NA	1 min
3A Cable Lunge and Press (p. 136)	3	10		4	NA		3	10		4	NA	
3B Barbell Bent-Over Row (p. 109)	3	12		7-8	3-4	1 min	3	12		7-8	3-4	1 min
4A Dead Bug Squeeze (p. 127)	3	10		5-7	NA		3	10		5-7	NA	
4B Goblet Squat With Lateral Rock (p. 201)	3	8		4-5	NA	1 min	3	8		4-5	NA	1 min
Day 2												
1A Eccentric Heel Drop (p. 201)	2	6		2-3	NA		3	6		2-3	NA	
1B Bench Leg Lift (p. 144)	2	8		4-5	NA	1 min	3	8		4-5	NA	1 min
2A Suitcase Carry (p. 122)	3	8		6-7	5-7		4	8		6-7	5-7	
2B Standing Horizontal Press (p. 93)	3	8-12		7-8	2-3	2 min	4	8-12		8-9	1-2	2 min
3A Dumbbell Goblet Squat (p. 62)	3	8		7-8	2-3		3	8		7-8	2-3	
3B Hanging Knee Raise (p. 142)	3	10		7-8	NA	1 min	3	10		7-8	NA	1 min
4A Hardstyle Plank (p. 146)	3	30 sec		7-8	NA		3	30 sec		6-8	NA	
4B Seated Row (p. 106)	3	8		3-4	NA	1 min	3	8		3-4	NA	1 min

	Exercises	WEEK 1						WEEK 2					
		Sets	Reps or time	Weight	RPE	RIR	Rest	Sets	Reps or time	Weight	RPE	RIR	Rest
Day 3													
1A	Ab Wheel Rollout (p. 145)	2	10		7-8	NA		3	10		7-8	NA	
1B	Dumbbell Pull-Over (p. 208)	2	10		3-4	NA	1 min	3	10		3-4	NA	1 min
2A	Dumbbell Goblet Squat (p. 62)	3	5		6-8	4-5		4	5		6-8	4-5	
2B	Angled Barbell Straight-Arm Rotation (p. 134)	3	8		6-8	NA	1 min	4	8		6-8	NA	1 min
3A	Lat Pulldown (p. 111)	3	8		6-8	4-5		3	8		6-8	4-5	
3B	Near Overhead Presses (p. 100)	3	8		6-8	4-5	1 min	3	8		6-8	4-5	1 min
4A	Wall Shoulder Slide and Lift-Off (p. 207)	3	8		4-5	NA		3	8		4-5	NA	
4B	Incline Bench Y Raise (p. 209)	3	8		3-4	NA	1 min	3	8		3-4	NA	1 min
Day 4													
1A	Plank Rotation (p. 128)	2	6		2-3	NA		3	6		2-3	NA	
1B	Sphinx Arm Slide (p. 206)	2	8		4-5	NA	1 min	3	8		4-5	NA	1 min
2A	Push-Up (p. 91)	3	6-10		6-7	2-5		4	6-10		6-7	2-5	
2B	Medicine Ball Standing Rotational Throw (p. 139)	3	8		6-7	5-7	1 min	4	8		6-7	5-7	1 min
3A	Barbell Deadlift (p. 75)	3	8		5-7	5-7		3	8		7-8	2-3	
3B	Goblet Squat With Lateral Rock (p. 201)	3	10		5-6	NA	1 min	3	10		5-6	NA	1 min
4A	Bird Dog (p. 126)	3	8		6-8	NA		3	8		6-8	NA	
4B	Dumbbell Goblet Squat (p. 62)	3	12		6-8	4-5	1 min	3	12		6-8	4-5	1 min

Table 10.11 Medium Everything Month 2, Weeks 3 and 4

	Exercises	WEEK 3						WEEK 4					
		Sets	Reps or time	Weight	RPE	RIR	Rest	Sets	Reps or time	Weight	RPE	RIR	Rest
Day 1													
1A	Medicine Ball Seated Rotation (p. 133)	3	8		6	NA		3	8		6	NA	
1B	Half-Kneeling Hip Flexion (p. 203)	3	6		4	NA	1 min	3	6		4	NA	1 min
2A	Dumbbell Goblet Squat (p. 62)	4	5		7-8	2-3		4	5		8-9	1-3	
2B	Suitcase Carry (p. 122)	4	8		7	NA	1 min	4	8		7	NA	1 min
3A	Cable Lunge and Press (p. 136)	3	10		4	NA		3	10		4	NA	
3B	Barbell Bent-Over Row (p. 109)	3	12		7-8	3-4	1 min	3	12		7-8	3-4	1 min
4A	Dead Bug Squeeze (p. 127)	3	10		5-7	NA		3	10		5-7	NA	
4B	Goblet Squat With Lateral Rock (p. 201)	3	8		4-5	NA	1 min	3	8		4-5	NA	1 min
Day 2													
1A	Eccentric Heel Drop (p. 201)	3	6		2-3	NA		3	6		2-3	NA	
1B	Bench Leg Lift (p. 144)	3	8		4-5	NA	1 min	3	8		4-5	NA	1 min
2A	Suitcase Carry (p. 122)	4	8		6-7	5-7		4	6		6-8	4-5	
2B	Standing Horizontal Press (p. 93)	4	8-12		8-9	1-2	2 min	4	8-12		8-9	1-2	2 min
3A	Dumbbell Goblet Squat (p. 62)	3	8		7-8	2-3		3	8		7-8	2-3	
3B	Hanging Knee Raise (p. 142)	3	10		7-8	NA	1 min	3	10		7-8	NA	1 min
4A	Hardstyle Plank (p. 146)	3	30 sec		6-8	NA		3	30 sec		6-8	NA	
4B	Seated Row (p. 106)	3	8		3-4	NA	1 min	3	8		3-4	NA	1 min

Exercises	WEEK 3						WEEK 4					
	Sets	Reps or time	Weight	RPE	RIR	Rest	Sets	Reps or time	Weight	RPE	RIR	Rest
Day 3												
1A Ab Wheel Rollout (p. 145)	3	10		7-8	NA		3	10		7-8	NA	
1B Dumbbell Pull-Over (p. 208)	3	10		3-4	NA	1 min	3	10		3-4	NA	1 min
2A Dumbbell Goblet Squat (p. 62)	4	5		6-8	4-5		5	3		6-8	4-5	
2B Angled Barbell Straight-Arm Rotation (p. 134)	4	8		6-8	NA	1 min	5	8		6-8	NA	1 min
3A Lat Pulldown (p. 111)	3	8		6-8	4-5		3	8		6-8	4-5	
3B Near Overhead Presses (p. 100)	3	8		6-8	4-5	1 min	3	8		6-8	4-5	1 min
4A Wall Shoulder Slide and Lift-Off (p. 207)	3	8		4-5	NA		3	8		4-5	NA	
4B Incline Bench Y Raise (p. 209)	3	8		3-4	NA	1 min	3	8		3-4	NA	1 min
Day 4												
1A Plank Rotation (p. 128)	3	6		2-3	NA		3	6		2-3	NA	
1B Sphinx Arm Slide (p. 206)	3	8		4-5	NA	1 min	3	8		4-5	NA	1 min
2A Push-Up (p. 91)	4	6-10		6-7	2-5		4	6-10		6-7	2-5	
2B Medicine Ball Standing Rotational Throw (p. 139)	4	8		6-7	5-7	1 min	4	8		6-7	5-7	1 min
3A Barbell Deadlift (p. 75)	4	5		7-9	2-3		4	5		7-9	1-3	
3B Goblet Squat With Lateral Rock (p. 201)	3	10		5-6	NA	1 min	3	10		5-6	NA	1 min
4A Bird Dog (p. 126)	3	8		6-8	NA		3	8		6-8	NA	
4B Dumbbell Goblet Squat (p. 62)	3	12		6-8	4-5	1 min	3	12		6-8	4-5	1 min

Table 10.12 Medium Everything Month 3, Weeks 1 and 2

Exercises	WEEK 1						WEEK 2					
	Sets	Reps or time	Weight	RPE	RIR	Rest	Sets	Reps or time	Weight	RPE	RIR	Rest
Day 1												
1A Cable Split Stance Chop (p. 137)	2	8		3	NA		3	8		3	NA	
1B Supported Squat Hip Pry (p. 203)	2	6		4	NA	1 min	3	6		4	NA	1 min
2A Dumbbell Goblet Squat (p. 62)	4	5		6-8	2-4		4	5		7-8	2-4	
2B Suitcase Carry (p. 122)	4	6		5	NA	1 min	4	8		4	NA	1 min
3A Bird Dog (p. 126)	3	10		4	NA		3	10		4	NA	
3B Pull-Up (p. 112)	3	12		5-7	5-7	1 min	3	12		8-9	1-2	1 min
4A Hanging Knee Raise (p. 142)	3	10		5-7	NA		3	10		5-7	NA	
4B Eccentric Heel Drop (p. 201)	3	8		4-5	NA	1 min	3	8		4-5	NA	1 min
Day 2												
1A Goblet Squat With Lateral Rock p. (201)	2	6		2-3	NA		3	6		2-3	NA	
1B Medicine Ball Seated Rotation (p. 133)	2	8		4-5	NA	1 min	3	8		4-5	NA	1 min
2A Trap Bar Deadlift (p. 74)	3	8		6-7	5-7		4	5		7-8	2-3	
2B Push-Up (p. 91)	3	6-10		6-7	5-7	2 min	4	6-10		6-7	5-7	2 min
3A Kneeling Bench T-Spine Stretch (p. 204)	3	8		2-3	NA		3	8		2-3	NA	
3B Medicine Ball Standing Rotational Throw (p. 139)	3	10		5-6	NA	1 min	3	10		5-6	NA	1 min

Exercises	WEEK 1						WEEK 2					
	Sets	Reps or time	Weight	RPE	RIR	Rest	Sets	Reps or time	Weight	RPE	RIR	Rest
Day 3												
1A Hardstyle Plank (p. 146)	2	30 sec		4-5	NA		3	30 sec		4-5	NA	
1B Wall Shoulder Slide and Lift-Off (p. 207)	2	10		3-4	NA	1 min	3	10		3-4	NA	1 min
2A Barbell Back Squat (p. 63)	3	5		6-8	4-5		4	5		6-8	4-5	
2B Medicine Ball Half-Kneeling Rotational Throw (p. 138)	3	8		3-4	4-5	1 min	4	8		3-4	NA	1 min
3A Pull-Up (p. 112)	3	8		6-8	4-5		3	8		6-8	4-5	
3B Barbell Bench Press (p. 96)	3	8		6-8	4-5	1 min	3	8		6-8	4-5	1 min
4A Incline Bench Y Raise (p. 209)	3	8		4-5	NA		3	8		4-5	NA	
4B Kneeling Active Ankle Rockback (p. 200)	3	8		3-4	NA	1 min	3	8		3-4	NA	1 min
5A Wall-Supported Knee to Chest (p. 202)	2	8		5-6	NA		2	8		5-6	3-4	
5B Ab Wheel Rollout (p. 145)	2	10		7-8	NA	1 min	2	10		7-8	3-4	1 min
Day 4												
1A Bench Leg Lift (p. 144)	3	6		2-3	NA		3	6		2-3	NA	
1B Half-Kneeling Wall T-spine Rotations (p. 205)	3	8		4-5	NA	1 min	3	8		4-5	NA	1 min
2A Dumbbell Bench Press (p. 94)	3	8		6-7	5-7		4	8		8-9	1-2	
2B Medicine Ball Slam (p. 140)	3	6		7-8	5-7	1 min	4	6		7-8	5-7	2 min
3A Barbell Deadlift (p. 75)	3	8		6-7	4-5		3	6		7-8	3-4	
3B Angled Barbell Straight-Arm Rotation (p. 134)	3	10		5-6	NA	1 min	3	10		5-6	NA	1 min
4A Cable Lunge and Press (p. 136)	3	6		6-8	NA		3	6		6-8	NA	
4B Dumbbell Goblet Squat (p. 62)	3	12		6-8	4-5	1 min	3	12		8-9	1-2	2 min

Table 10.13 Medium Everything Month 3, Weeks 3 and 4

	Exercises	WEEK 3						WEEK 4					
		Sets	Reps or time	Weight	RPE	RIR	Rest	Sets	Reps or time	Weight	RPE	RIR	Rest
Day 1													
1A	Cable Split Stance Chop (p. 137)	3	8		3	NA		3	8		3	NA	
1B	Supported Squat Hip Pry (p. 203)	3	6		4	NA	1 min	3	6		4	NA	1 min
2A	Dumbbell Goblet Squat (p. 62)	4	5		7-8	2-3		4	5		8-9	1-3	
2B	Suitcase Carry (p. 122)	4	8		4	NA	1 min	4	8		4	NA	1 min
3A	Bird Dog (p. 126)	3	10		4	NA		3	10		4	NA	
3B	Pull-Up (p. 112)	3	12		8-9	1-2	1 min	3	12		8-9	1-2	1 min
4A	Hanging Knee Raise (p. 142)	3	10		5-7	NA		3	10		5-7	NA	
4B	Eccentric Heel Drop (p. 201)	3	8		5-7	NA	1 min	3	8		4-5	NA	1 min
Day 2													
1A	Goblet Squat With Lateral Rock (p. 201)	3	6		2-3	NA		3	6		2-3	NA	
1B	Medicine Ball Seated Rotation (p. 133)	3	8		4-5	NA	1 min	3	8		4-5	NA	1 min
2A	Trap Bar Deadlift (p. 74)	4	5		7-8	2-3		4	5		7-8	2-3	
2B	Push-Up (p. 91)	4	6-10		6-7	5-7	2 min	4	6-10		8-9	1-2	2 min
3A	Kneeling Bench T-Spine Stretch (p. 204)	3	8		2-3	NA		3	8		2-3	NA	
3B	Medicine Ball Standing Rotational Throw (p. 139)	3	10		5-6	NA	1 min	3	10		5-6	NA	1 min

	Exercises	WEEK 3						WEEK 4					
		Sets	Reps or time	Weight	RPE	RIR	Rest	Sets	Reps or time	Weight	RPE	RIR	Rest
Day 3													
1A	Hardstyle Plank (p. 146)	3	30 sec		4-5	NA		3	30 sec		4-5	NA	
1B	Wall Shoulder Slide and Lift Off (p. 207)	3	10		3-4	NA	1 min	3	10		2-3	NA	1 min
2A	Barbell Back Squat (p. 63)	4	5		6-8	4-5		5	3		6-8	4-5	
2B	Medicine Ball Half-Kneeling Rotational Throw (p. 138)	4	8		3-4	NA	1 min	5	8		3-4	NA	1 min
3A	Pull-Up (p. 112)	3	8		6-8	4-5		3	8		6-8	4-5	
3B	Barbell Bench Press (p. 96)	3	8		6-8	4-5	1 min	3	8		6-8	4-5	1 min
4A	Incline Bench Y Raise (p. 209)	3	8		4-5	NA		3	8		4-5	NA	
4B	Kneeling Active Ankle Rockback (p. 200)	3	8		3-4	NA	1 min	3	8		3-4	NA	1 min
5A	Wall Supported Knee to Chest (p. 202)	2	8		5-6	3-4		2	8		5-6	3-4	
5B	Ab Wheel Rollout (p. 145)	2	10		7-8	3-4	1 min	2	10		7-8	3-4	1 min
Day 4													
1A	Bench Leg Lift (p. 144)	3	6		2-3	NA		3	6		2-3	NA	
1B	Half-Kneeling Wall T-Spine Rotation (p. 205)	3	8		4-5	NA	1 min	3	8		4-5	NA	1 min
2A	Dumbbell Bench Press (p. 94)	4	8		8-9	1-2		5	3		8-9	1-2	
2B	Medicine Ball Slam (p. 140)	4	6		7-8	5-7	2 min	5	6		7-8	5-7	2 min
3A	Barbell Deadlift (p. 75)	4	5		8-9	1-2		4	3		8-9	1-2	
3B	Angled Barbell Straight-Arm Rotation (p. 134)	4	10		5-6	NA	1 min	4	10		5-6	NA	1 min
4A	Cable Lunge and Press (p. 136)	3	6		6-8	NA		3	6		6-8	NA	
4B	Dumbbell Goblet Squat (p. 62)	3	12		8-9	1-2	2 min	3	12		8-9	1-2	2 min

Table 10.14   Medium Everything Month 3, Week 5, Deload Week

| | Exercises | Sets | Reps or time | WEEK 5 DELOAD | | | |
				Weight	RPE	RIR	Rest
Day 1							
1A	Cable Split Stance Chop (p. 137)	2	8		3	NA	
1B	Supported Squat Hip Pry (p. 203)	2	6		4	NA	1 min
2A	Dumbbell Goblet Squat (p. 62)	2	5		6-7	3-5	
2B	Suitcase Carry (p. 122)	2	8		4	NA	1 min
3A	Bird Dog (p. 126)	2	10		4	NA	
3B	Pull-Up (p. 112)	2	12		6-7	3-5	1 min
4A	Hanging Knee Raise (p. 142)	3	10		5-7	NA	
4B	Eccentric Heel Drop (p. 201)	3	8		4-5	NA	1 min
Day 2							
1A	Goblet Squat With Lateral Rock (p. 201)	2	6		2-3	NA	
1B	Medicine Ball Seated Rotation (p. 133)	2	8		4-5	NA	1 min
2A	Trap Bar Deadlift (p. 74)	2	5		6-8	3-4	
2B	Push-Up (p. 91)	2	6-12		6-7	4-5	2 min
3A	Kneeling Bench T-Spine Stretch (p. 204)	3	8		2-3	NA	
3B	Medicine Ball Standing Rotational Throw (p. 139)	3	10		5-6	NA	1 min

WEEK 5 DELOAD

	Exercises	Sets	Reps or time	Weight	RPE	RIR	Rest
Day 3							
1A	Hardstyle Plank (p. 146)	2	30 sec		4-5	NA	
1B	Wall Shoulder Slide and Lift Off (p. 207)	2	10		3-4	NA	1 min
2A	Barbell Back Squat (p. 63)	3	3		6-7	3-5	
2B	Medicine Ball Half-Kneeling Rotational Throw (p. 138)	3	8		3-4	NA	1 min
3A	Pull-Up (p. 112)	2	8		6-7	3-5	
3B	Barbell Bench Press (p. 96)	2	8		6-7	3-5	1 min
4A	Incline Bench Y Raise (p. 209)	3	8		4-5	NA	
4B	Kneeling Active Ankle Rockback (p. 200)	3	8		3-4	NA	1 min
Day 4							
1A	Bench Leg Lift (p. 144)	2	6		2-3	NA	
1B	Half- Kneeling Wall T-Spine Rotation (p. 205)	2	8		4-5	NA	1 min
2A	Dumbbell Bench Press (p. 94)	3	3		8-9	1-2	
2B	Medicine Ball Slam (p. 140)	3	6		6-7	5-7	2 min
3A	Barbell Deadlift (p. 75)	2	5		6-8	3-4	
3B	Angled Barbell Straight-Arm Rotation (p. 134)	2	10		5-6	NA	1 min
4A	Cable Lunge and Press (p. 136)	3	6		6-8	NA	
4B	Dumbbell Goblet Squat (p. 62)	3	12		8-9	1-2	2 min

Table 10.15 Unrestricted Everything Month 1, Weeks 1 and 2

Exercises	WEEK 1						WEEK 2					
	Sets	Reps or time	Weight	RPE	RIR	Rest	Sets	Reps or time	Weight	RPE	RIR	Rest
Day 1												
1A Plank Rotation (p. 128)	2	8		3	NA		3	8		3	NA	
1B Half-Kneeling Hip Flexion (p. 203)	2	6		4	NA	1 min	3	6		4	NA	1 min
2A Barbell Front Squat (p. 64)	3	8		5-7	5-7		4	8		5-7	5-7	
2B Suitcase Carry (p. 122)	3	30 sec		4	NA	1 min	4	30 sec		4	NA	1 min
3A Lat Pulldown (p. 111)	3	10		5	5-7		3	10		6	5-7	
3B Half-Kneeling Wall T-Spine Rotation (p. 205)	3	12		5-7	NA	1 min	3	12		5-7	NA	1 min
Day 2												
1A Pull-Up (p. 112)	2	6		6-7	3-4		3	6		6-7	3-4	
1B Ab Wheel Rollout (p. 145)	2	8		4-5	NA	1 min	3	8		4-5	NA	1 min
2A Suitcase Carry (p. 122)	3	8		6-7	5-7		4	8		6-7	5-7	
2B Barbell Overhead Press (p. 99)	3	6-10		6-7	5-7	1 min	4	6-10		6-7	5-7	1 min
3A Kneeling Bench T-Spine Stretch (p. 204)	3	8		2-3	NA		3	8		2-3	NA	
3B Angled Barbell Straight-Arm Rotation (p. 134)	3	10		5-6	NA	1 min	3	10		5-6	NA	1 min

	Exercises	WEEK 1						WEEK 2					
		Sets	Reps or time	Weight	RPE	RIR	Rest	Sets	Reps or time	Weight	RPE	RIR	Rest
Day 3													
1A	Hardstyle Plank (p. 146)	2	30 sec		4-5	NA		3	30 sec		4-5	NA	
1B	Barbell Bent-Over Row (p. 109)	2	10		6-7	4-5	1 min	3	10		6-7	4-5	1 min
2A	Barbell Back Squat (p. 63)	3	5		6-8	4-5		4	5		6-8	4-5	
2B	Cable Lunge and Press (p. 136)	3	8		5-6	NA	1 min	4	8		5-6	NA	1 min
3A	Push-Up (p. 91)	3	8		6-8	4-5		3	8		6-8	4-5	
3B	Ab Wheel Rollout (p. 145)	3	8		6-8	4-5	1 min	3	8		6-8	4-5	1 min
Day 4													
1A	Medicine Ball Slam (p. 140)	2	6		2-3	NA		3	6		2-3	NA	
1B	Half-Kneeling Wall T-Spine Rotation (p. 205)	2	8		4-5	NA	1 min	3	8		4-5	NA	1 min
2A	Barbell Overhead Press (p. 99)	3	8		6-7	5-7		4	8		6-7	5-7	
2B	Dumbbell Goblet Squat (p. 62)	3	6-10		6-7	5-7	1 min	4	6-10		6-7	5-7	1 min
3A	Barbell Deadlift (p. 75)	3	8		6-7	4-5		3	8		6-7	4-5	
3B	Seated Row (p. 106)	3	10		7-8	3-4	1 min	3	10		7-8	3-4	1 min

Table 10.16 Unrestricted Everything Month 1, Weeks 3 and 4

		WEEK 3						WEEK 4					
	Exercises	Sets	Reps or time	Weight	RPE	RIR	Rest	Sets	Reps or time	Weight	RPE	RIR	Rest
Day 1													
1A	Plank Rotation (p. 128)	3	8		3	NA		3	8		3	NA	
1B	Half-Kneeling Hip Flexion (p. 203)	3	6		4	NA	1 min	3	6		4	NA	1 min
2A	Barbell Front Squat (p. 64)	4	8		5-7	5-7		4	6		6-8	4-5	
2B	Suitcase Carry (p. 122)	4	30 sec		6	NA	1 min	4	30 sec		6	NA	1 min
3A	Lat Pulldown (p. 111)	3	10		7	4-5		3	10		8	2-3	
3B	Half-Kneeling Wall T-Spine Rotation (p. 205)	3	12		5-7	NA	1 min	3	12		5-7	NA	1 min
Day 2													
1A	Pull-Up (p. 112)	3	6-8		6-7	3-4		3	6-8		6-7	3-4	
1B	Ab Wheel Rollout (p. 145)	3	8		4-5	NA	1 min	3	8		4-5	NA	1 min
2A	Suitcase Carry (p. 122)	4	8		6-7	4-5		4	6		6-8	4-5	
2B	Barbell Overhead Press (p. 99)	4	6-10		6-7	4-5	1 min	4	6-10		6-7	4-6	1 min
3A	Kneeling Bench T-Spine Stretch (p. 204)	3	8		2-3	NA		3	8		2-3	NA	
3B	Angled Barbell Straight-Arm Rotation (p. 134)	3	10		5-6		1 min	3	10		5-7	NA	1 min

Sample Programs

	Exercises	WEEK 3						WEEK 4					
		Sets	Reps or time	Weight	RPE	RIR	Rest	Sets	Reps or time	Weight	RPE	RIR	Rest
Day 3													
1A	Hardstyle Plank (p. 146)	3	30 sec		4-5	NA		3	30 sec		4-5	NA	
1B	Barbell Bent-Over Row (p. 109)	3	10		7-8	2-3	1 min	3	10		7-8	2-3	1 min
2A	Barbell Back Squat (p. 63)	4	5		6-8	4-5		5	3		6-8	2-3	
2B	Cable Lunge and Press (p. 136)	4	8		5-6	NA	1 min	5	8		5-6	NA	1 min
3A	Push-Up (p. 91)	3	8		6-8	4-5		3	8		6-8	4-5	
3B	Ab Wheel Rollout (p. 145)	3	8		6-8	4-5	1 min	3	8		6-8	4-5	1 min
Day 4													
1A	Medicine Ball Slam (p. 140)	3	6		2-3	NA		3	6		2-3	NA	
1B	Half-Kneeling Wall T-Spine Rotation (p. 205)	3	8		4-5	NA	1 min	3	8		4-5	NA	1 min
2A	Barbell Overhead Press (p. 99)	4	8		6-7	5-7		4	5		7-8	4-5	
2B	Dumbbell Goblet Squat (p. 62)	4	6-10		7-8	2-3	1 min	4	6-10		7-8	2-3	1 min
3A	Barbell Deadlift (p. 75)	4	5		7-8	2-3		4	5		7-8	2-3	
3B	Seated Row (p. 106)	3	10		7-8	3-4	1 min	3	10		7-8	3-4	1 min

Table 10.17 Unrestricted Everything Month 2, Weeks 1 and 2

	Exercises	WEEK 1						WEEK 2					
		Sets	Reps or time	Weight	RPE	RIR	Rest	Sets	Reps or time	Weight	RPE	RIR	Rest
Day 1													
1A	Bench Leg Lift (p. 144)	2	8		5-6	NA		3	8		3	NA	
1B	Half-Kneeling Hip Flexion (p. 203)	2	6		4	NA	1 min	3	6		4	NA	1 min
2A	Dumbbell Goblet Squat (p. 62)	4	5		6-8	2-4		4	5		7-8	2-4	
2B	Dead Bug Squeeze (p. 127)	4	6		5	NA	1 min	4	8		4	NA	1 min
3A	Medicine Ball Seated Rotation (p. 133)	3	10		4	NA		3	10		4	NA	
3B	Lat Pulldown (p. 111)	3	12		5-7	4-5	1 min	3	12		5-7	4-5	1 min
4A	Hardstyle Plank (p. 146)	3	30 sec		4-5	NA		3	30 sec		5-7	NA	
4B	Kneeling Active Ankle Rockback (p. 200)	3	8		4-5	NA	1 min	3	8		4-5	NA	1 min
Day 2													
1A	Goblet Squat with Lateral Rock (p. 201)	2	6		2-3	NA		3	6		2-3	NA	
1B	Cable Lunge and Press (p. 136)	2	8		4-5	NA	1 min	3	8		4-5	NA	1 min
2A	Trap Bar Deadlift (p. 74)	3	8		6-7	4-5		4	8		6-7	4-5	
2B	Standing Horizontal Press (p. 93)	3	8		6-7	4-5	2 min	4	8		6-7	4-5	2 min
3A	Barbell Front Squat (p. 64)	3	8		2-3	NA		3	8		2-3	NA	
3B	Medicine Ball Slam (p. 140)	3	10		5-6	NA	1 min	3	10		5-6	NA	1 min
4A	Farmer's Carry (p. 121)	3	30 sec		7-8	NA		3	30 sec		7-8	NA	
4B	Dumbbell Row (p. 108)	3	8		3-	NA	1 min	3	8		3-4	NA	1 min

Exercises	WEEK 1						WEEK 2					
	Sets	Reps or time	Weight	RPE	RIR	Rest	Sets	Reps or time	Weight	RPE	RIR	Rest
Day 3												
1A Rack Carry (p. 123)	2	30 sec		4-5	NA		3	30 sec		4-5	NA	
1B Push-Up (p. 91)	2	10		3-4	NA	1 min	3	10		3-4	NA	1 min
2A Dumbbell Goblet Squat (p. 62)	3	5		6-8	4-5		4	5		6-8	4-5	
2B Hanging Knee Raise (p. 142)	3	8		3-4	NA	1 min	4	8		3-4	NA	1 min
3A Barbell Deadlift (p. 75)	3	8		6-8	4-5		3	8		6-8	4-5	
3B Barbell Bench Press (p. 96)	3	8		6-8	4-5	1 min	3	8		6-8	4-5	1 min
4A Dumbbell Pull-Over (p. 208)	3	8		4-5	NA		3	8		4-5	NA	
4B Kneeling Active Ankle Rockback (p. 200)	3	8		3-4	NA	1 min	3	8		3-4	NA	1 min
Day 4												
1A Medicine Ball Half-Kneeling Rotational Throw (p. 138)	2	6		4-5	NA		3	6		2-3	NA	
1B Sphinx Arm Slide (p. 206)	2	8		4-5	NA	1 min	3	8		4-5	NA	1 min
2A Dumbbell Bench Press (p. 94)	3	8		6-7	4-5		4	8		6-7	4-5	
2B Angled Barbell Straight-Arm Rotation (p. 134)	3	6-8		6-7	4-5	1 min	4	6-8		6-7	4-5	1 min
3A Seated Row (p. 106)	3	8		6-7	4-5		3	8		6-7	4-5	
3B Eccentric Heel Drop (p. 201)	3	10		5-6	NA	1 min	3	10		5-6	NA	1 min
4A Barbell Overhead Press (p. 99)	3	6		6-8	3-4		3	6		6-8	3-4	
4B Barbell Bent-Over Row (p. 109)	3	12		6-8	4-5	1 min	3	12		6-8	4-5	1 min

Table 10.18 Unrestricted Everything Month 2, Weeks 3 and 4

	Exercises	WEEK 3						WEEK 4					
		Sets	Reps or time	Weight	RPE	RIR	Rest	Reps or time	Sets	Weight	RPE	RIR	Rest
Day 1													
1A	Bench Leg Lift (p. 144)	3	8		3	NA		8	3		3	NA	
1B	Half-Kneeling Hip Flexion (p. 203)	3	6		4	NA	1 min	6	3		4	NA	1 min
2A	Dumbbell Goblet Squat (p. 62)	4	5		7-8	2-3		5	4		8-9	1-3	
2B	Dead Bug Squeeze (p. 127)	4	8		4	NA	1 min	8	4		4	NA	1 min
3A	Medicine Ball Seated Rotation (p. 133)	3	10		4	NA		10	3		4	NA	
3B	Lat Pulldown (p. 111)	3	12		5-7	4-5	1 min	12	3		5-7	4-5	1 min
4A	Hardstyle Plank (p. 146)	3	30 sec		5-7	NA		30 sec	3		5-7	NA	
4B	Kneeling Active Ankle Rockback (p. 200)	3	8		4-5	NA	1 min	8	3		4-5	NA	1 min
Day 2													
1A	Goblet Squat With Lateral Rock (p. 201)	3	6		2-3	NA		6	3		2-3	NA	
1B	Cable Lunge and Press (p. 136)	3	8		4-5	NA	1 min	8	3		4-5	NA	1 min
2A	Trap Bar Deadlift (p. 74)	4	8		6-7	4-5		6	4		6-8	4-5	
2B	Standing Horizontal Press (p. 93)	4	8		6-7	4-5	2 min	12	4		6-7	5-7	2 min
3A	Barbell Front Squat (p. 64)	3	8		2-3	NA		8	3		2-3	NA	
3B	Medicine Ball Slam (p. 140)	3	10		5-6	NA	1 min	10	3		5-6	NA	1 min
4A	Farmer's Carry (p. 121)	3	30 sec		7-8	NA		30 sec	3		7-8	NA	
4B	Dumbbell Row (p. 108)	3	8		3-4	NA	1 min	8	3		3-4	NA	1 min

Exercises	WEEK 3						WEEK 4					
	Sets	Reps or time	Weight	RPE	RIR	Rest	Sets	Reps or time	Weight	RPE	RIR	Rest
Day 3												
1A Rack Carry (p. 123)	3	30 sec		4-5	NA		3	30 sec		4-5	NA	
1B Push-Up (p. 91)	3	10		3-4	NA	1 min	3	10		3-4	NA	1 min
2A Dumbbell Goblet Squat (p. 62)	4	5		6-8	4-5		5	3		6-8	4-5	
2B Hanging Knee Raise (p. 142)	4	8		3-4	NA	1 min	5	8		3-4	NA	1 min
3A Barbell Deadlift (p. 75)	3	8		6-8	4-5		3	8		6-8	4-5	
3B Barbell Bench Press (p. 96)	3	8		6-8	4-5	1 min	3	8		6-8	4-5	1 min
4A Dumbbell Pull-Over (p. 208)	3	8		4-5	NA		3	8		4-5	NA	
4B Kneeling Active Ankle Rockback (p. 200)	3	8		3-4	NA	1 min	3	8		3-4	NA	1 min
Day 4												
1A Medicine Ball Half-Kneeling Rotational Throw (p. 138)	3	6		2-3	NA		3	6		2-3	NA	
1B Sphinx Arm Slide (p. 206)	3	8		4-5	NA	1 min	3	8		4-5	NA	1 min
2A Dumbbell Bench Press (p. 94)	4	8		6-7	4-5		4	5		7-8	3-4	
2B Angled Barbell Straight-Arm Rotation (p. 134)	4	6-8		6-7	4-5	1 min	4	6-8		6-7	4-5	1 min
3A Seated Row (p. 106)	4	10		7-8	NA		4	10		7-8	4-5	
3B Eccentric Heel Drop (p. 201)	3	10		5-6	NA	1 min	3	10		5-6	NA	1 min
4A Barbell Overhead Press (p. 99)	3	6		6-8	3-4		3	6		6-8	3-4	
4B Barbell Bent-Over Row (p. 109)	3	12		6-8	4-5	1 min	3	12		6-8	4-5	1 min

Table 10.19 Unrestricted Everything Month 3, Weeks 1 and 2

	WEEK 1						WEEK 2					
Exercises	Sets	Reps or time	Weight	RPE	RIR	Rest	Sets	Reps or time	Weight	RPE	RIR	Rest
Day 1												
1A Medicine Ball Half-Kneeling Rotational Throw (p. 138)	2	8		5	NA		3	8		5	NA	
1B Supported Squat Hip Pry (p. 203)	2	6		4	NA	1 min	3	6		4	NA	1 min
2A Dumbbell Goblet Squat (p. 62)	4	5		6-8	2-4		4	5		7-8	2-4	
2B Dead Bug Squeeze (p. 127)	4	6		5	NA	1 min	4	8		4	NA	1 min
3A Bird Dog (p. 126)	3	10		4	NA		3	10		4	NA	
3B Dumbbell Row (p. 108)	3	12		5-7	4-5	1 min	3	12		8-9	1-2	1 min
4A Farmer's Carry (p. 121)	3	30 sec		5-	NA		3	30 sec		5-7	NA	
4B Eccentric Heel Drop (p. 201)	3	8		4-5	NA	1 min	3	8		4-5	NA	1 min
Day 2												
1A Wall Shoulder Slide and Liftoff (p. 207)	2	8		3-4	NA		3	8		3-4	NA	
1B Medicine Ball Slam (p. 140)	2	8		4-5	NA	1 min	3	8		4-5	NA	1 min
2A Kettlebell Deadlift (p. 73)	3	8		6-7	4-5		4	8		6-7	4-5	
2B Standing Horizontal Press (p. 93)	3	8-12		6-7	4-5	2 min	4	8-12		6-7	4-5	2 min
3A Half-Kneeling Wall T-Spine Rotation (p. 205)	3	8		2-3	NA		3	8		3-4	NA	
3B Hanging Knee Raise (p. 142)	3	10		5-6	NA	1 min	3	10		5-6	NA	1 min

	Exercises	WEEK 1						WEEK 2					
		Sets	Reps or time	Weight	RPE	RIR	Rest	Sets	Reps or time	Weight	RPE	RIR	Rest
Day 3													
1A	Plank Rotation (p. 128)	2	8		4-5	NA		3	8		5-6	NA	
1B	Wall Supported Knee to Chest (p. 202)	2	10		3-4	NA	1 min	3	10		4-	NA	1 min
2A	Dumbbell Goblet Squat (p. 62)	3	5		6-8	4-5		4	5		6-8	3-4	
2B	Angled Barbell Straight-Arm Rotation (p. 134)	3	8		4-5	NA	1 min	4	8		4-5	NA	1 min
3A	Pull-Up (p. 112)	3	5-8		6-8	2-3		3	5-8		6-8	2-3	
3B	Barbell Overhead Press (p. 99)	3	8		6-8	4-5	1 min	3	8		6-8	3-4	1 min
4A	Incline Bench Y Raise (p. 209)	3	8		4-5	NA		3	8		4-5	NA	
4B	Goblet Squat With Lateral Rock (p. 201)	3	8		3-4	NA	1 min	3	8		4-5	NA	1 min
5A	Half-Kneeling Wall T-Spine Rotation (p. 205)	2	8		4-5	NA		2	8		4-5	NA	
5B	Medicine Ball Half-Kneeling Rotational Throw (p. 138)	2	6		7-8	NA	1 min	2	6		7-8	2-3	1 min
Day 4													
1A	Cable Split Stance Chop (p. 137)	3	6		3-4	NA		3	6		3-4	NA	
1B	Kneeling Bench T-Spine Stretch (p. 204)	3	8		4-5	NA	1 min	3	8		4-5	NA	1 min
2A	Near Overhead Presses (p. 100)	3	8		6-7	4-5		4	8		8-9	1-2	
2B	Ab Wheel Rollout (p. 145)	3	10		6-7	4-5	1 min	4	10		6-7	4-5	2 min
3A	Barbell Deadlift (p. 75)	3	8		3-4	NA		3	8		3-4	NA	
3B	Barbell Bent-Over Row (p. 109)	3	10		5-7	NA	1 min	3	10		5-6	NA	1 min
4A	Rack Carry (p. 123)	3	30 sec		6-8	NA		3	30 sec		6-8	NA	
4B	Dumbbell Goblet Squat (p. 62)	3	12		6-8	4-5	1 min	3	12		8-9	1-2	1 min

Table 10.20 Unrestricted Everything Month 3, Weeks 3 and 4

	Exercises	WEEK 3						WEEK 4					
		Sets	Reps or time	Weight	RPE	RIR	Rest	Sets	Reps or time	Weight	RPE	RIR	Rest
Day 1													
1A	Medicine Ball Half-Kneeling Rotational Throw (p. 138)	3	8		5	NA		3	8		5	NA	
1B	Supported Squat Hip Pry (p. 203)	3	6		4	NA	1 min	3	6		4	NA	1 min
2A	Dumbbell Goblet Squat (p. 62)	4	5		7-8	2-3		4	5		8-9	1-3	
2B	Dead Bug Squeeze (p. 127)	4	8		4	NA	1 min	4	8		4	NA	1 min
3A	Bird Dog (p. 126)	3	10		4	NA		3	10		4	NA	
3B	Dumbbell Row (p. 108)	3	12		8-9	1-2	1 min	3	12		8-9	1-3	1 min
4A	Farmer's Carry (p. 121)	3	30 sec		5-7	NA		3	30 sec		5-7	NA	
4B	Eccentric Heel Drop (p. 201)	3	8		4-6	NA	1 min	3	8		4-5	NA	1 min
Day 2													
1A	Wall Shoulder Slide and Liftoff (p. 207)	3	8		3-4	NA		3	8		3-4	NA	
1B	Medicine Ball Slam (p. 140)	3	8		4-5	NA	1 min	3	8		4-5	NA	1 min
2A	Kettlebell Deadlift (p. 73)	4	8		6-7	3-4		4	6		6-8	3-4	
2B	Standing Horizontal Press (p. 93)	4	8-12		6-7	3-4	2 min	4	8-12		8-9	1-3	2 min
3A	Half-Kneeling Wall T-Spine Rotation (p. 205)	3	8		3-4	NA		3	8		3-4	NA	
3B	Hanging Knee Raise (p. 142)	3	10		5-6	NA	1 min	3	10		5-6	NA	1 min

Exercises	Week 3 Sets	Reps or time	Weight	RPE	RIR	Rest	Week 4 Sets	Reps or time	Weight	RPE	RIR	Rest
Day 3												
1A Plank Rotation (p. 128)	3	8		4-5	NA		3	8		4-5	NA	
1B Wall-Supported Knee to Chest (p. 202)	3	10		4-5	NA	1 min	3	10		4-5	NA	1 min
2A Dumbbell Goblet Squat (p. 62)	4	5		6-8	3-4		5	3		6-8	4-5	
2B Angled Barbell Straight-Arm Rotation (p. 134)	4	8		4-5	NA	1 min	5	8		4-5	NA	1 min
3A Pull-Up (p. 112)	3	5-8		6-8	2-3		3	5-8		6-8	2-3	
3B Barbell Overhead Press (p. 99)	3	8		6-8	3-4	1 min	3	8		6-8	3-4	1 min
4A Incline Bench Y Raise (p. 209)	3	8		4-5	NA		3	8		4-5	NA	
4B Goblet Squat With Lateral Rock (p. 201)	3	8		4-5	NA	1 min	3	8		4-5	NA	1 min
5A Half-Kneeling Wall T-Spine Rotation (p. 205)	2	8		4-5	NA		2	8		4-5	NA	
5B Medicine Ball Half-Kneeling Rotational Throw (p. 138)	2	6		7-8	2-3	1 min	2	6		7-8	3-4	1 min
Day 4												
1A Cable Split Stance Chop (p. 137)	3	6		4-5	NA		3	6		3-4	NA	
1B Kneeling Bench T-Spine Stretch (p. 204)	3	8		4-5	NA	1 min	3	8		4-5	NA	1 min
2A Near Overhead Presses (p. 100)	4	8		8-9	1-2		5	3		8-9	1-2	
2B Ab Wheel Rollout (p. 145)	4	10		6-7	4-5	2 min	4	10		6-7	4-5	2 min
3A Barbell Deadlift (p. 75)	4	5		4-5	NA		4	5		2-3	NA	
3B Barbell Bent-Over Row (p. 109)	4	10		5-6	NA	1 min	4	10		5-6	NA	1 min
4A Rack Carry (p. 123)	3	30 sec		6-8	NA		3	30 sec		6-8	NA	
4B Dumbbell Goblet Squat (p. 62)	3	12		8-9	1-2	1 min	3	12		8-9	1-2	1 min

Table 10.21   Unrestricted Everything Month 3, Week 5, Deload Week

	Exercises	Sets	Reps or time	WEEK 5 DELOAD Weight	RPE	RIR	Rest
Day 1							
1A	Medicine Ball Half-Kneeling Rotational Throw (p. 138)	2	8		5	NA	
1B	Supported Squat Hip Pry (p. 203)	2	6		4	NA	1 min
2A	Dumbbell Goblet Squat (p. 62)	2	5		6-7	3-5	
2B	Dead Bug Squeeze (p. 127)	2	8		4	NA	1 min
3A	Bird Dog (p. 126)	2	10		4	NA	
3B	Dumbbell Row (p. 108)	2	12		6-7	3-5	1 min
4A	Farmer's Carry (p. 121)	3	30 sec		5-6	NA	
4B	Eccentric Heel Drop (p. 201)	3	8		4-5	NA	1 min
Day 2							
1A	Wall Shoulder Slide and Liftoff (p. 207)	2	6		4-5	NA	
1B	Medicine Ball Slam (p. 140)	2	8		4-5	NA	1 min
2A	Kettlebell Deadlift (p. 73)	2	6		6-8	3-4	
2B	Standing Horizontal Press (p. 93)	2	8-12		6-7	4-5	2 min
3A	Half- Kneeling Wall T-Spine Rotation (p. 205)	3	8		4-5	NA	
3B	Hanging Knee Raise (p. 142)	3	10		5-6	NA	1 min

	Exercises	Sets	Reps or time	Weight	RPE	RIR	Rest
WEEK 5 DELOAD							
Day 3							
1A	Plank Rotation (p. 128)	2	8		4-5	NA	
1B	Wall-Supported Knee to Chest (p. 202)	2	10		4-5	NA	1 min
2A	Dumbbell Goblet Squat (p. 62)	3	3		6-8	3-5	
2B	Angled Barbell Straight-Arm Rotation (p. 134)	3	8		3-4	NA	1 min
3A	Pull-Up (p. 112)	2	5-8		6-7	2-3	
3B	Barbell Overhead Press (p. 99)	2	8		6-7	3-5	1 min
4A	Incline Bench Y Raise (p. 209)	3	8		4-5	NA	
4B	Goblet Squat With Lateral Rock (p. 201)	3	8		4-5	NA	1 min
Day 4							
1A	Cable Split Stance Chop (p. 137)	2	6		4-5	NA	
1B	Kneeling Bench T-Spine Stretch (p. 204)	2	8		4-5	NA	1 min
2A	Near Overhead Presses (p. 100)	3	3		8-9	1-2	
2B	Ab Wheel Rollout (p. 145)	3	10		6-7	4-5	2 min
3A	Barbell Deadlift (p. 75)	2	5		4-5	NA	
3B	Barbell Bent-Over Row (p. 109)	2	10		5-6	NA	1 min
4A	Rack Carry (p. 123)	3	30 sec		6-8	NA	
4B	Dumbbell Goblet Squat (p. 62)	3	12		8-9	1-2	1 min

References

Preface

1. Winett RA, Carpinelli RN. Potential health-related benefits of resistance training. *Prev Med.* 2001 Nov;33(5):503-513. doi:10.1006/pmed.2001.0909. PMID: 11676593.

2. Shailendra P, Baldock KL, Li LSK, Bennie JA, Boyle T. Resistance Training and Mortality Risk: A Systematic Review and Meta-Analysis. *Am J Prev Med.* 2022 Aug;63(2):277-285. doi:10.1016/j.amepre.2022.03.020. Epub 2022 May 20. PMID: 35599175.

3. Westcott WL. Resistance training is medicine: effects of strength training on health. *Curr Sports Med Rep.* 2012 Jul-Aug;11(4):209-216. doi:10.1249/JSR.0b013e31825dabb8. PMID: 22777332.

4. Saeidifard F, Medina-Inojosa JR, West CP, Olson TP, Somers VK, Bonikowske AR, Prokop LJ, et al. The association of resistance training with mortality: A systematic review and meta-analysis. *Eur J Prev Cardiol.* 2019 Oct;26(15):1647-1665. doi:10.1177/2047487319850718. Epub 2019 May 19. PMID: 31104484.

5. Schroeder EC, Franke WD, Sharp RL, Lee DC. Comparative effectiveness of aerobic, resistance, and combined training on cardiovascular disease risk factors: A randomized controlled trial. *PLoS One.* 2019 Jan 7;14(1):e0210292. doi:10.1371/journal.pone.0210292. PMID: 30615666; PMCID: PMC6322789.

6. Clark JE. Diet, exercise or diet with exercise: comparing the effectiveness of treatment options for weight loss and changes in fitness for adults (18-65 years old) who are overfat or obese; systematic review and meta-analysis. *J Diabetes Metab Disord.* 2015 Apr 17;14:31. doi:10.1186/s40200-015-0154-1. Erratum in: *J Diabetes Metab Disord.* 2015;14:73. PMID: 25973403; PMCID: PMC4429709.

7. Sherrington C, Fairhall NJ, Wallbank GK, Tiedemann A, Michaleff ZA, Howard K, Clemson L, et al. Exercise for preventing falls in older people living in the community. *Cochrane Database Syst Rev.* 2019 Jan 31;1(1):CD012424. doi:10.1002/14651858.CD012424.pub2. PMID: 30703272; PMCID: PMC6360922.

8. Marquez DX, Aguiñaga S, Vásquez PM, Conroy DE, Erickson KI, Hillman C, Stillman CM, et al. A systematic review of physical activity and quality of life and well-being. *Transl Behav Med.* 2020 Oct 12;10(5):1098-1109. doi:10.1093/tbm/ibz198. PMID: 33044541; PMCID: PMC7752999.

9. Coelho-Junior H, Marzetti E, Calvani R, Picca A, Arai H, Uchida M. Resistance training improves cognitive function in older adults with different cognitive status: a systematic review and meta-analysis. *Aging Ment Health.* 2022 Feb;26(2):213-224. doi:10.1080/13 607863.2020.1857691. Epub 2020 Dec 16. PMID: 33325273.

10. Lamb SE, Mistry D, Alleyne S, Atherton N, Brown D, Copsey B, Dosanjh S, et al. Aerobic and strength training exercise programme for cognitive impairment in people with mild to moderate dementia: the DAPA RCT. *Health Technol Assess.* 2018 May;22(28):1-202. doi:10.3310/hta22280. PMID: 29848412; PMCID: PMC5994643.

11. Wang L, Ye H, Li Z, Lu C, Ye J, Liao M, Chen X. Epidemiological trends of low back pain at the global, regional, and national levels. *Eur Spine J.* 2022 Apr;31(4):953-962. doi:10.1007/s00586-022-07133-x. Epub 2022 Feb 26. PMID: 35217914.

12. Lauersen JB, Bertelsen DM, Andersen LB. The effectiveness of exercise interventions to prevent sports injuries: a systematic review and meta-analysis of randomised controlled trials. *Br J Sports Med.* 2014 Jun;48(11):871-877. doi:10.1136/bjsports-2013-092538. Epub 2013 Oct 7. PMID: 24100287.

13. Cunha PM, Werneck AO, Nunes JP, Stubbs B, Schuch FB, Kunevaliki G, Zou L, Cyrino ES. Resistance training reduces depressive and anxiety symptoms in older women: a pilot study. *Aging Ment Health.* 2022 Jun;26(6):1136-1142. doi:10.1080/13607863.2021 .1922603. Epub 2021 May 18. PMID: 34003711.

References

Chapter 1

1. Grier T, Brooks RD, Solomon Z, Jones BH. Injury risk factors associated with weight training. *J Strength Cond Res*. 2022 Feb 1;36(2):e24-e30. doi:10.1519/JSC.0000000000003791. PMID: 32796416.

2. Prieto-González P, Martínez-Castillo JL, Fernández-Galván LM, Casado A, Soporki S, Sánchez-Infante J. Epidemiology of sports-related injuries and associated risk factors in adolescent athletes: an injury surveillance. *Int J Environ Res Public Health*. 2021 May 2;18(9):4857. doi:10.3390/ijerph18094857. PMID: 34063226; PMCID: PMC8125505.

3. Keogh JW, Winwood PW. The epidemiology of injuries across the weight-training sports. *Sports Med*. 2017 Mar;47(3):479-501. doi:10.1007/s40279-016-0575-0. PMID: 27328853.

4. Batterson AM, Froelich RK, Schleck CD, Laskowski ER. Injury rate and patterns in group strength-endurance training classes. *Mayo Clin Proc*. 2020 Mar;95(3):468-475. doi:10.1016/j.mayocp.2019.03.032. Epub 2019 Dec 5. PMID: 31813529.

5. Aasa U, Svartholm I, Andersson F, Berglund L. Injuries among weightlifters and powerlifters: a systematic review. *Br J Sports Med*. 2017 Feb;51(4):211-219. doi:10.1136/bjsports-2016-096037. Epub 2016 Oct 4. PMID: 27707741.

6. Requa, RK, DeAvilla, LN, and Garrick, JG. Injuries in recreational adult fitness activities. *Am J Sports Med*. 1993 May-Jun;21(3):461-467.

7. Finucane LM, Downie A, Mercer C, Greenhalgh SM, Boissonnault WG, Pool-Goudzwaard AL, Beneciuk JM, et al. International framework for red flags for potential serious spinal pathologies. *J Orthop Sports Phys Ther*. 2020 Jul;50(7):350-372. doi:10.2519/jospt.2020.9971. Epub 2020 May 21. PMID: 32438853.

8. Siewe J, Rudat J, Röllinghoff M, Schlegel UJ, Eysel P, Michael JW. Injuries and overuse syndromes in powerlifting. *Int J Sports Med*. 2011 Sep;32(9):703-711. doi:10.1055/s-0031-1277207. Epub 2011 May 17. PMID: 21590644.

9. Patel DR, Kinsella E. Evaluation and management of lower back pain in young athletes. *Transl Pediatr*. 2017 Jul;6(3):225-235. doi:10.21037/tp.2017.06.01. PMID: 28795014; PMCID: PMC5532202.

10. Wilk KE, Macrina LC, Reinold MM. Non-operative rehabilitation for traumatic and atraumatic glenohumeral instability. *N Am J Sports Phys Ther*. 2006 Feb;1(1):16-31.

11. Factor D, Dale B. Current concepts of rotator cuff tendinopathy. *Int J Sports Phys Ther*. 2014 Apr; 9(2): 274-288. www.ncbi.nlm.nih.gov/pmc/articles/PMC4004132.

12. Snyder GM, Mair SD, Lattermann C. Tendinopathy of the long head of the biceps. *Med Sport Sci*. 2012;57:76-89. doi:10.1159/000328880. Epub 2011 Oct 4. PMID: 21986047.

13. Auge WK, Fischer RA. Arthroscopic distal clavicle resection for isolated atraumatic osteolysis in weight lifters. *Am J Sports Med*. 1998 Mar-Apr;26(2):189-192. doi:10.1177/03635465980260020701. PMID: 9548111.

14. DeFroda SF, Nacca C, Waryasz GR, Owens BD. Diagnosis and management of distal clavicle osteolysis. *Orthopedics*. 2017 Mar 1;40(2):119-124. doi:10.3928/01477447-20161128-03. Epub 2016 Dec 7. PMID: 27925640.

15. Stanborough RO, Bestic JM, Peterson JJ. Shoulder osteoarthritis. *Radiol Clin North Am*. 2022 Jul;60(4):593-603. doi:10.1016/j.rcl.2022.03.003. PMID: 35672092.

16. Plachel F, Akgün D, Imiolczyk JP, Minkus M, Moroder P. Patient-specific risk profile associated with early-onset primary osteoarthritis of the shoulder: is it really primary? *Arch Orthop Trauma Surg*. 2023 Feb;143(2):699-706. doi:10.1007/s00402-021-04125-2. Epub 2021 Aug 18. PMID: 34406506; PMCID: PMC9925503.

17. Willy RW, Meira EP. Current concepts in biomechanical interventions for patellofemoral pain. *Int J Sports Phys Ther*. 2016 Dec;11(6):877-890. PMID: 27904791; PMCID: PMC5095941.

18. Reinking MF. Current concepts in the treatment of patellar tendinopathy. *Int J Sports Phys Ther*. 2016 Dec;11(6):854-866. PMID: 27904789; PMCID: PMC5095939.

19. Chirichella, PS, Jow, S, Iacono, S, Wey, HE, Malanga, GA. Treatment of knee meniscus pathology: rehabilitation, surgery, and orthobiologics. *PM&R*. 2018. doi:10.1016/j.pmrj.2018.08.384

20. Woo SL, Abramowitch SD, Kilger R, Liang R. Biomechanics of knee ligaments: injury, healing, and repair. *J Biomech.* 2006;39(1):1-20. doi:10.1016/j.jbiomech.2004.10.025. Epub 2005 Jan 7. PMID: 16271583.

21. Amin S, Goggins J, Niu J, Guermazi, A, Grigoryan, M, Hunter, DJ, Genant, HK, Felson, DT. Occupation-related squatting, kneeling, and heavy lifting and the knee joint: a magnetic resonance imaging–based study in men. *J Rheumatol.* 2008;35(8):1645-1649.

22. Szajkowski S, Dwornik M, Pasek J, Cieślar G. Risk factors for injury in CrossFit®: a retrospective analysis. *Int J Environ Res Public Health.* 2023 Jan 26;20(3):2211. doi:10.3390/ijerph20032211. PMID: 36767578; PMCID: PMC9916303.

23. Gabbett TJ. The training–injury prevention paradox: should athletes be training smarter and harder? *Br J Sports Med.* 2016;50:273-280.

24. Loudon JK. Biomechanics and pathomechanics of the patellofemoral joint. *Int J Sports Phys Ther.* 2016 Dec;11(6):820-830. PMID: 27904787; PMCID: PMC5095937.

25. Belavý DL, Quittner MJ, Ridgers N, Ling Y, Connell D, Rantalainen T. Running exercise strengthens the intervertebral disc. *Sci Rep.* 2017 Apr 19;7:45975. doi:10.1038/srep45975. PMID: 28422125; PMCID: PMC5396190.

26. Bohm S, Mersmann F, Arampatzis A. Human tendon adaptation in response to mechanical loading: a systematic review and meta-analysis of exercise intervention studies on healthy adults. *Sports Med Open.* 2015 Dec;1(1):7. doi:10.1186/s40798-015-0009-9. Epub 2015 Mar 27. PMID: 27747846; PMCID: PMC4532714.

27. Kujala UM, Kaprio J, Sarna S. Osteoarthritis of weight-bearing joints of lower limbs in former élite male athletes [published correction appears in BMJ 1994 Mar 26;308(6932):819]. *BMJ.* 1994;308(6923):231-234. doi:10.1136/bmj.308.6923.231

28. Mikesky AE, Mazzuca SA, Brandt KD, Perkins SM, Damush T, Lane KA. Effects of strength training on the incidence and progression of knee osteoarthritis. *Arthritis Rheum.* 2006;55(5):690-699. doi:10.1002/art.22245

29. Hamlin MJ, Wilkes D, Elliot CA, Lizamore CA, Kathiravel Y. Monitoring training loads and perceived stress in young elite university athletes. *Front Physiol.* 2019 Jan 29;10:34. doi:10.3389/fphys.2019.00034

30. Finan, PH, Goodin, BR, Smith, MT. The association of sleep and pain: an update and a path forward. *J Pain.* 2013 Dec; 14(12): 1539-1552.

31. Lindell M, Grimby-Ekman A. Stress, nonrestorative sleep, and physical inactivity as risk factors for chronic pain in young adults: a cohort study. *PLoS One.* 2022 Jan 21;17(1):e0262601. doi:10.1371/journal.pone.0262601. PMID: 35061825; PMCID: PMC8782303.

32. Gledhill A, Forsdyke D, Murray E. Psychological interventions used to reduce sports injuries: a systematic review of real-world effectiveness. *Br J Sports Med.* 2018 Aug;52(15):967-971. doi:10.1136/bjsports-2017-097694. Epub 2018 Feb 20. PMID: 29463497.

33. Huang K, Ihm J. Sleep and injury risk. *Curr Sports Med Rep.* 2021 Jun 1;20(6):286-290. doi:10.1249/JSR.0000000000000849. PMID: 34099605.

34. Martin S, Johnson U, McCall A, Ivarsson A. Psychological risk profile for overuse injuries in sport: an exploratory study. *J Sports Sci.* 2021 Mar 31:1-10. doi:10.1080/02640414.2021.1907904. Epub ahead of print. PMID: 33787453.

35. Bonilla-Jaime H, Sánchez-Salcedo JA, Estevez-Cabrera MM, Molina-Jiménez T, Cortes-Altamirano JL, Alfaro-Rodríguez A. Depression and pain: use of antidepressants. *Curr Neuropharmacol.* 2022;20(2):384-402. doi:10.2174/1570159X19666210609161447. PMID: 34151765; PMCID: PMC9413796.

36. Michaelides A, Zis P. Depression, anxiety and acute pain: links and management challenges. *Postgrad Med.* 2019 Sep;131(7):438-444. doi:10.1080/00325481.2019.1663705. Epub 2019 Sep 12. PMID: 31482756.

37. Lim JA, Choi SH, Lee WJ, Jang JH, Moon JY, Kim YC, Kang DH. Cognitive-behavioral therapy for patients with chronic pain: implications of gender differences in empathy. *Medicine (Baltimore).* 2018 Jun;97(23):e10867. doi:10.1097/MD.0000000000010867. PMID: 29879022; PMCID: PMC5999451.

38. Li S, Wu Q, Chen Z. Effects of psychological interventions on the prevention of sports injuries: a meta-analysis. *Orthop J Sports Med.* 2020 Aug 25;8(8):2325967120928325. doi:10.1177/2325967120928325. PMID: 32923493; PMCID: PMC7450469.

39. Griffin KL, Knight KB, Bass MA, Valliant MW. Predisposing risk factors for stress fractures in collegiate cross-country runners. *J Strength Cond Res.* 2021 Jan 1;35(1):227-232. doi:10.1519/JSC.0000000000002408. PMID: 29239997.

40. Papadopoulou SK. Rehabilitation nutrition for injury recovery of athletes: the role of macronutrient intake. *Nutrients.* 2020 Aug 14;12(8):2449. doi:10.3390/nu12082449. PMID: 32824034; PMCID: PMC7468744.

41. Fulton J, Wright K, Kelly M, Zebrosky B, Zanis M, Drvol C, Butler R. Injury risk is altered by previous injury: a systematic review of the literature and presentation of causative neuromuscular factors. *Int J Sports Phys Ther.* 2014 Oct;9(5):583-595. PMID: 25328821; PMCID: PMC4196323.

42. Whalan, M, Lovell, R, Sampson, JA. Do niggles matter? Increased injury risk following physical complaints in football (soccer). *Science and Medicine in Football.* 2019 Dec 23;4(3):216-224. https://doi.org/10.1080/24733938.2019.1705996.

43. Stephenson SD, Kocan JW, Vinod AV, Kluczynski MA, Bisson LJ. A comprehensive summary of systematic reviews on sports injury prevention strategies. *Orthop J Sports Med.* 2021 Oct 28;9(10):23259671211035776. doi:10.1177/23259671211035776. PMID: 34734094; PMCID: PMC8558815.

44. Mueller MJ, Maluf KS, Tissue adaptation to physical stress: a proposed "physical stress theory" to guide physical therapist practice, education, and research, *Phys Ther.* 2002 Apr;82(4):383-403.

45. Alentorn-Geli E, Samuelsson K, Musahl V, Green CL, Bhandari M, Karlsson J. The association of recreational and competitive running with hip and knee osteoarthritis: a systematic review and meta-analysis. *J Orthop Sports Phys Ther.* 2017 Jun;47(6):373-390. doi:10.2519/jospt.2017.7137. Epub 2017 May 13. PMID: 28504066.

46. Kolk, BA. van der (2014). *The Body Keeps the Score: Brain, Mind, and Body in the Healing of Trauma.* Viking; 2014.

47. Bliddal, H, Leeds, AR, Christensen, R. Osteoarthritis, obesity and weight loss: evidence, hypotheses and horizons—a scoping review. *Obes Rev.* 2014 Jul;15(7):578-86. doi: 10.1111/obr.12173. Epub 2014 Apr 22. PMID: 24751192; PMCID: PMC4238740.

Chapter 2

1. Bassey EJ, Morgan K, Dallosso HM, Ebrahim SB. Flexibility of the shoulder joint measured as range of abduction in a large representative sample of men and women over 65 years of age. *Eur J Appl Physiol Occup Physiol.* 1989;58(4):353-360. doi:10.1007/BF00643509. PMID: 2920713.

2. Medeiros HB, de Araújo DS, de Araújo CG. Age-related mobility loss is joint-specific: an analysis from 6,000 Flexitest results. *Age (Dordr).* 2013 Dec;35(6):2399-407. doi:10.1007/s11357-013-9525-z. Epub 2013 Mar 27. PMID: 23529505; PMCID: PMC3824991.

3. McKean MR, Dunn PK, Burkett BJ. The lumbar and sacrum movement pattern during the back squat exercise. J Strength Cond Res. 2010 Oct;24(10):2731-2741. doi:10.1519/JSC.0b013e3181e2e166. Erratum in: *J Strength Cond Res.* 2012 May;26(5):1454. PMID: 20885195.

4. Swank AM, Funk DC, Durham MP, Roberts S. Adding weights to stretching exercise increases passive range of motion for healthy elderly. *J Strength Cond Res.* 2003 May;17(2):374-378. doi:10.1519/1533-4287(2003)017<0374:awtsei>2.0.co;2. PMID: 12741881.

5. Alizadeh S, Daneshjoo A, Zahiri A, Anvar SH, Goudini R, Hicks JP, et al. Resistance training induces improvements in range of motion: a systematic review and meta-analysis. *Sports Med.* 2023 Mar;53(3):707-722. doi:10.1007/s40279-022-01804-x. Epub 2023 Jan 9. PMID: 36622555; PMCID: PMC9935664.

6. Thomas E, Bianco A, Paoli A, Palma A. The Relation between stretching typology and stretching duration: the effects on range of motion. *Int J Sports Med.* 2018 Apr;39(4):243-254. doi:10.1055/s-0044-101146. Epub 2018 Mar 5. PMID: 29506306.

7. Krause, DA, Youdas, JW, Hollman, JH, Smith, J. Abdominal muscle performance as measured by the double leg-lowering test. *Arch Phys Med Rehabil.* 2005 Jul;86(7):1345-8. doi: 10.1016/j.apmr.2004.12.020. PMID: 16003662.

Chapter 3

1. D'Lima DD, Urquhart AG, Buehler KO, Walker RH, Colwell CW Jr. The effect of the orientation of the acetabular and femoral components on the range of motion of the hip at different head-neck ratios. *J Bone Joint Surg Am.* 2000 Mar;82(3):315-321
2. Zalawadia A, Ruparelia S, Shah S, Parekh D, Patel S, Rathod S, et al. Study of femoral neck anteversion of adult dry femora in Gujarat region. *NJIRM.* 2010 July-Sept.; 1(3).
3. Ross, J R, Nepple, JJ, Philippon, MJ, Kelly, BT, Larson, CM, Bedi, A, Giveans, MR. Effect of changes in pelvic tilt on range of motion to impingement and radiographic parameters of acetabular morphologic characteristics. *Am J Sports Med.* 2014 Oct;42(10):2402-2409. doi:10.1177/0363546514541229. Epub 2014 Jul 24.
4. Laborie, LB, Lehmann, TG, Engesæter, I Ø, Sera, F, Engesæter, LB, Rosendahl, K. (2014). The alpha angle in cam-type femoroacetabular impingement. *Bone Joint J.* 2014 Apr;96-B(4):449-454. doi:10.1302/0301-620X.96B4.32194.
5. Widmer, K-H. and Zurfluh, B. Compliant positioning of total hip components for optimal range of motion. *J Orthop Res.* 2004;22: 815-821. doi: 10.1016/j.orthres.2003.11.001. PMID: 15183439.
6. Bhise, SA, Patil, NK. Dominant and nondominant leg activities in young adults. *IntJ Ther Rehab Res.* 2016;5(4), 257-264.
7. Shaw, CN., Stock, JT. Habitual throwing and swimming correspond with upper limb diaphyseal strength and shape in modern human athletes. *Am J Phys Anthropol.* 2009;140:160-172.
8. Hales, M. (Improving the deadlift: understanding biomechanical constraints and physiological adaptations to resistance exercise. *Strength Cond J.* 2010 Aug;32(4):44-51.
9. Cholewa JM, Atalag O, Zinchenko A, Johnson K, Henselmans M. Anthropometrical determinants of deadlift variant performance. *J Sports Sci Med.* 2019 Aug 1;18(3):448-453.

Chapter 4

1. Krause, D, Dueffert, L, Postma, J, Vogler, E, Walsh, A, Hollman, J. Influence of body position on shoulder and trunk muscle activation during resisted isometric shoulder external rotation. *Sports Health.* 2018;10(4):355-360.
2. Moll JM, Wright V. Normal range of spinal mobility: an objective clinical study. *Ann Rheum Dis.* 1971 Jul;30(4):381-386.
3. Wang JC, Shapiro MS. Changes in acromial morphology with age. *J Shoulder Elbow Surg.* 1997 Jan-Feb;6(1):55-59.
4. Balke M, Schmidt C, Dedy N, Banerjee M, Bouillon B, Liem D. Correlation of acromial morphology with impingement syndrome and rotator cuff tears. *Acta Orthop.* 2013 Apr;84(2):178-183.
5. Escamilla, R., Yamashiro, K., Paulos, L., Andrews, J. Shoulder muscle activity and function in common shoulder rehabilitation exercises. *Sports Med.* 2009; 39(8): 663-685.
6. Król H, Gołaś A. Effect of barbell weight on the structure of the flat bench press. J *Strength Cond Res.* 2017 May;31(5):1321-1337.
7. Mier, C., Amasay, T., Capehart, S., and Garner, H. Differences between men and women in percentage of body weight supported during push-up exercise. *I J Exercise Science.* 2014;7(2):161-8.
8. Ji-Hyun L, Heon-seock C, Chung-Hwi Y, Oh-yun K, Tae-Lim Y. Predictor variables for forward scapular posture including posterior shoulder tightness. *J Bodywork & Movement Ther.* 2015;19(2):253-260.
9. Baker, D, Newton, R. An analysis of the ratio and relationship between upper body pressing and pulling strength. *J Strength Conditioning Res.* 2004 Aug;18(3):594-598.
10. Noteboom, L, Belli, I, Hoozemans, MJM, Seth, A, Veeger, HEJ, Van Der Helm, FCT. Effects of bench press technique variations on musculoskeletal shoulder loads and potential

References

injury risk. *Front Physiol.* 2024 Jun;15:1393235. doi: 10.3389/fphys.2024.1393235. PMID: 38974522; PMCID: PMC11224528.

Chapter 5

1. Shengyao, L, Kim, G, Kim, L, He, S, Nasnoor, J, Congxin, D, Xiuwen, Z. Effects of core training on skill performance among athletes: a systematic review. *Front Physiol* 2022;13(6).
2. Saeterbakken, A, Stien, N, Andersen, V, Scott, S, Cumming, K, Behm, D, Granacher, U, Preiske, O. The effects of trunk muscle training on physical fitness and sport-specific performance in young and adult athletes: a systematic review and meta-analysis. *Sports Med.* 2022;52:1599-1622.
3. Olivia-Lozano, J, Muyor, JM. Core muscle activity during physical fitness exercises: a systematic review. *Int J Environ Res. Pub Health.* 2020;17:4306.
4. Duong, A, Wójcicki, TR, Carnes, AJ. The effects of unilateral resistance training on muscular strength, power, and measures of core stability in resistance trained individuals. *Int J Strength Cond.* 2022;2(1).
5. Smrcina Z, Woelfel S, Burcal C. A systematic review of the effectiveness of core stability exercises in patients with non-specific low back pain. *Int J Sports Phys Ther.* 2022 Aug 1;17(5):766-774. doi:10.26603/001c.37251. PMID: 35949382; PMCID: PMC9340836.
6. Shiri R, Coggon D, Falah-Hassani K. Exercise for the prevention of low back pain: systematic review and meta-analysis of controlled trials. *Am J Epidemiol.* 2018 May 1;187(5):1093-1101. doi:10.1093/aje/kwx337. PMID: 29053873.
7. McGill, SM, Marshall, L, and Andersen, J. Low back loads while walking and carrying: comparing the load carried in one hand or in both hands. *Ergonomics.* 2013;56(2):293-302.
8. McGill, SM, McDermott, A, and Fenwick, CM. Comparison of different strongman events: trunk muscle activation and lumbar spine motion, load, and stiffness. J Strength Cond Res. 2009;23(4):1148-1161.
9. McGill, SM, Marshall, L, and Andersen, J. Low back loads while walking and carrying: comparing the load carried in one hand or in both hands. *Ergonomics.* 2013;56(2):293-302.
10. Santana, JC, McGill, S, Brown, L. Anterior and posterior serape: the rotational core. *Strength Cond J.*2015 Oct;37(5):8-13.

Chapter 6

1. Lee, DH, Rezende, LFM, Joh, HK, Keum, N, Ferrari, G, Rey-Lopez, JP, Rimm, EB, et al. Long-term leisure-time physical activity intensity and all-cause and cause-specific mortality: a prospective cohort of US adults. *Circulation.* 2022 Jul 25;146(7): 523-534.
2. Carvalho L, Junior RM, Barreira J, Schoenfeld BJ, Orazem J, Barroso R. Muscle hypertrophy and strength gains after resistance training with different volume-matched loads: a systematic review and meta-analysis. *Appl Physiol Nutr Metab.* 2022 Apr;47(4):357-368.
3. Schoenfeld BJ, Grgic J, Ogborn D, Krieger JW. Strength and hypertrophy adaptations between low vs. high-load resistance training: a systematic review and meta-analysis. *J Strength Cond Res.* 2017 Dec;31(12):3508-3523. doi:10.1519/JSC.0000000000002200. PMID: 28834797.
4. Schoenfeld BJ, Contreras B, Krieger J, Grgic J, Delcastillo K, Belliard R, Alto A. Resistance training volume enhances muscle hypertrophy but not strength in trained men. *Med Sci Sports Exerc.* 2019 Jan;51(1):94-103.
5. Schoenfeld BJ. The mechanisms of muscle hypertrophy and their application to resistance training. *J Strength Cond Res.* 2010 Oct;24(10):2857-2872.
6. Schoenfeld BJ, Grgic J, Van Every DW, Plotkin DL. Loading recommendations for muscle strength, hypertrophy, and local endurance: a re-examination of the repetition continuum. *Sports (Basel).* 2021 Feb 22;9(2):32.
7. Wilk M, Zajac A, Tufano JJ. The influence of movement tempo during resistance training on muscular strength and hypertrophy responses: a review. *Sports Med.* 2021 Aug;51(8):1629-1650.

8. Włodarczyk M, Adamus P, Zieliński J, Kantanista A. Effects of velocity-based training on strength and power in elite athletes: a systematic review. *Int J Environ Res Pub Health*. 2021 May 14;18(10):5257.

9. Collins BW, Pearcey GEP, Buckle NCM, Power KE, Button DC. Neuromuscular fatigue during repeated sprint exercise: underlying physiology and methodological considerations. *Appl Physiol Nutr Metab*. 2018 Nov;43(11):1166-1175.

10. Halperin I, Emanuel A. Rating of perceived effort: methodological concerns and future directions. *Sports Med*. 2020 Apr;50(4):679-687.

11. Remmert JF, Robinson ZP, Pelland JC, John TA, Dinh S, Hinson SR, Elkins E, et al. Changes in intraset repetitions in reserve prediction accuracy during six weeks of bench press training in trained men. *Percept Mot Skills*. 2023 Oct;130(5):2139-60. doi: 10.1177/00315125231189098. Epub 2023 Jul 12. PMID: 37436724.

12. Halperin I, Malleron T, Har-Nir I, Androulakis-Korakakis P, Wolf M, Fisher J, Steele J. Accuracy in predicting repetitions to task failure in resistance exercise: a scoping review and exploratory meta-analysis. *Sports Med*. 2022 Feb;52(2):377-390. doi:10.1007/s40279-021-01559-x. Epub 2021 Sep 20.

13. Häkkinen K. Neuromuscular fatigue in males and females during strenuous heavy resistance loading. *Electromyogr Clin Neurophysiol*. 1994 Jun;34(4):205-214.

14. Thomas K, Brownstein CG, Dent J, Parker P, Goodall S, Howatson G. Neuromuscular fatigue and recovery after heavy resistance, jump, and sprint training. *Med Sci Sports Exerc*. 2018 Dec;50(12):2526-2535.

15. Wang J, Shapiro M. Changes in acromial morphology with age. *J Shoulder Elbow Surg*. 1997 Jan-Feb; 6(1):55-59.

16. Nicolson G, Goodman D, Flatow E, Bigliani L. The acromion: morphologic condition and age-related changes. A study of 420 scapulas. *J Shoulder Elbow Surg*. 1996 Jan-Feb;5(1):1-11.

17. Black L, Allen P, Morris S, Stone P, Suki B. Mechanical and failure properties of extra-cellular matrix sheets as a function of structural protein composition. *Biophys J*. 2008 Mar 1; 94(5):1916-1929.

18. Wenger M, Bozec, L, Horton M, Mesquida P. Mechanical properties of collagen fibrils. *Biophys J*. 2007 Aug 15;93(4): 1255-1263.

19. JP Janssens, JC Pache, LP Nicod. Physiological changes in respiratory function associated with ageing. *Eur Resp J*. 1999; 13:197-205.

20. Ogawa T, Spina R, Martin W, Kohrt W, Schechtman K, Holloszy J, Ehsani A. Effects of aging, sex, and physical training on cardiovascular responses to exercise. *Circulation*. 1992;86(2): 494-503.

Chapter 8

1. Keogh JW, Winwood PW. The epidemiology of injuries across the weight-training sports. *Sports Med*. 2017 Mar;47(3):479-501. doi:10.1007/s40279-016-0575-0. PMID: 27328853

2. Whalan, M, Lovell, R, Sampson, JA. Do niggles matter? Increased injury risk following physical complaints in football (soccer). *Science and Medicine in Football*. 2019 Dec 23;4(3):216-224. https://doi.org/10.1080/24733938.2019.1705996.

3. Wilke J, Behringer M. Is "delayed onset muscle soreness" a false friend? The potential implication of the fascial connective tissue in post-exercise discomfort. *Int J Mol Sci*. 2021 Aug 31;22(17):9482. doi:10.3390/ijms22179482. PMID: 34502387; PMCID: PMC8431437.

4. Cheung K, Hume P, Maxwell L. Delayed onset muscle soreness: treatment strategies and performance factors. *Sports Med*. 2003;33(2):145-164. doi:10.2165/00007256-200333020-00005. PMID: 12617692.

5. Miles MP, Clarkson PM. Exercise-induced muscle pain, soreness, and cramps. *J Sports Med Phys Fitness*. 1994 Sep;34(3):203-216. PMID: 7830383.

6. Sluka, KA. *Mechanisms and Management of Pain for the Physical Therapist,* Second Edition.

7. Khan KM, Scott A. Mechanotherapy: how physical therapists' prescription of exercise promotes tissue repair. *Br J Sports Med*. 2009 Apr;43(4):247-252. doi:10.1136/bjsm.2008.054239. Epub 2009 Feb 24. PMID: 19244270; PMCID: PMC2662433.

8. Louw, Adriaan, Puentedura, Emilio Therapeutic Neuroscience Education 2013 International Spine and Pain Institute

9. Milton K, Gomersall SR, Schipperijn J. Let's get moving: the Global Status Report on Physical Activity 2022 calls for urgent action. *J Sport Health Sci.* 2023 Jan;12(1):5-6. doi:10.1016/j.jshs.2022.12.006. Epub 2022 Dec 14. PMID: 36528290; PMCID: PMC9923423.

10. Noteboom, L, Belli, I, Hoozemans, MJM, Seth, A, Veeger, HEJ, Van Der Helm, FCT. Effects of bench press technique variations on musculoskeletal shoulder loads and potential injury risk. *Front Physiol.* 2024 Jun;15:1393235. doi: 10.3389/fphys.2024.1393235. PMID: 38974522; PMCID: PMC11224528.

Chapter 9

1. Rogers DL, Tanaka MJ, Cosgarea AJ, Ginsburg RD, Dreher GM. How mental health affects injury risk and outcomes in athletes. *Sports Health.* 2023 Jun 16:19417381231179678. doi:10.1177/19417381231179678. Epub ahead of print. PMID: 37326145.

2. Hamlin MJ, Wilkes D, Elliot CA, Lizamore CA, Kathiravel Y. Monitoring training loads and perceived stress in young elite university athletes. *Front Physiol.* 2019 Jan 29;10:34. doi:10.3389/fphys.2019.00034

3. Gabbett TJ. The training–injury prevention paradox: should athletes be training smarter and harder? *Br J Sports Med.* 2016;50:273-280.

4. Keogh JW, Winwood PW. The epidemiology of injuries across the weight-training sports. *Sports Med.* 2017 Mar;47(3):479-501. doi:10.1007/s40279-016-0575-0. PMID: 27328853.

5. Finan PH, Goodin BR, Smith MT. The association of sleep and pain: an update and a path forward. *J Pain.* 2013 Dec; 14(12):1539-1552.

6. Lindell M, Grimby-Ekman A. Stress, non-restorative sleep, and physical inactivity as risk factors for chronic pain in young adults: a cohort study. *PLoS One.* 2022 Jan 21;17(1):e0262601. doi:10.1371/journal.pone.0262601. PMID: 35061825; PMCID: PMC8782303.

7. Griffin KL, Knight KB, Bass MA, Valliant MW. Predisposing risk factors for stress fractures in collegiate cross-country runners. *J Strength Cond Res.* 2021 Jan 1;35(1):227-232. doi:10.1519/JSC.0000000000002408. PMID: 29239997.

8. Papadopoulou SK. Rehabilitation nutrition for injury recovery of athletes: the role of macronutrient intake. *Nutrients.* 2020 Aug 14;12(8):2449. doi:10.3390/nu12082449. PMID: 32824034; PMCID: PMC7468744.

9. Vitale KC, Owens R, Hopkins SR, Malhotra A. Sleep hygiene for optimizing recovery in athletes: review and recommendations. *Int J Sports Med.* 2019;40(8):535-543. doi:10.1055/a-0905-3103

10. Whalan, M, Lovell, R, Sampson, JA. Do niggles matter? Increased injury risk following physical complaints in football (soccer). *Science and Medicine in Football.* 2019 Dec 23; 4(3):216-224. https://doi.org/10.1080/24733938.2019.1705996.

11. Guidi J, Lucente M, Sonino N, Fava GA. Allostatic load and its impact on health: a systematic review. *Psychother Psychosom.* 2021;90(1):11-27. doi:10.1159/000510696. Epub 2020 Aug 14. PMID: 32799204.

12. Tomes C, Schram B, Orr R. Relationships between heart rate variability, occupational performance, and fitness for tactical personnel: a systematic review. *Front Public Health.* 2020 Nov 9;8:583336. doi:10.3389/fpubh.2020.583336. PMID: 33240835; PMCID: PMC7680786.

13. Miller DJ, Sargent C, Roach GD. A validation of six wearable devices for estimating sleep, heart rate and heart rate variability in healthy adults. *Sensors (Basel).* 2022 Aug 22;22(16):6317. doi:10.3390/s22166317. PMID: 36016077; PMCID: PMC9412437.

14. Huang K, Ihm J. Sleep and injury risk. *Curr Sports Med Rep.* 2021 Jun 1;20(6):286-290. doi:10.1249/JSR.0000000000000849. PMID: 34099605.

15. Williams S, Booton T, Watson M, Rowland D, Altini M. Heart rate variability is a moderating factor in the workload-injury relationship of competitive CrossFit™ athletes. *J Sports Sci Med.* 2017 Dec 1;16(4):443-449. PMID: 29238242; PMCID: PMC5721172.

About the Authors

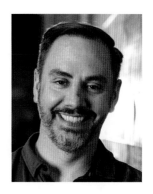

Dean Somerset is a personal trainer and certified exercise physiologist who specializes in postrehabilitation fitness. He has worked with clients recovering from joint replacements, sports injuries, spinal cord injuries, cancer, and cardiac surgery. He also trains healthy individuals—in person and virtually—to help them reach their strength, flexibility, and fitness goals. Somerset has developed and taught courses and seminars all around the world on the topics of postrehabilitation fitness, mobility, hip and shoulder health, client assessment, and core training. He has also written for and been featured in *Muscle & Fitness*, *Men's Health*, *Men's Journal*, Bodybuilding.com, and T Nation. Somerset has presented on numerous occasions for the National Strength and Conditioning Association (NSCA) and canfitpro and is a contributor to *Developing the Core, Second Edition,* and *NSCA's Essentials of Personal Training, Third Edition*.

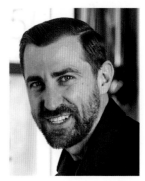

Dan Pope, DPT, is a physical therapist and strength coach with over 20 years of experience in getting strength and fitness athletes out of pain and returning them to a high level of performance. He is also the owner of Fitness Pain Free, a continuing education company that has helped thousands of other coaches and clinicians learn how to do the same. He has also been blessed to be able to travel around the world, speaking on the topics of injury prevention and rehabilitation.

Pope is a big believer in practicing what he preaches; he has been a CrossFit regional qualifier, a strongman national champion, and a collegiate pole vaulter.

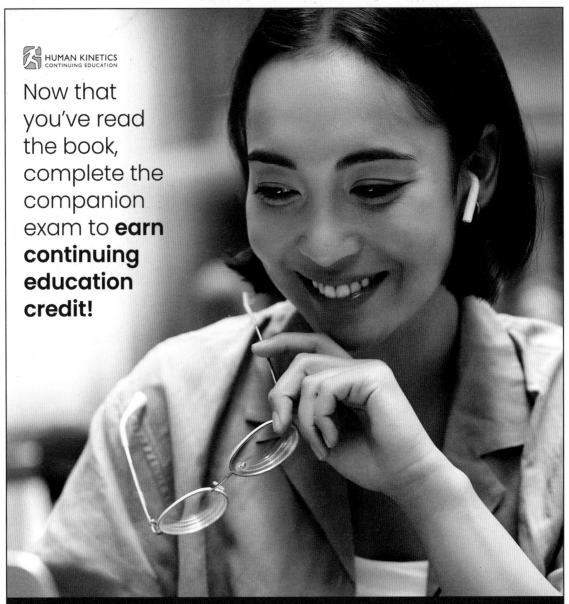
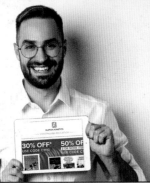